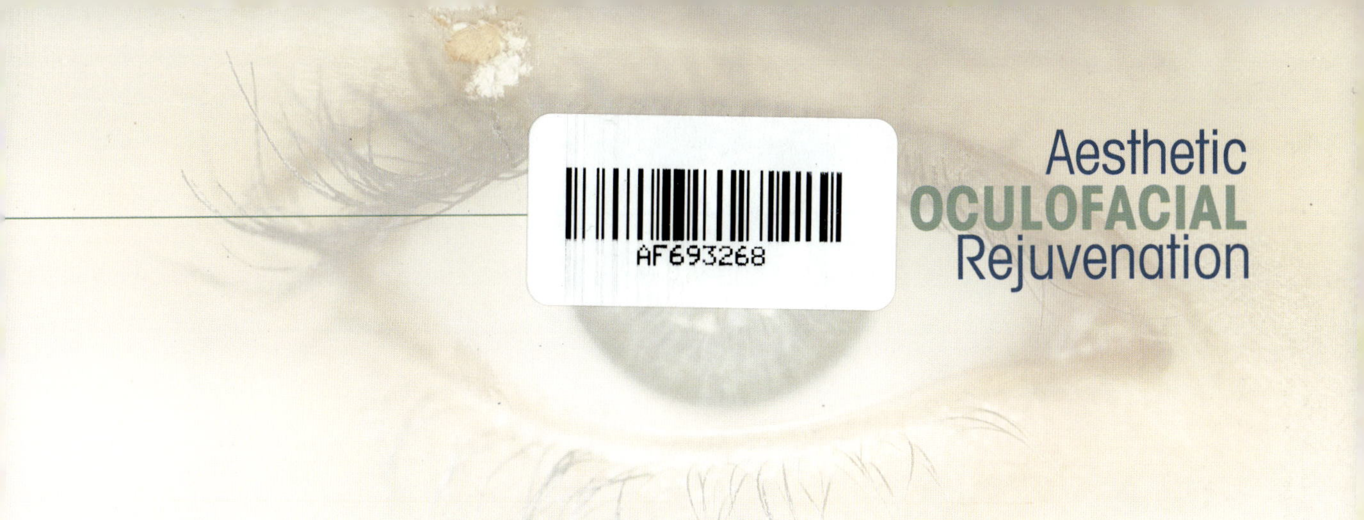

Aesthetic
OCULOFACIAL
Rejuvenation

DVD ROM CONTENTS

Ch/Clip no.	Clip Title	Video contributor/s
4.1	Lower Lid Peel	Richard H. Bensimon
4.2	Periorbital Peeling	Marina Landau
5.1	Lasers: Ablative/Pearl™	Alessandra Haddad
5.2	Lasers: Intense Pulsed Light/Limelight™	Alessandra Haddad
6.1	Photodynamic Therapy: PDT	Alessandra Haddad
7.1	Radiofrequency Devices: Radiage™	Reynaldo Javate
7.2	Infrared Devices: Titan™	Alessandra Haddad
8.1	Botulinum Toxin - Treatment 1	Alessandra Haddad
8.2	Botulinum Toxin - Treatment 2	Alessandra Haddad
8.3	Botulinum Toxin - Treatment 3	Alessandra Haddad
9.1	Tear Trough Correction	Marian Cantisano-Zilkha, Alessandra Haddad
9.2	Perioral, Nasolabial Fold Correction and Lips Enhancement	Marian Cantisano-Zilkha, Alessandra Haddad
9.3	Facial Dystrophy Correction	Marian Cantisano-Zilkha, Alessandra Haddad
9.4	Lower Face and Perioral Rejuvenation	Marian Cantisano-Zilkha, Alessandra Haddad
11.1	Dark Circles: A Combined Approach	Doris M. Hexsel, Taciana Dal´Forno
12.1	Laser Lipolysis: The Technique	Bruce Katz, Jason McBean
13.1	Skin Rejuvenation with Platelet Rich Plasma	Maria Angelo-Khattar
14.1	Stretchmarks: Intradermal Injection of CO2 Gas to Improve Stretchmarks - Tutorial	Philippe Cadic
14.2	Localized-Adiposities: Localized Subdermal Injection - Modification of the Appearance of the Skin and Gas Diffusion	Philippe Cadic
14.3	Periocular Rejuvenation: Upper and Lower Lid Intradermal and Subcutaneous Injection of CO2 to Improve Wrinkles	Philippe Cadic

Approximate runtime 80 minutes

Aesthetic Oculofacial Rejuvenation

Elsevier DVD-ROM Licence Agreement

Commissioning Editor: Russell Gabbedy
Development Editor: Sharon Nash
Project Manager: Glenys Norquay
Design: Kirsteen Wright
Illustration Manager: Merlyn Harvey
Illustrator: EPS Inc
Marketing Manager(s) (UK/USA): Clara Toombs/Helena Mutak

Aesthetic Oculofacial Rejuvenation

Marian Cantisano-Zilkha MD PhD
Center for Integrative and Aesthetic Medicine
New York, NY, USA
Center of Oculoplastic Esthetic and
Reconstructive Surgery of Ipanema
Ipanema, RJ, Brazil

Alessandra Haddad MD
Chief of Laser and Skin Care Section
Plastic Surgery Division
Federal University of São Paulo
Haddad Clinic Med & Surg
São Paulo, SP, Brazil

SAUNDERS
ELSEVIER

SAUNDERS
ELSEVIER

SAUNDERS is an imprint of Elsevier Inc.

Notices

Knowledge and best practice in this field are constantly changing. As new research and experience broaden our understanding, changes in research methods, professional practices, or medical treatment may become necessary. Practitioners and researchers must always rely on their own experience and knowledge in evaluating and using any information, methods, compounds, or experiments described herein. In using such information or methods they should be mindful of their own safety and the safety of others, including parties for whom they have a professional responsibility.

With respect to any drug or pharmaceutical products identified, readers are advised to check the most current information provided (i) on procedures featured or (ii) by the manufacturer of each product to be administered, to verify the recommended dose or formula, the method and duration of administration, and contraindications. It is the responsibility of practitioners, relying on their own experience and knowledge of their patients, to make diagnoses, to determine dosages and the best treatment for each individual patient, and to take all appropriate safety precautions.

To the fullest extent of the law, neither the Publisher nor the authors, contributors, or editors, assume any liability for any injury and/or damage to persons or property as a matter of products liability, negligence or otherwise, or from any use or operation of any methods, products, instructions, or ideas contained in the material herein.

Saunders

British Library Cataloguing in Publication Data
Aesthetic oculofacial rejuvenation
1. Facelift 2. Dermatologic agents - Therapeutic use
3. Rejuvenation
I. Cantisano-Zilkha, Marian II. Haddad, Alessandra
617.5'2

ISBN-13: 9780702033650

Library of Congress Cataloging in Publication Data
A catalog record for this book is available from the Library of Congress

Printed in China
Last digit is the print number: 9 8 7 6 5 4 3 2 1

Contents

Foreword vii
Preface ix
Contributors xi
Dedication xiii
Acknowledgment xiv

1 Overview of the Aesthetic Approach **1**
i) Current concepts in oculofacial aging 1
Marian Cantisano-Zilkha, Alessandra Haddad
ii) Economic impact of non-invasive technologies in plastic surgery 4
Lydia Masako Ferreira, Marcel Vinicius de Aguiar Menezes

2 Combining Non-Invasive Therapies **9**
i) A step by step guide 9
Marian Cantisano-Zilkha, Alessandra Haddad
ii) Anatomy of the periorbital area 17
Ioannis P Glavas

3 Skincare **21**
Eckart Haneke

4 Chemical Peels **29**
Marina Landau, Richard H Bensimon

5 Lasers and Intense Light Sources **39**
Eckart Haneke

6 Photodynamic Treatment **57**
Eckart Haneke

7 Skin Tightening Devices **67**
i) Radiofrequency and infrared technologies 67
Alessandra Haddad, Marian Cantisano-Zilkha
ii) Radiofrequency technology 74
Reynaldo M Javate, Nikolaos Trakos, Raul T Cruz Jr
iii) Bipolar radiofrequency 82
Neil S Sadick

8 Botulinum Toxin for Oculofacial Aesthetic Rejuvenation **85**
Doris M Hexsel, Luitgard Wiest, Mariana Soirefmann

9 Facial Fillers and Volumizers **97**
Marian Cantisano-Zilkha, Alessandra Haddad

10 Fat Transfer **119**
Luiz Alexandre Lorico Tissiani

11 Dark Circles: A Combination Approach **127**
Doris M Hexsel, Taciana Dal'Forno, Alessandra Haddad, Marian Cantisano-Zilkha

12 Minimally Invasive Laser Lipolysis for Facial and Neck Rejuvenation **133**
Bruce E Katz, Jason C McBean

13 Mesotherapy **141**
i) Mesotherapy 141
Alexander Kulick
ii) Skin rejuvenation with platelet-rich plasma 149
Maria Angelo-Khattar

14 Carbon Dioxide Therapy: Face and Body Rejuvenation **155**
Philippe Cadic

15 Cosmetic Dentistry of the Perioral Area – The Odontological Point of View **179**
Luiz Gustavo Nascimento de Melo, Marcelo Pereira Nunes, Marcelo Wolff Fernandes, Luciane Magalhães Antonini, Maria Beatriz RG de Oliveira

16 The Importance of the Aesthetician in a Cosmetic Practice **189**
Susanne S Warfield

17 From the Inside Out: A Psychotherapist's Views on Aesthetic Enhancement **195**
Michael Colberg

18 The Future of Oculofacial Rejuvenation: A Perspective **203**
Sterling Baker, Erin L Holloman

Index 205

Foreword

Head Professor of the Post-Graduate Courses in Plastic Surgery of the Pontifical Catholic University of Rio de Janeiro and the Carlos Chagas Post-Graduate Medical Institute. Member of the Brazilian Society of Plastic Surgery, the Brazilian National Academy of Medicine, and the Brazilian Academy of Letters. Visiting professor, I.S.A.P.S. FACS, FICS.

Throughout the history of mankind, great value has been given to physical appearance. Self-esteem is enhanced when an individual projects an image of youthfulness, vitality and health. Inevitably, aging brings about changes that are undesirable, and, more than ever, patients are increasingly seeking to correct alterations due to senescence. Motivation for treatment spans different aspects, such as personal, social and professional reasons.

The approach to the medical treatment of the signs of facial aging may be divided into surgical and non-surgical. It is important to understand that these modalities are many times complementary; the results from a formal face-lift operation may be greatly enhanced by skin management, either before or following surgery. Furthermore, the non-invasive procedures demand minimal recovery, allowing for a quick return to work.

In this book, Aesthetic Oculofacial Rejuvenation, written by Dr Zilkha and co-authored by Dr Haddad, non-surgical procedures are emphasized, the aim of which is to correct rhytids, discromia, skin irregularities and other acquired alterations. Each modality is systematically explained in detail, with guest authors describing their experience. Readers of this book will include plastic surgeons, dermatologists, and all medical specialists who are involved in the aesthetic enhancement of the face. I congratulate the authors for the excellence of their work, as I am sure it will prove to be an invaluable contribution to this ever-expanding area of cosmetic medicine.

Prof Ivo Pitanguy

Preface

Aesthetic Facial Plastic Surgery has drastically changed in the last 30 years. No longer skin-pulling and lifting procedures is the gold standard of Oculofacial Rejuvenation. The current aging concept of facial volume loss has yielded a new three-dimensional approach of tissue repositioning. This missing link once understood, has led to the phenomenal development of newer and safer technology for volume replacement, skincare and skin tightening in the eternal search of beauty and harmony, for the ultimate well-being.

On this book, we compiled the experience of different experts in different fields of true beautification and we hope we can convey that knowledge in an enthusiastic fashion. The concept has become simpler but the approach has become more technological. Nowadays, we count on safer and sophisticated technology making this a very exciting field that evolves very rapidly.

We hope you find this to be useful for you and your patients and that you enjoy it as much as we did, from the very beginning to the end. This has been a very exciting project for us.

Yours sincerely,
Marian and Alessandra

List of Contributors

Maria Angelo-Khattar PhD
Director, Aesthetica Clinic, Dubai Healthcare City, Dubai, UAE

Luciane Magalhães Antonini DDS
Student of Esthetics and Restorative Dentistry, School of Professional Improvement (EAPGOIÁS), Goiânia, Brazil

Sterling S Baker MD
Assistant Clinical Professor, Department of Ophthalmology, Adjunct Clinical Professor, Department of Dermaology, College of Medicine, University of Oklahoma, Oklahoma City, OK, USA

Richard H Bensimon MD
Director of Plastic Surgery, Pearl Women's Center, Portland, OR, USA

Philippe Cadic MD
Medical Aesthetic Doctor and Laser Physician, Private Practice, Orleans, France

Michael Colberg JD LCSW MFT
Private Practice, Clinical Instructor, Department of Child and Adolescent Psychiatry, NYU/Langone Medical Center, New York, NY, USA

Raul T Cruz Jr MD
Consultant, Department of Ophthalmology, Orbital, Lacrimal and Oculofacial Plastic Surgery Section, University of Santo Tomas Hospital, Manila, Philippines

Taciana Dal'Forno MD PhD
Professor of Dermatology, Brazilian Lutheran University, Dermatologist, Hexsel Dermatologic Clinic, Porto Alegre, RS, Brazil

Maria Beatriz RG de Oliveira DDS
Professor of Esthetics and Restorative Dentistry, School of Professional Improvement (EAPGOIÁS), Goiânia, Brazil

Marcel Vinicius de Aguiar Menezes MD
Resident, Plastic Surgery Department, Federal University of São Paulo, São Paulo, SP, Brazil

Luiz Gustavo Nascimento de Melo DDS PHD
Professor of Implantology, School of Professional Improvement (EAPGOIÁS), Goiânia, Brazil

Marcelo Wolff Fernandes DDS
Private Practice, São Paulo, SP, Brazil

Lydia Masako Ferreira MD
Full Professor and Chairwoman, Plastic Surgery Division, Federal University of São Paulo, São Paulo, SP, Brazil

Ioannis P Glavas
Clinical Assistant Professor, NYU School of Medicine, Boston, MA, USA

Alessandra Haddad MD
Chief of Laser and Skin Care Section, Plastic Surgery Division, Federal University of São Paulo, Haddad Clinic Med & Surg, São Paulo, SP, Brazil

Eckart Haneke MD PHD
Professor of Dermatology, Department of Dermatology, University of Bern, Bern, Switzerland

Doris Maria Hexsel MD
Formerly Professor of Dermatology, School of Medicine, University of Passo Fundo, Porto Alegre, RS, Brazil

Erin L Holloman MD
Private Practice, Oklahoma City, OK, USA

Reynaldo M Javate MD
Professor and Chairman, Department of Ophthalmology, Chief, Orbital, Lacrimal and Oculofacial Plastic Surgery Section, University of Santo Tomas Hospital, Manila, Philippines

Bruce E Katz MD
Clinical Professor of Dermatology, Mount Sinai School of Medicine, Director, JUVA Skin & Laser Center, Director, Cosmetic Surgery & Laser Clinic, Mount Sinai Medical Center, New York, NY, USA

Alexander Kulick MD
Department of Family Practice, Beth Israel Medical Center, New York, NY, USA

Marina Landau MD
Senior Dermatologist, Wolfson Medical Center, Holon, Israel

Jason C McBean MD
Dermatologist in Private Practice, Fairfield, CT, USA

Marcelo Pereira Nunes DDS
Professor of Periodontics, Paulista Association of Surgeon-Dentists (APCD), Paulista, Brazil

Neil S Sadick MD
Clinical Professor of Dermatology, Department of Dermatology, Weill Medical College of Cornell University, New York, NY, USA

Mariana Soirefmann MD
Investigator, Brazilian Center for Studies in Dermatology, Porto Alegre; Preceptor of Cosmetic Dermatology at the Department of Dermatology, Pontificia Universidade do Rio Grande do Sul, Porto Alegre, Brazil

Luiz Alexandre L Tissiani MD
Attending Surgeon, Division of Plastic Surgery, Mandaqui Hospital, São Paulo, SP, Brazil

Nikolaos Trakos MD PhD
Director of Aesthetic and Reconstructive Ophthalmic Plastic Surgery, Orasis Hellenic Ophthalmologic Center, Athens, Greece

Susanne S Warfield
Licensed Esthetician, Ridgewood, NJ, USA

Luitgard G Wiest MD
Private Practice, Munich, Germany

Marian Cantisano-Zilkha MD PHD
Center for Integrative and Aesthetic Medicine, New York, NY, USA, Center of Oculoplastic Esthetic and Reconstructive Surgery of Ipanema, Ipanema, RJ, Brazil

To our patients – our eternal source of inspiration.
To our colleagues for sharing our passion and art.
To our close friends and family, for the continuous support.

Acknowledgment

To all of our contributors for the enthusiasm on sharing this project with us.
To the editorial staff of Elsevier for their extreme professionalism and camaraderie
To our office staff,
Thank you!

1 Overview of the Aesthetic Approach

Current concepts in oculofacial aging

Marian Cantisano-Zilkha, Alessandra Haddad

INTRODUCTION

The growing demand for facial aesthetic enhancement without extended recovery time has fueled technologic advances that have made non-invasive facial rejuvenation a reality. Improvement of facial skin texture, pigmentation, tone, wrinkling and facial contour can now be accomplished using a combination of non-surgical therapeutic modalities, including botulinum toxins (Botox®, Dysport® and Myoblock®), injectable fillers and volumizers (Restylane®, Perlane®, Juvederm®, Juvederm Plus®, Cosmoderm®, Cosmoplast®, Sculptra® and Radiesse®), chemical peeling agents (glycolic and trichloracetic acids), intense pulsed light, photodynamic therapy, light-emitting diode devices, non-ablative and fractionated lasers, and skin tightening technologies (radiofrequency and infrared). These techniques usually require several treatment sessions, which are scheduled at intervals that allow the body to recover and respond appropriately. In most cases, these non-invasive procedures are not stand-alone therapies. They complement each other and have a cumulative effect. This multidimensional approach offers an acceptable trade-off for patients who want to avoid the lengthy healing time or potential risks required by many surgical approaches to aesthetic enhancement.

The purpose of this book is to inform physicians of the variety of non-surgical approaches to facial rejuvenation that are currently available, to provide information on how each of these individual components is applied and to demonstrate how each modality compliments the other. Used in combination, these non-invasive aesthetic enhancement techniques can often achieve results that exceed expectations. The wide range of currently available technology for facial rejuvenation is directed toward achieving improvements in three general categories:

- skin texture and pigmentation
- wrinkle removal
- skin tightening

A new approach to facial aging takes into consideration a three-dimensional level for rejuvenation, considering not only the epidermal photodamage or the dermal changes, what could be considered as a bi-dimensional concept, but also facial contour modifications and volume changes in facial structure.

Epidermal changes include textural modifications, dischromias, mottled hyperpigmentation, loss of shine and hydration level. Dermal changes represent loss of elasticity in combination with continuous muscle action, creating wrinkles related to muscular activity or dynamic wrinkles. The dermis becomes thinner and its functions as a connective and supportive tissue are reduced.

The facial fat compartments undergo a migration in the caudal direction, leading to fat atrophy in the orbital, frontal, buccal, temporal and perioral regions, while the submental, lateral malar regions of nasolabial fold will present an excess of redundant and ptotic tissue (festoons). The superficial musculoaponeurotic system (SMAS) becomes thinner and longer. The zygomatic bones have horizontal insertions in SMAS attachments; for this reason the superior and inferomedial aspects of face do not suffer all the gravity action. Atrophy of the malar and maxilla bones, reduction of mandibular angle, and reduction of the inferior orbit and chin projections are also associated with facial contour alterations.

The first step in evaluating patients who are seeking facial aesthetic enhancement is to discuss what bothers them about their appearance. Good rapport and open and uninhibited communication between physician and patients are essential. Patients have their own opinions about what they like and dislike about their appearance, so before making treatment recommendations it is a good idea to sit down and look in the mirror with them, and listen to their comments about their appearance. Encourage patients to specify which flaws or deformities they want to correct and then conduct a physical examination to identify the source of the patient's complaint. They usually notice that their eyes are not the same[1] and they notice bags, wrinkles, skin laxity and eyebrow changes but they do not see behind the symptoms the cardinal signs of the aging process: volume displacement, loss of skin elasticity and muscle hyperactivity. Some patients request the surgeon to pull sinking brows and lids up and out, unaware that this can exacerbate the effects of volume loss, or worse leave them with an artificial tailored look. Any patient who does not have gross dropping of the eyelids is a good candidate for minimally invasive techniques.

Clinical evaluation begins by examining the position and arching of the eyebrows, the muscle activity of the forehead, the heaviness of the upper eyelids and the upper eyelid skin texture, checking for drooping of the upper eyelid muscles and narrowing of the palpebral apertures (ptosis), excessive skin and prolapsing fat or prominent lacrimal glands. The lower lids should be examined for position of the lower lid margin-lower lid retraction or inferior scleral show. They should also be checked for skin texture as well as changes in pigmentation and vascular pooling, creating dark circles, prolapsing fat, creating shadows and contour irregularities, and laxity of the lateral canthal tendons and lower eyelid margin. The presence of extra folds of skin, muscle or fat on the cheek is known as a 'bag on a bag' (a *malar festoon*).

Aging changes of the mid-face are manifest by skin laxity, loss of bony contours, less prominent cheek bones, soft tissue loss and deepening of nasolabial folds.[2] The lower face shows the presence of more prominent jowls, deepening 'marionette lines' (melo-mental folds), submental skin redundancy and fatty deposition, creating a double chin. The lips lose volume and disappear, and the corners of the mouth may droop (Figs 1.1 and 1.2, Table 1.1).

Once the source of the patient's complaints has been identified, the patient and physician must decide what procedures are most appropriate for the patient and what alterations are most compatible with his or her face. They must agree on how much downtime is acceptable and balance that with how much improvement they will be satisfied with. The objective is to achieve a natural look. Reviewing old photographs can be helpful in tailoring the procedure to individual patients.

Patients should be informed of the available non-surgical options for correcting or improving their appearance, and presented with the pros and cons of each approach. It is important that patients have realistic expectations about the limitations of the recommended procedures and what the outcomes can be. They need to be made aware of the variability in healing and the important differences in the tone and texture of each person's skin. Patients

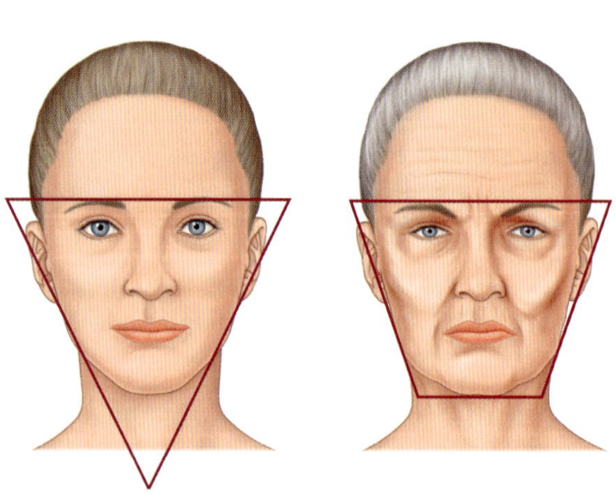

Fig. 1.1 Facial contour changes with age.

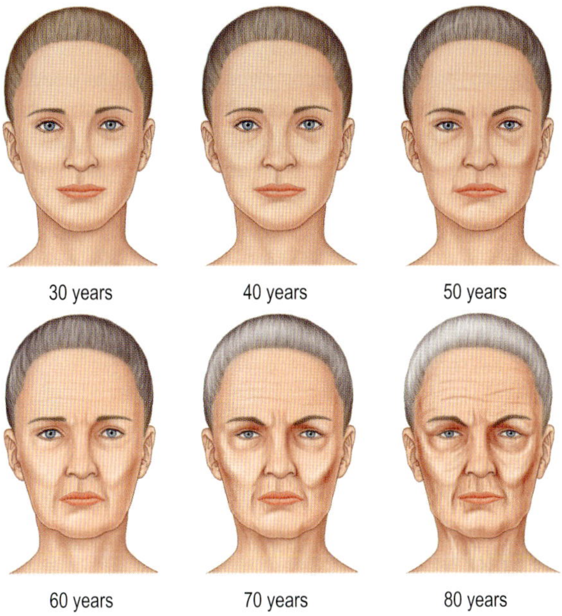

Fig. 1.2 Aging facial changes by decades of life.

Table 1.1 Histologic changes of human skin due to intrinsic aging

Epidermal	Dermal	Cutaneous adnexa
Flattening of the dermo-epidermal junction	Atrophy (loss of dermal volume)	Greying of hair
Reduction of thickness	Few fibroblasts	Hair loss
Different cellular sizes and shapes	Fewer mast cells	Change of terminal and vellus hair
Occasional nuclear atypia	Reduced vascularity	Abnormal nail plate
Reduction of melanocytes	Shorter capillaries	Fewer glands
Fewer Langerhans cells	Abnormal nerve endings	

also need to understand that, although cosmetic enhancement can make them look better and feel better about themselves, it is unrealistic to expect their lives to change dramatically.[3,4]

OVERVIEW OF NON-INVASIVE THERAPIES

As mentioned previously, the available non-surgical aesthetic enhancement procedures are not stand-alone therapies. The sum of their effects yields a result that exceeds their individual effects. Currently available therapies include intense pulsed light (and enhanced effect with amino-levulinic acid and photodynamic therapy), botulinum toxins, injectable soft tissue fillers, chemical peeling agents, volumetric radio frequency tissue heating instrumentation, and non-ablative and fractionated lasers.

Intense pulsed light, first introduced in the mid-1990s, is a well-recognized treatment modality for improving the appearance of the photoaged face. Photoaging refers to the clinical changes to facial and other sun-exposed skin caused by chronic exposure to ultraviolet light, including the appearance of telangectasias (red lesions in the skin caused by permanent dilation of preexisting small blood vessels), rough texture, fine and coarse wrinkles, yellow and mottled pigmentation, brown age spots or 'liver spots'.[1]

Injections of botulinum toxin type A are the most commonly used cosmetic enhancement procedures in the USA, and are used to relax facial muscles and diminish their secondary wrinkle-producing effects. Understanding the anatomy and balance of facial muscles will allow botulinum toxin, in addition to relaxing the dynamic rhytides, to be used to achieve facial symmetry by elevating brows, compensating for blepharoptosis and subtly adjusting a downturned mouth. It works by binding to the nerve endplate and blocking the release of acetylcholine. The bond is permanent until the nerve develops a new endplate that begins releasing acetylcholine again.[2–5]

Injectable fillers and volumizers are used to add volume to the facial structure, filling in wrinkles and furrows, replacing lost facial volume and accentuating bony contours. Purified bovine collegen and autogenous fat are two FDA-approved fillers that have been successfully used in the USA for more than 20 years. The ease of use and the lack of adverse reactions and longer-lasting effect have made hyaluronic acids the most widely used fillers. They are available in an increasingly wide variety of viscosities and differing characteristics.[3,4]

Chemical peels are an effective therapeutic option for reversing photoaging. They are recommended for treating a variety of superficial conditions involving the epidermis and superficial dermis, including mild sun damage, superficial wrinkling and pigmentary disorders, actinic keratoses (growths caused by excessive exposure to the sun) and active acne. They are available in a wide variety of strengths. Some strengths can be used without any downtime. More potent varieties require several days of healing.

Radiofrequency volumetric heating technology, or *thermage*, uses high-frequency electrical current to heat the deeper layers of the skin while cooling the surface; this minimizes downtime and enhances the effectiveness of the treatment. It is primarily a lifting, tightening and contouring procedure.

Infrared volumetric heating technology (i.e. Titan lasers and ALMA Lasers™) uses infrared properties to heat the deep dermis and promote a lifting effect.

Laser resurfacing is performed using a beam of laser energy. Three types of lasers – ablative, non-ablative and fractionated – are used for skin resurfacing. *Ablative lasers* stimulate collagen regeneration by removing the epidermis and heating the papillary dermis. *Non-ablative lasers* are less intense and require little or no healing time. They work by treating the papillary dermis, causing the skin to respond by regenerating as if repairing a wound. Lasers that use chromophores (tissues that have a color that attracts laser light of a specific wavelength) are used for treating telangiectasias, hemangiomas, vascular lesions, hair removal and abnormal skin pigmentation. *Fractionated lasers*, which are adaptations of ablative lasers, are designed to improve skin texture with a minimum of downtime and without anesthesia. They have the unique ability to create microthermal zones of tissue treatment between untouched areas of skin. They are used to improve skin texture, erase unwanted brown spots and improve wrinkles around the eyes and mouth.[6]

Mesotherapy and *carbon dioxide insufflation* are helpful tools for minimally invasive face and body rejuvenation.

CONCLUSION

This textbook will summarize and address what is available in the technologies of minimally invasive facial and oculoplastic rejuvenation and how these technologies have enriched and revolutionized the field of plastic surgery.

REFERENCES

1 Perkins SW, Batniji RK. Rejuventaion of the lower eyelid complex. *Facial Plast Surg*. 2005;21(4):279–285.
2 Mandelson BC, Hartley W, Scott M, McNab A, Granzow JW. Age related changes of the orbit and mid cheek and the implications for facial rejuvenation. *Aesthetic Plast Surg*. 2007;31(5): 419–423.
3 Glavas IP, Purewall BK. Non invasive techniques in periorbital rejuvenation. *Facial Plast Surg*. 2007;23(3):162–167.
4 Finn JC, Cox S. Fillers in periorbital complex. *Facial Plast Surg Clin North Am*. 2007;15(1):123–132, VII.
5 Lee CJ, Kim SG, Han JY. The results of periorbital rejuvenation with botulinum toxin A using two different protocols. *Aesthetic Plast Surg*. 2006;30(1):65–70.
6 Shook BA, Heuza GJ. Periorbital ablative and non ablative resurfacing. *Facial Plast Surg Clin North Am*. 2005;13 (4):571–582, VII.

Economic impact of non-invasive technologies in plastic surgery

Lydia Masako Ferreira, Marcel Vinicius de Aguiar Menezes

INTRODUCTION

Less or non-invasive technologies have been progressively used and sought after in medical and surgical procedures.[1] Over the years they have gained popularity in the surgical world, probably for being less harmful to the organism or because of the technical ease of their application.[2] New technology developments in plastic surgery have followed this tendency, which aims to shorten surgical time and downtime as much as possible by employing procedures that produce equivalent results to invasive procedures. In some cases, they may even delay invasive plastic surgeries.[3]

To develop minimally invasive surgical procedures, several improved techniques have been incorporated into plastic surgery, such as pharmacology, cosmetology and diversified technologies, for example fillers and volumizers, botulinum toxins, lasers and radiofrequency tightening devices.[3] Video-endoscopy was introduced to plastic surgery in 1991 and quickly became popular as a less invasive choice.[4]

Products and technologies in the plastic surgery field associated with media influence or that are perceived as being straightforward have been responsible for the explosion in aesthetic procedures when compared to traditional plastic surgery procedures.[5,6] This growth is evident in the number of aesthetic procedures taking place annually in the USA:[5–7] 11.7 million in 2007[6] against 11.5 million in 2006.[7]

The most commonly used non-invasive techniques are currently botulinum toxin injections, hyaluronic acid fillers, laser hair removal, facial resurfacing and microdermabrasion.[6,7]

Table 1.2 Procedures most frequently performed in 2007

Procedure	Number performed
Surgical	
Liposuction	456 828
Breast augmentation	399 440
Blepharoplasty	240 763
Abdominoplasty	185 335
Breast reduction	53 087
Non-surgical	
Botulinum toxin	2 775 176
Hyaluronic acid injection	1 448 716
Laser hair removal	1 412 657
Microdermabrasion	829 658
Laser resurfacing	647 707

IMPACT OF MINIMALLY INVASIVE PROCEDURES

According to the American Society of Aesthetic Plastic Surgery (ASAPS), the four most common cosmetic surgeries performed are liposuction, breast augmentation, blepharoplasty and breast reduction.[6,7] Liposuction is by far the most popular of these, totaling 456 828 procedures in 2007, compared with 176 863 in 1996.[6,7]

The popularity of plastic surgery and aesthetic non-invasive procedures is rapidly increasing and these aesthetic non-invasive procedures are gaining acceptance, as indicated by comparing the number of procedures performed in 1997 (1 126 177) with that in 2006 (9 533 980) (Table 1.2).[7] Botulinum toxin injection was the non-invasive procedure performed most often in 2007, with a total of 2 775 176 applications.[7]

NON-INVASIVE TECHNOLOGIES IN PLASTIC SURGERY

Economic Impact

The intense growth in the use of new non-invasive procedures has generated questions about their economic impact, and if they delay, or even avoid, more extensive surgical procedures.[3,5,8] In North America, US$13 billion was spent in aesthetic procedures in 2007, of which US$8.3 billion was on surgical procedures and US$4.7 billion was on non-surgical ones.[6]

The use of botulinum toxin and facial fillers has indirectly reduced the rate of growth in facial surgeries.[9,10] Statistical data show a significant rise in the number of treatments with botulinum toxin in women when comparing data collected between 1997 and 2006, while procedures such as rhytidoplasty and blepharoplasty, while still growing in popularity, did so at a much slower pace in the same period for the same group (40 and 30%, respectively).[7] However, it is well known that botulinum toxin and facial fillers, although efficient and practical, are of a transient nature. For example, the effect of botulinum toxin application is good for 6 months on average and then the procedure has to be repeated. This option has an average cost of US$500 per treatment (labor only, excluding the cost of material) while a procedure like blepharoplasty costs only US$2882. Another example illustrating this discrepancy is lip augmentation surgery, which has long-lasting results with a cost around US$1726. Using filling substances such as hyaluronic acid costs an average of US$512 per treatment, but the temporary results last only 6 to 8 months.

Table 1.3 Number of surgical and non-surgical procedures performed: 10-year comparison, 1997–2008

Procedure	Number performed	
	1997	2008
Liposuction (lipoplasty)	176 863	403 684
Breast augmentation	101 176	383 836
Eyelid surgery (blepharoplasty)	159 232	209 999
Botox	65 157	3 181 592
Chemical peel	481 227	338 432
Laser skin resurfacing	154 153	576 309

As previously stated, the large number of non-invasive procedures performed, because they are simpler in nature and application, is delaying classical and invasive surgery (Table 1.3).[11]

The growth in the use of non-invasive technologies has attracted professionals from other medical specialities, and they are now increasingly using these procedures.[12,13] In North America dermatologists (48%), plastic surgeons (38%), general surgery professionals (>4%), otorhinolaryngologists (>3%), ophthalmologists (>3%), family doctors (<1%), pediatricians (<1%) and general clinicians (<1%) are involved in these treatments.[12] The professionals in these specialities are attracted by the immediate results and the high financial returns provided by less invasive technologies.[12] However, as a result unsatisfactory results are increasingly being observed, which are related to technically and scientifically unqualified medical or, even worse, non-medical professionals.[14]

Botulinum Toxin

The application of botulinum toxin is the minimally invasive procedure performed most often in the USA.[6,7,13] During 2007, it comprised 23.7% of all cosmetic non-invasive procedures in that country.[6]

Botulinum toxin blocks the transmission of nervous stimuli through muscle synapses, resulting in a temporary, but reversible, paralysis.[14] Clinically, its effects last from 3 to 6 months and its use has been expanded to various medical specialities, for example the treatment of achalasia,[14,15] blepharospasm, hyperidrosis, spasmodic dysphonia and, commonly, in the context of plastic surgery as an aesthetic procedure.[13,14,16]

The rate of success in botulinum toxin therapy is heavily dependent on a knowledge of anatomy, which also minimizes the incidence of complications and adverse side effects.[14] Knowledge of the functional facial musculature may make the difference between two professional treatments when the toxin application is performed by a skilled medical professional or a just a technician or even by a medical professional who is not skilled in cosmetics and facial balance.[14]

Botulinum toxin applications on the face are most frequently done in the glabella, frontal and orbital regions in the neck, nasolabial groove, peri-oral lines and mentum.[9,10,14] Facial rejuvenation using the toxin requires new applications in programmed periods because of its temporary effects,[10,13,14] therefore to the initial cost of treatment the patient must add the cost of future applications in order to ensure durable results and prolonged effects.[5,6,9,10,13,14]

Economic Impact

As already stated, botulinum toxin has become very popular, and in 2007 a total of 2 775 176 procedures were performed in the USA, representing 23% of all non-invasive procedures and costing a total of US$1 054 566 736.[6]

Lasers

Laser beams have several applications in plastic surgery, for example hair removal, facial resurfacing, as an adjuvant in post-surgery periods and in the correction of unaesthetic scars.[6,17] Laser technology for facial resurfacing has been a valuable addition to the techniques of therapeutic plastic surgery. Its accuracy and broad spectrum allow different depths of penetration to be achieved and it can be tailored to treat a variety of skin types for the removal of devitalized and aged tissue. A more natural tissue renewal is then possible with collagen remodelling.[18,19]

Before the 1990s, lasers had only one wavelength per machine, were highly selective for treatment performance and besides being expensive were also big, which made their indication, purchase, accommodation and maintenance difficult. They have evolved into compact pieces of equipment and intense pulsed light has extended the use of the technology and reduced the cost. In addition, the advent of multiple platforms or stations as bases holding several types of lasers has made this technique more popular, widespread and accessible.

Economic Impact

The number of laser-based procedures in plastic surgery has been increasing in recent years. In 1997 in the USA there were 154 000 applications for facial resurfacing, while in 2007 this number was up to 509 591, which is an increase of 230.8% and is greater than the total number of liposuctions performed in 2007. The revenue generated from the use of lasers in facial resurfacing in 2006 was over US$600 000, which, if added to the use of laser for hair removal, reaches US$1 100 000.

Hyaluronic Acid

Hyaluronic acid is a polymer with viscous-elastic properties that is safely used for facial fillings.[20] Because of its characteristics, its popularity has increased in recent years.[6] It is a good option for skin rejuvenation since it has low tissue reactivity and shows longer-lasting results than injections of at or collagen.[21] However, like other non-invasive procedures, several studies have shown that it has limited duration and has to be reapplied every 3 to 6 months. Although in some cases the results may last for 12 months, there is still a cumulative cost to users.[20–22] The products available in the market may have various origins, such as animal, avian or bacterial fermentation. Each product has properties that should be known by the professional using it.[22]

Economic Impact

In 2007 1 448 715 applications of hyaluronic acid were performed in the USA at a global cost of US$834 460 585.[6] The average application cost was US$532 in 2006 and US$576 in 2007. Patients using hyaluronic acid will need more applications in the future, leading to a cumulative cost of US$2500 dollars in 10 years if applications are made every 2 years. If used for lip augmentation, hyaluronic acid therapy is more expensive than conventional surgery (around US$1776) over 10 years, as the results of conventional surgery last much longer.[6,21]

Microdermabrasion

This is a common procedure in plastic surgery, consisting of a superficial skin abrasion to regain cutaneous youthfulness.[23] It may be used for hyperchromia clearing, facial scars and in facial rejuvenation in cases of photo-induced injuries.[23]

The rejuvenation effect of cutaneous dermoabrasion is based on collagen remodeling, which decreases small facial wrinkles.[23]

Economic Impact

A total of 829 638 microdermabrasion were performed in the USA in 2007 at a total cost of US $10 785 294. The average cost is US$130 per treatment, making it the least expensive non-invasive procedure.

CONCLUSION

It is obvious that the use of non-invasive technology in plastic surgery is growing at an intensive rate. Its popular appeal is notorious and the literature documents its results very well. The economic impact of these procedures may be high because in many cases the applications must be periodically renewed to obtain results comparable to those for longer-lasting conventional surgery. Thus, in absolute values, economic investment in this market is favorable to non-invasive technologies when compared to conventional surgeries.

It is highly possible that lower immediate costs and rapid results attract more and more patients to non-invasive procedures, although the relatively short result durations do not mean less cost to the patient if the treatment is evaluated as a long-term investment. Finally, we would like to clarify that these procedures are not substitutes for but may delay and supplement conventional plastic surgery, addressing problems that conventional invasive techniques cannot.

REFERENCES

1 Wollina U, Goldman A, Berger U, Abdel-Naser MB. Esthetic and cosmetic dermatology. *Dermatol Ther*. 2008;21(2):118–130.

2 Aust MC, Fernandes D, Kolokythas P, Kaplan HM, Vogt PM. Percutaneous collagen induction therapy: an alternative treatment for scars, wrinkles, and skin laxity. *Plast Reconstr Surg*. 2008; 121:1421.

3 Grunwald T, Krummel T, Sherman R. Advanced technologies in plastic surgery: how new innovations can improve our training and practice. *Plast Reconstr Surg*. 2004;114:1556.

4 Vasconez LO, Monteroz AE. História da cirurgia videoendoscópica corporal. In: *Videoendoscopia no Contorno Corporal e Procedimentos Complementares*. Rio de Janeiro: Edit Revinter; 2007: P03, 5.

5 McCollough EG. Minimally invasive – minimally effective. *Arch Facial Plast Surg*. 2007;9(4).

6 *American Society for Aesthetic Plastic Surgery. Cosmetic Surgery National Data Bank Statistics*. extraído do site, www.surgery.org; 2007. no dia 15/05/08.

7 *American Society for Aesthetic Plastic Surgery. Cosmetic Surgery National Data Bank Statistics*. extraído do site, www.surgery.org; 2006. no dia 28/02/08.

8 Lasalvia CG, Pereira LDES, Da Cunha MC, Kitadai SP. Costs and efficacy of type A botulinum toxin for the treatment of essential blepharospasm and hemifacial spasm. *Arq Bras Oftalmol*. 2006;69(5):701–705.

9 De Maio M. The minimal approach: an innovation in facial cosmetic procedures. *Aesth Plast Surg*. 2004;28:295–300.

10 Ferreira LM, Ferreira LF, Blanes L. Toxina botulínica. In: *Cirurgia Plástica: Guias de medicina ambulatorial e Hospitalar UNIFESP- Escola Paulista de Medicina*. São Paulo: Edit Manole; 2007:817, 822.

11 Alsarraf R, Alsarraf NW, Larrabee WF, Johnson Jr CM. Cosmetic surgery procedures as luxury goods: measuring price and demand in facial plastic surgery. *Arch Facial Plast Surg*. 2002;4:105–110.

12 Housman TS, Hancox JG, Mir MR. What specialties perform the most common outpatient cosmetic procedures in the United States? *Dermatol Surg*. 2008;34(1):1–8 doi:10.1111/j.1524-4725.2007.34000.

13 Lee H, Saladi RN, Fox JL. Cohort study on patient response to botulinum toxin cosmetic therapy. *J Cosmet Dermatol*. 2008; 7(1):39–42.

14 Kane MAC. Botulinum toxin. In: *Grabb and Smith's Plastic Surgery*. 6th ed. 2007:475.

15 Lake JM, Wong RK. Review article: the management of achalasia: a comparison of different treatment modalities. *Aliment Pharmacol Ther*. 2006;24(6):909–918.

16 Glaser DA, Hebert AA, Pariser DM, Solish N. Facial hyperhidrosis: best practice recommendations and special considerations. *Cutis*. 2007;79(suppl 5):29–32.

17 Cavaliere CM. Lasers em cirurgia plástica. In: Livros Di, ed. *Manual de Cirurgia Plástica de Mishigan*. vol. 10: Rio de Janeiro: Di Livros; 2006:55.

18 Ferreira LM, Horibe EK, Haddad A, Zanata F. Cosmiatria. In: *Cirurgia Plástica: Guias de medicina ambulatorial e Hospitalar UNIFESP – Escola Paulista de Medicina*. São Paulo: Edit Manole; 2007:783, 815.

19 Ruiz-Esparza J, Gomez JB. The medical face lift: a noninvasive, nonsurgical approach to tissue tightening in facial skin using nonablative radiofrequency. *Dermatol Surg*. 2003;29(4)Ç:335.

20 Rohrich RJ, Ghavami A, Crosby MA. The role of hyaluronic acid fillers (restylane) in facial cosmetic surgery: review and technical considerations. *Plast Reconstr Surg*. 2007;120(suppl):41S.

21 Barbosa MVJ, Nahas FX, Ferreira LM. Cirurgia Plástica: Biomateriais injetáveis. In: *Guias de medicina ambulatorial e Hospitalar UNIFESP – Escola Paulista de Medicina*. São Paulo: Edit Manole; 2007:823–830.

22 Kurtz ES, Spencer JM. Approaches to document the efficacy and safety of microdermabrasion procedure. *Dermatol Surg*. 2006; 32:1353–1357.

23 Karimipour DJ, Kangs Johnson TM, Orringer JS, Hamilton T, Hammerbergc G, Fisher G. Microdermabrasion with and without aluminum oxide crystal *abrasion*: A comparative molecularanalysis of dermal remodeling. *J Am Acad Dermatol*. 2005;52:215–223.

2 Combining Non-Invasive Therapies

A step by step guide

Marian Cantisano-Zilkha, Alessandra Haddad

INTRODUCTION

A better comprehension of the facial aging process and the introduction of safer, longer-lasting materials for restoring volume to facial structures has given a new dimension to non invasive facial rejuvenation. Since the introduction of injectable bovine collagen for improving or eliminating facial wrinkles, many new agents with safer and more effective properties have been introduced. These newer injectable fillers, when used in combination with other minimally invasive therapies for the skin – such as microdermabrasion, chemical peels, botulinum toxin and radiofrequency-based and light-based treatments – have increased and prolonged the degree of aesthetic results and the level of satisfaction for patients and physicians. The appropriate procedures, when skillfully performed, can dramatically improve the patient's appearance with little or no downtime. Before considering the many options, the physician has to be highly qualified and knowledgeable about how to combine the different resources to optimize the final result.

A multidimensional approach, using a combination of modalities, can improve facial skin texture, pigmentation, tone, rhytidosis and facial contour. It is important to understand that alterations can be assessed in three levels: superficial, medium and deep. Concerns at the deep level involve muscular laxity or hyperactivity, fat migration, bone reabsorption and deep dermal laxity. In general, these alterations are considered a manifestation of intrinsic aging because they are more related to genetic inheritance than external ambiental factors. Problems at the medium level include deterioration of the integument marked by dermal atrophy, loss of turgor and thickness, which is externally manifested by wrinkles. Epidermal changes at the superficial level include textural and vascular alterations, mottled pigmentation and fine wrinkles. These changes are usually related to photodamage or ambiental influence into the skin (extrinsic aging).[1] Non-invasive rejuvenation requires a three-dimensional approach, always starting from the deeper level to the superficial one.

The main purpose of this chapter is to suggest a step-by-step guide to standardize the diagnostics for individualizing patient needs and to propose a logical sequence of procedures.

DEEP LEVEL

The options for facial rejuvenation at the deep level include:

I. volume replacement
II. skin tightening
III. muscle relaxation (facial balance)
IV. surgery

I Volume Replacement

Although we will describe fillers for deep level volumetric correction, changing the presentation of the product and the level of application allows its use for the intermediate level of correction.

Filling in the convex and concave areas of the face, which reflect light and shadows, can lead to a notable rejuvenating effect. The volume replacement is usually performed with fillers, implants or autologus fat. Prior to the advent of modern soft tissue fillers, the anatomical changes of the aging face were primarily surgically addressed (rhytidectomy, brow lift and mid-facelift) or by using ablative (carbon dioxide, CO_2) lasers or peelings (fenol). Although these more invasive techniques are associated with an increased morbidity (infection, bleeding and increased downtime), they are still valuable tools in the cosmetic surgeon's armamentarium for advanced facial antiaging. Combination therapies using soft tissue fillers, chemo-denervation, non-ablative laser and light sources provide a more appealing option to patients and surgeons, and can address many of the mild to moderate signs of aging.[2]

There are many classifications of fillers, but they can be categorized based on their source as follows:

- autogenic: fat (see Chapter 10), autologous plasma (see Chapter 13), autologous collagen (see Chapter 9)
- allogenic: cadaveric collagen, human fibroblast cell culture
- xenogenic: collagen, mostly from bovine or porcine sources, and hyaluronic acid products from rooster combs or bacterial fermentation
- synthetic: silicone products, polymethylmethacrylate (PMMA), hydroxylapatite, poly-L-lactic acid, polyacrylamide.

They can also be classified according to their durability after being injected in biodegradables and non-biodegradables (see Chapter 9). Some authors classify them according to their fibroblastic properties (poly-L-lactic acid, hydroxylapatite and, in a lower scale, hyaluronic acid fillers)[3] if they are just passive fillers (collagen) or if they are permanent (silicone, PMMA). Pathologists do not always agree with this classification because it is their belief that every time a foreign body is introduced into the dermis it causes some degree of inflammatory reaction. That reaction can be mild or almost imperceptible (e.g. collagen) or moderate, with consequent fibroblastic activity associated (e.g. poly-L-lactic acid, hydroxylapatite or hyaluronic acid)[3] or severe inflammatory response, generally related to clinical problems such as foreign body granulomatous reaction or even true troublesome tuberculoid granulomas.

II Skin Tightening

The development of CO_2 lasers demonstrated that heat can promote long-term collagen remodeling.[4,5] Because of the long healing time and since patient selection is limited to fair skin types, the technology had to develop in another direction. The advent of radiofrequency (RF) technology opened up a new path for skin tightening without epidermal damage.

Radiofrequency energy is different from optical energy because it depends on the electrical properties of the skin, rather than on the levels of pigmentation, for the selective thermal destruction of targeted areas, which is known as electro-thermolysis. In 2004 the FDA approved RF dermal heating with simultaneous epidermal cooling as a tool to stimulate new collagen formation and, consequently, improve skin laxity. Thermage® (Thermage Inc., CA) was the first RF device launched, and today many devices promise to tighten the skin in a non-ablative way.[6]

Systems using RF current alone, have achieved good results for skin tightening, with comparable efficacy to laser resurfacing and potentially more rapid healing. However, because of the high depth of penetration, the procedure can be more painful. A technology that integrates RF energy with optical energy – using a lower intensity of both – has also shown efficacy in hair removal and wrinkle reduction for all hair colors and skin types. In addition, these dual systems may reduce the risk of the side effects associated with either RF or optical treatments alone.[7]

RF technology, using high frequency current in the range of 0.3 to 10 megahertz (MHz), produces a pure thermal effect on biological tissue that has made it useful for both electrosurgery and various dermatologic applications. Electrical conductivity relies on the frequency of electrical current, and the type and temperature of tissue. The distribution of electrical current depends on how the electrodes are configured. Typical configurations used in medicine are unipolar and bipolar. Although they differ in the way the RF current is controlled and directed at the target tissue, there is no difference in the final tissue effect at the same RF frequency.[8]

One of the problems with RF technology is that some of the devices do not produce enough heat to cause collagen remodeling. Achieving a true skin-tightening effect in the dermal level (1 to 3 mm under the surface) requires a sustained volumetric dermal heating in one area, for a prescribed amount of time,[9] without exposing fat, cartilage and nerves to residual heat. Inappropriate use of RF can paradoxically reduce fat in that area.

Another FDA-approved RF device for treating wrinkles and rhytids is the Accent XL® (Alma Lasers, Caesarea, Israel). It combines two RF modes in a single device. Each proprietary mode – bipolar and unipolar – is delivered by a discrete handpiece to distribute therapeutic heat at different tissue depths within the body. The bipolar handpiece creates local, superficial dermal heating on delicate areas, such as the face. The unipolar and larger handpieces provide deep dermal and subdermal heating of larger areas.

The latest application, currently in the final 544 Investigational Protocol FDA process, is able to penetrate to a depth of 100 mm. This device, the Lipotron® (RevecoMED International, Anaheim, CA), unlike its predecessors, will be used not only for wrinkle reduction, rejuvenation of the face and cellulite smoothing, but also for body contouring. The most significant feature of the Lipotron®, with its depth of heat penetration, is that it affects the visceral fat as well as the subcutaneous fat. It operates at 0.5 MHz and feels like a warm massage to the patient.

Other modalities, such as infrared devices (Titan®, Cutera Inc., CA) and ST Near Infrared handpiece (Alma Laser, Caesarea, Israel) are being used worldwide with a high level of patient satisfaction and few reports of collateral effects. Good candidates for these procedures are patients with light to moderate laxity, hidden mandibular arch, submental laxity, prominent nasolabial fold due to skin laxity and suborbicularis oculi fat (SOOF) pad descend (more than due to dermal atrophy), ptosis of eyebrow secondary to skin laxity of the upper third of the face, and thin skin, with little or no subcutaneous fat deposit, below the targeted area.

When using skin-tightening devices, perhaps the most critical point is making sure that the patient has realistic expectations of the limited potential of these non-invasive techniques. They should understand that they will not achieve the same results as with plastic surgery but they will have less risk, no scars or recovery time, and no interruption of their social or work activities. The key is to identify the critical areas that will elicit a pull or a lifting effect, distally to the vector force of the areas, and treat them in the same direction as in a facelift. Some practitioners even re-treat the area with multiple passes over the 'anchoring points' along the frontal hairline, zygomatic bone and pre auricular sulcus areas or any area where the skin is barely movable over the deep structures.

III Muscle Relaxation and Facial Balance

Botulinum toxin injection is the most widely performed non-invasive procedure. It is the 'gold standard' treatment, especially for the upper third of the face. Botulinum toxin type A is a protein complex that is produced by the bacterium *Clostridium botulinum*, a powerful neurotoxin that causes muscle paralysis. In a medical setting, small doses of an injectable form of sterile, purified botulinum toxin are used to block the release of acetylcholine, which signals muscle contractions in the face. By selectively blocking the muscles' ability to contract, botulinum toxin can soften the vertical frown lines between the eyebrows (glabellar lines) that tend to make individuals look tired, angry or old.[10]

In 1989, the FDA approved botulinum toxin type A (Botox®) to treat two eye muscle disorders: blepharospasm (uncontrollable blinking) and strabismus (misaligned eyes). The toxin was subsequently approved to treat certain types of dystonia, a neurological disorder that causes severe contractions of the muscles, and hyperhidrosis, severe sweating of the armpits. During the course of these treatments, physicians noticed that Botox® softened the glabellar lines. In April 2002, after placebo-controlled, multicenter, randomized clinical studies demonstrated that botulinum toxin markedly improved these frown lines, the FDA approved Botox® for cosmetic use to temporarily improve the appearance of moderate to severe glabellar lines.

The cosmetic uses of the botulinum toxin are thoroughly discussed in Chapter 8.

Botox® in Combination Therapy

There are a number of areas where combining botulinum toxin with other modalities produces improved and longer-lasting results. In patients with deep glabellar frown lines that persist even at rest, using an injectable soft tissue filler gives an immediate improvement that is accentuated after the botulinum toxin effect is apparent, and this improvement lasts longer than when either modality is used alone.[11,12] Although injectable fillers can improve marionette lines and oral commissures, the patient and physician often view the improvement as unsatisfactory. The outcome can be greatly improved by injecting the depressor anguli oris muscle with botulinum toxin to raise the corners of the mouth and reduce the muscular ridge descending from the corner of the mouth.[13]

Botulinum injections are also used as pretreatment for intense pulsed light (IPL), non-ablative laser and photomodulation therapies. Using IPL not only improves skin texture, but also makes the effect of botulinum toxin treatment more striking. In addition, botulinum toxin seems to enhance the skin texture improvement achieved with non-ablative lasers and may also augment the effects of non-thermal, non-ablative photomodulation using light-emitting diodes.

Botulinum toxin injection is a standard pretreatment procedure for laser resurfacing and its effect is crucial during the period of collagen remodeling.[14] Ideally, patients are treated 2 weeks prior to the laser resurfacing procedure. This allows sufficient time for additional touch-up injections when needed. Botulinum toxin pretreatment also improves the effect of facial RF technology.[15]

Botulinum toxin injection is a non-invasive therapy that has dramatically and safely changed the process of facial rejuvenation. Table 2.1 summarizes the benefits of combining several aesthetic enhancement treatments.[16]

IV The Surgical Approach

Although it is not the intention of this book to discuss surgical alternatives, the surgical approach has also changed dramatically because of the evolution and awareness of the physiology of the skin and the aging process. For many years, the classic surgical facelift with large incisions – eye, neck and brow lifts, bi-coronal pre- and retroauricular incisions – has been the only option for treating wrinkles associated with the skin's loss of elasticity. Society's growing interest in maintaining a youthful appearance has resulted in a greater awareness of the physiology of the skin and how to treat it in a more efficient way. Consequently, the incision size has decreased, sutures can be more effectively placed and the endoscopic approach is a reality. For periocular rejuvenation, the gold standard surgical approach is the transcutaneous approach to the

Table 2.1 Benefits of specific combination therapies

Combination therapy	Benefits
Botulinum toxin and fillers	Combines the treatment of dynamic and static wrinkles for a more complete and long-lasting effect than either treatment by itself
Botulinum toxin and IPL	Improves the surface of the skin while addressing the dynamic cause of many facial wrinkles and enhancing the effects of IPL treatment
IPL and microdermabrasion	Work together to superficially resurface and tone the outer layers of skin with minimal downtime and risk. If the skin is not too sensitive, using microdermabrasion the day after a superficial IPL treatment speeds up the clearing of mottled pigmentation
Microdermabrasion and peels	Both therapies address the outer layers of skin, using different techniques – chemical and mechanical – to improve the skin's appearance. Performing microdermabrasion first enhances the depth of the peel but does not address wrinkles caused by volume loss or facial expression
Skincare, microdermabrasion, chemical peels, botulinum toxin, injectable soft fillers, IPL, CO_2 laser	A good skincare regimen at home is essential for maximizing the effects of aesthetic enhancement procedures. The better the condition of the skin, the greater the effect of other non-invasive therapies
Fillers and IPL	Fillers restore volume to the face, and IPL tones and refines the texture of the outer layers of skin and improves its appearance

Cantisano-Zilkha, M. Contemporary Aesthetic Enhancement. Handbooks in Health Care Company, 2008.

upper lids and transconjunctival for the lower lids (CO_2 laser-assisted or not) combined with resurfacing techniques (ablative, fractional lasers or chemical peels). The need for plastic surgery still exists, but non-invasive alternatives can complement surgery and often allow the patient to postpone surgery and bring longer-lasting results.

SUPERFICIAL AND MEDIUM LEVELS

The overall appearance of aging skin is primarily related to the effects of sun exposure over time. Signs of photoaging are becoming evident in younger people, especially those who regularly participate in outdoor activities that expose them to increasingly high levels of UV radiation. When epidermal damage, or photodamage, is predominant, the treatment must include cosmeceuticals, microdermabrasion, IPL photorejuvenation and, in more severe cases where precancerous lesions such as actinic keratosis are present, the use of photodynamic therapy and fractionated lasers. These therapies are discussed in Chapter 4.

The Glogau Wrinkle Scale (Table 2.2), developed by Richard G. Glogau, MD, a clinical professor of dermatology at the University of California, San Francisco, USA, provides a method for physicians to quickly categorize patients' faces, based on photoaging, and match them to the appropriate therapy.[16]

The following therapies are used to treat superficial and medium-depth, age-related changes. Table 2.3 suggests therapies for photodamaged skin, based on the Glogau photodamage scale.[16]

I Chemical Peels

Alpha-hydroxyl Acid Peels

Alpha-hydroxyl acid peels are useful in the management of mild rhytidosis and dyspigmentation. They are available in varying strengths. We usually begin with a 50% glycolic buffered solution applied for a maximum of 10 minutes. A 70% buffered solution is much more potent. The strength of the peel is increased during subsequent sessions according to patient's tolerance and therapeutical response.[1]

Trichloracetic Acid Peels

Trichloracetic acid peels are useful in the management of mild-to-moderate rhytidosis and dyspigmentation. Trichloracetic acid (TCA) can be used as a superficial (20 or 25%) or medium (30 or 35%) depth peel depending on the concentration used and the number of layers applied.[1]

II Microdermabrasion

This procedure should not be confused with the classic dermabrasion. It is a superficial technique for minor skin problems that is effective in smoothing out mild skin blemishes, such as fine wrinkles, age spots and light acne scars. In addition, it stimulates the body to produce new skin cells and increased collagen, which improves the skin's elasticity and makes it look fresher. Because of its simplicity, microdermabrasion has become one of the most popular cosmetic treatments in the USA.

Microdermabrasion gradually removes the upper layers of skin using a tool that rapidly sprays tiny aluminum oxide crystals at the skin's surface, removing one layer at a time. A vacuum device, which is used simultaneously, takes away the separated skin and blasting particles. To achieve the desired effect, a series of 5 to 12 microdermabrasion treatments, spaced a few weeks apart, are usually needed. Periodic treatments every few months can maintain the appearance of the rejuvenated skin. Although the treatment process is long, each treatment is fairly quick and painless, and the recovery is undemanding. This type of treatment is generally performed by a well-trained aesthetician, and does not require a physician. Care should be taken in patients with rosacea, diffuse red background pigmentation of the face or telangiectasias, since it could worsen the condition.

III Dermabrasion and Dermaplaning

When dermabrasion was first developed more than 100 years ago, it was primarily used to improve scars caused by acne, chicken pox, accidents or diseases. Over the last few decades, this resurfacing technique has been refined and grown in popularity. Today, dermabrasion is most often used to treat other skin conditions, including defects in pigmentation, fine facial wrinkles, sun damage, liver spots and certain types of skin lesions (e.g. precancerous growths), and for tattoo removal. Dermaplaning is most commonly used to treat deep acne scars.

Dermabrasion and dermaplaning help to renew the skin's top layers using different methods of controled scraping. Both procedures can be performed on the entire face or on selected small anatomic

Table 2.2 Glogau photoaging classification		
Skin type	**Approximate age**	**Findings**
I. 'No wrinkles' (Fig. 2.1) 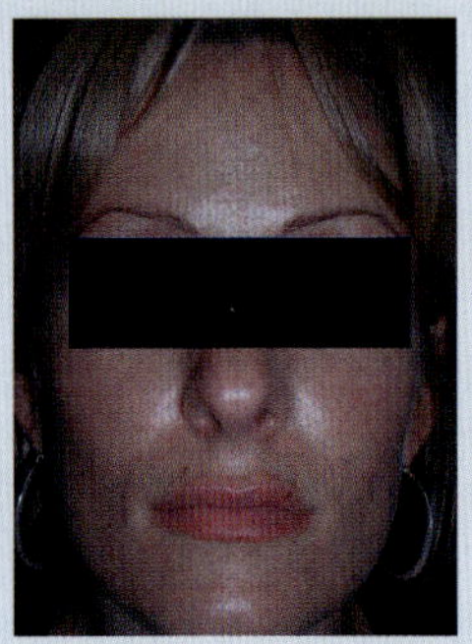	20s to 30s	• Mild pigmentary changes • No keratoses • Minimal wrinkles • Patient wears minimal or no make-up
II. 'Wrinkles in motion' (Fig. 2.2) 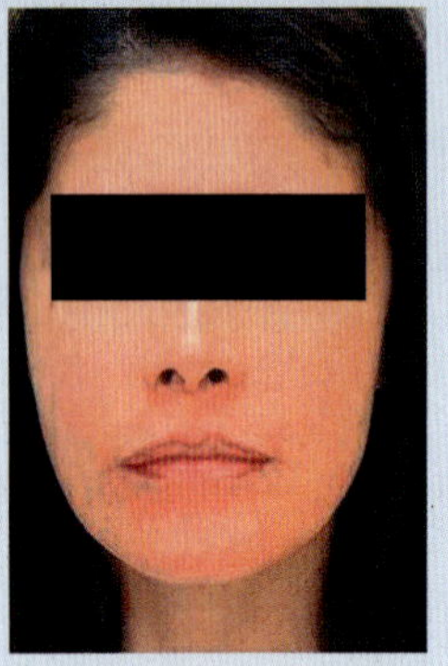	Late 30s or 40s	• Visible early senile lentigines • Palpable but not visible keratoses • Parallel smile lines beginning to appear lateral to mouth • Patient usually wears some foundation
III. 'Wrinkles at rest' (Fig. 2.3) 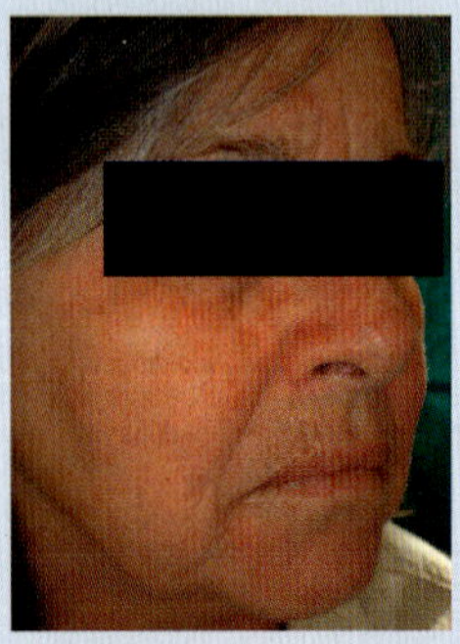	50s or older	• Obvious dyschromia and telangiectasias • Visible keratoses • Wrinkles even when not moving facial muscles • Patient always wears heavy foundation
IV. 'Only wrinkles' (Fig. 2.4) 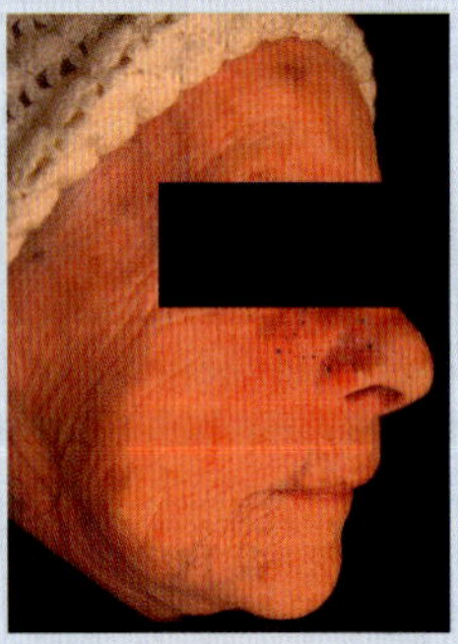	60s or 70s	• Yellow-gray skin color • Prior skin malignancies • Wrinkled throughout; no normal skin • Patient cannot wear make-up because it 'cakes' or 'cracks'

Cantisano-Zilkha, M. Contemporary Aesthetic Enhancement. Handbooks in Health Care Company, 2008.

Table 2.3 Suggested combination treatments for photoaging skin based on the Glogau scale

Goglau wrinkle scale	Treatments
Level I	• Light moisturizers • Sunscreen • Topical and internal antioxidants
Level II	• Sunscreen • Moisturizers • Sensitive clarifying lotion with Kojic acid* and retinoids • Retinoids • AHA peels • Prophylactic botulinum toxin to prevent progression of dynamic wrinkling • IPL
Level III	• Sunscreen • Moisturizers • Clarifying lotion with hydroquinone* and retinoids • AHA peels • IPL series or PDT • TCA peel • Erbium laser peel • Fractional devices
Level IV	• Sunscreen • Moisturizers • Nourishing cream • Clarifying lotion with extra-strength retinoids and extra-strength hydroquinone • PDT or TCA peel • Phenol peel • CO_2 laser resurfacing

*A skin-lightening agent. AHA, alpha-hydroxy acid; TCA, trichloroacetic.

subunits. With dermabrasion, the outer layer of skin is scraped away with a rough wire brush, a burr or a fraise containing diamond particles and attached to a motorized handle. The surgeon continues scraping until the safest level that will make the scar or wrinkle less visible is reached. With dermaplaning, the surgeon uses a hand-held instrument resembling an electric razor (dermatome) with an oscillating blade that moves back and forth to evenly remove the surface layers of skin that surround the facial defect until the lowest point of the scar becomes more level with the surrounding skin. Depending on the size of the area of skin that is to be treated, the procedure can take from a few minutes to an hour and a half to perform. In cases where scarring is deep or a large area of skin is involved, the procedure may be performed in stages or more than once.

IV Intense Pulsed Light

IPL is administered by a flash lamp device emitting light of multiple wavelengths. Cutoff filters are used to enhance the preferential absorption by blood vessels or pigment.[17] IPL is an increasingly popular non-ablative light modality. Unlike lasers, it is a non-collimated, non-coherent light source that penetrates the dermis to generate collagen and cause skin to contract and tighten. IPL emits a spectrum of wavelengths in the 515 to 1200 nm range, and allows for variation of pulse length and mode, delay between pulses and change in the amount of power delivered. Because cutoff filters eliminate the lower range of wavelength of light emitted, patients with darker skin types (Fitzpatrick III to IV) can be safely treated. IPL has been successfully used to treat unwanted and ingrown hair, rosacea, telangiectasias (permanently dilated facial blood vessels), freckles and skin darkening, sun damage, wrinkles, scars, acne and tattoos. It is also used in combination with photodynamic therapy (PDT) as the light source to activate the photosensitizing agent in the tissue to be treated.

V Photodynamic Therapy

PDT dates from 1400BC, when a variety of botanicals where used to improve phototherapy.[17] It is defined as the selective destruction of malignant or fast-growing cells by light activation of a photosensitizing agent, in the presence of oxygen. It treats specific areas of the skin without damaging surrounding tissue. In the early 1960s, Lipson and Schwartz, at the Mayo Clinic, injected hematoporphyrins into a patient undergoing surgery and they noted a fluorescence in the neoplastic tumor that demonstrated the localization of photosensitizing agent into the tumors. Although used in dermatology to treat basal cell carcinoma, multiple actinic keratoses (AKs) and sebaceous disorders, such as acne and sebaceous hyperplasia, PDT has been found to have a variety of cosmetic benefits and has become one of the ideal treatment options to treat patients with signs of chronic aging, such as wrinkling, irregular thinning of the epidermis, blotchy hyperpigmentation, telangectasias and premalignant AKs with little downtime.

Clinicians should be aware of the bright future of this non-invasive modality and should be ready for the way it may not only change how certain malignant or premalignant conditions of the skin and acne conditions are treated, but also open up another level in skin rejuvenation.

Lasers and non-lasers, such as blue light, IPL (560–590 filters) or pulsed dye lasers, can be successfully used in PDT for dermatologic conditions.[17]

VI Non-ablative Lasers

Non-ablative lasers include the 1064-nm neodymium: yttrium–aluminum garnet (Nd:YAG) laser, which is useful for vessel ablation and hair removal (Cool Glide®), and the 1320-nm Nd:Yag (Cool Touch®) laser, which is used for collagen stimulation.

VII Fractionated Laser Devices

Fractional resurfacing, or fractional laser therapy (FLT) represents a technology that seeks to address the limitations of both ablative resurfacing and non-ablative treatments. Many companies now offer versions of fractionated erbium or carbon dioxide lasers. The Fraxel™ and the Pixel™ lasers are both adaptations of the erbium laser that were designed to improve skin texture with a minimum of downtime and without anesthesia. Both of these lasers have the unique ability to create microthermal zones of tissue treatment between untouched areas of skin. Side effects are generally limited to a sunburn-like redness, which disappears in a few days.[17]

More recently, CO_2 fractionated lasers, such as Ellipse Juvia® (Ellipse A/S Hørsholm, Denmark) and Pixel CO_2 Omnifit® (Alma Lasers, Caesarea, Israel), have also been developed and approved. They are supposed to have the ideal wavelength for treating wrinkles, poor skin texture, large pores, sun spots, brown spots, scars and uneven pigmentation. Multiple treatments are required for a desirable result, but discomfort is minimal and there is little healing downtime.

CONCLUSIONS

Non-invasive approaches for improving facial skin texture and contours are becoming increasingly popular, but physicians and patients must understand that one treatment modality alone is not the answer. Non-invasive facial rejuvenation is an effective modality with few complications and little recovery time. Our patients have experienced significant improvement with combined approaches to rejuvenation. When multiple therapies are used in combination, the outcome can exceed the expectations, and the final result can be more than the sum of the individual components (see Table 2.4).

Table 2.4 Recommended techniques by facial area
Forehead and eyebrows
Skin-tightening techniques Botulinum toxin IPL/PDT/chemical peels Micropigmentation for eyebrows
Glabella
Botulinum toxin Avoid fillers; if needed, carefully fill residual depressions using serial puncture or linear threading techniques
Upper eyelids
Botulinum toxin for retraction Skin tightening devices Micropigmentation for cosmetic purposes
Lower eyelids
Relax and flatten the pretarsal orbicularis muscle with one to two units of Botox For rhytids, use fractional devices, resurfacing techniques, peels For laxity and/or retraction, perform lateral canthal tendon plication
Malar eminences
Skin-tightening devices IPL/PDT/chemical peels Volumetric replacement with high-density hyaluronic acid, Sculptra, Radiesse
Nasolabial folds
Fillers Skin-tightening devices
Melomental folds
Botulinum toxin at depressor angulii oris muscles Skin-tightening devices Fillers
Lower facial contours
Skin-tightening devices Platysma treatment with Botulinum toxin
Lips
Fillers Neuromodulation Resurfacing, peels or fractional devices Micropigmentation

REFERENCES

1 Cantisano-Zilkha M. Patient home care regimens. *Ophthalmol Clin N Am*. 2005.

2 Bosniak S, Cantisano-Zilkha M, Glavas IP. Injectable fillers. In: *Minimally Invasive Techniques of Oculofacial Rejuvenation*. Theime Publishers; 2005:41–53.

3 Carruthers J, Carruthers A. *Soft Tissue Augmentation*. 2nd ed., Vol. 7. Elsevier Inc; 2008:84–87.

4 Kirsch KM, Zelickson BD, Zachary CB, et al. *Ultrastructure of collagen thermally denatured by microsecond domain pulsed CO_2 laser*. Paper presented at the 17th Annual Meeting of the American Society of Lasers in Medicine and Surgery, Phoenix, April 1997.

5 Fitzpatrick RE, Rostan EF, Marchell N. Collagen tighetening induced by carbon dioxide laser versus erbium:YAG laser. *Lasers Surg Med*. 2000;27(5):395–4003.

6 Zelickson BD, Kist D, Bernstein E, et al. Histological and ultrastructural evaluation of the effects of a radiofrequency-based nonablative dermal remodeling device. *Arch Dermatol*. 2004;140:204–209.

7 Bitter Jr R, Mulholland S. Report of a new technique for enhanced non-invasive skin rejuvenation using a dual mode pulsed light and radio-frequency energy source: Selective radiothermolysis. *J Cosmet Dermatol*. 2002;1:142–143.

8 Sadick NS. Selective electro-thermolysis in aesthetic medicine: a review. *Lasers Surg Med*. 2004;34:91–97.

9 Narins RS, Tope WD, Pope K, Ross EV. Effects associated with a radiofrequency tissue tightening device: rare, preventable, and correctable with subcision and autologous fat transfer. *Dermatol Surg*. 2006;32:115–121.

10 Bosniak S, Cantisano-Zilkha M. Neuromodulation and management of facial rhytidosis. In: *Minimally Invasive Techniques of Oculofacial Rejuvenation*. New York, NY: Thieme; 2005.

11 Bosniak S, Cantisano-Zilkha M. Hyaluronic acid gel injections for facial rejuvenation: a 3-year clinical experience. *Operative Techniques in Oculoplastic, Orbital, and Reconstructive Surgery*. 1999;2:177–181.

12 Carruthers J, Carruthers A. A prospective randomized, parallel group study analyzing the effect of BTX-A (Botox) and nonanimal sources hyaluronic acid (NASHA, Restylane) in combination compared with NASHA (Restylane) alone in severe glabellar rhytides in adult female subjects: treatment of severe glabellar rhytides with hyaluronic acid derivative compared with the derivative and BTX-A. *Dermatol Surg*. 2003;29:802–809.

13 Bosniak S, Cantisano-Zilkha M, Rinaldi P, et al. Lip and perioral rejuventation: a multidisciplinary approach. *Operative Techniques in Oculoplastic, Orbital, and Reconstructive Surgery*. 2001;4:104–108.

14 Bosniak S, Cantisano-Zilkha M. *Cosmetic Blepharoplasty and Facial Rejuvenation*. Philadelphia: Lippincott-Raven Publishers; 1999.

15 Bosniak S, Cantisano-Zilkha M. Neuromodulation and management of facial rhytidosis. In: *Minimally Invasive Techniques of Oculofacial Rejuvenation*. New York, NY: Thieme; 2005.

16 Cantisano-Zilkha M. *Combining aesthetic enhancement therapies*. In: *Contemporary Aesthetic Enhancement*. Handbooks in Health Care Company. www.hhcbooks.com; 2008.

17 Cantisano-Zilkha M. *Understanding skin resurfacing-mechanical devices, lasers and other modalities. Contemporary Aesthetic Enhancement*. Handbooks in Health Care Company. www.hhcbooks.com; 2008.

Anatomy of the periorbital area

Ioannis P Glavas

INTRODUCTION

The upper and lower eyelids are two complex and thin flaps covering the eye. Knowledge of their anatomy is important for the cosmetic surgeon for several reasons. The eyelids protect the eyes from the outside world and play an important role in the production, distribution and drainage of the tears (eyelid lacrimal pump mechanism). From an aesthetic aspect, it is the anatomic characteristics of the eyelids and their relationship with the surrounding tissues (orbital fat and suborbicularis oculi fat) and structures (brows and midface) that define the ethnic identity of a person. They also contribute to the appearance of the 'eye' that people perceive as beautiful or not. The level and shape of the eyelid margin and crease, the amount and position of orbital fat, the degree of skin rhytidosis and the underlying vascularity are factors that contribute to the appearance of the eyelids and may be modified using surgical or non-surgical procedures.

Gender and ethnic variations should be taken into account when evaluating the eyelids. Male upper eyelids are fuller and their crease is lower

3 Skincare

Eckart Haneke

INTRODUCTION

The skin, our biggest organ, is the outer layer of the body and protects us against noxious influences from our environment. It also has very important immunologic and defense functions and is our largest sensory organ. It maintains the body's external shape and exhibits important direct and indirect social functions. Genetic and hormonal factors, sex, lifestyle and gender characteristics are responsible for determining differing tolerances of exogenous factors and for influencing skin structure and function.

The skin is made up of three layers:

- the epidermis
- the dermis
- the subcutis.

The epidermis is the outermost layer of our skin. It is made up of:

- the basal layer, with cells in continuous division to allow lifelong renewal
- the spinous layer, the thickest of the epidermal layers
- the granular layer, which prepares the epidermis for cornification (or keratinization)
- the outermost stratum corneum or horny layer.

The stratum corneum is functionally the most important layer as it prevents the skin and thus the body from losing its water content. Without this layer, which is just a few microns thick but consists of many layers of horn cells, we would not be able to live outside an aqueous environment. The stratum corneum is also very important in controling the penetration of substances into the skin, including drugs and cosmetics.

Hair and nails are derived from the epidermis, as are sweat and apocrine glands.

Melanocytes populate the basal layer. Female hormones have an influence on the biochemical composition of the horny layer and improve its quality.[1] Skin pigmentation is lighter in women than in men,[2] but is subject to female hormonal influences.

The dermis is the carrier layer of the epidermis and is a tough and resistant layer of connective tissue. It is made up of collagen and elastic fibers embedded in the so-called ground substance of glycosaminoglycans, of which the most important is hyaluronic acid. Hyaluronic acid is able to bind water, and functions both as a lubricant for the collagen and elastic fibers and as a volume-giving substance for the skin.

The skin is less thick in women than in men,[3] and that discrepancy increases noticeably with age. Estrogen therapy over a 12-month period leads to a thickening of the dermis.[4]

The subcutaneous fat is both a mechanical and thermal insulator, as well as an energy storage organ. Its distribution over the body is determined by gender-specific hormonal influences and by genetic factors. Its total amount depends greatly on the calories consumed and used every day. Although most people do not like fat in their bodies, it is important for thermal insulation and for the shape of the face and the rest of the body. However, once the body has accumulated excess adipose tissue it tends not to lose it again. This tendency is what makes weight loss so difficult. Fat is unique and contains approximately 5000 stem cells per gram, and since it can be easily grafted from a donor site of the body to a receptor site, fat transplantation is probably also a 'stem cell transfer'.[5]

The cutaneous fat layer is thicker in women than in men[6] and it has architectural differences, particularly where it is the thickest – so-called cellulite.[7] The difference in fat distribution is the probable reason that women's tolerance to cold is superior to men's.[8]

All three skin layers are equally important for good shape and health. There are many myths about skincare that are supposed to guarantee beautiful skin. Although beautiful skin is healthy skin, the reverse is not always true. When the epidermis is not healthy it may become red, rough, sallow, dry, scaly, spotty or lose its luster and smooth texture. It develops large pores and dilated blood vessels, and a variety of benign and precancerous lesions as well as cancers. When the dermis gets old and/or sun-damaged, it loses its turgor and elasticity, takes on a yellowish color and develops wrinkles and folds.

BASIC SKINCARE

Beautiful skin has a smooth and shiny surface, is evenly pigmented and has a silky touch – it is like babies' skin. Traditional knowledge tells us that prevention is better than treatment. The best protection from the harmful effects of ultraviolet (UV) rays are UV-proof clothes (hats, shirts, trousers), avoidance of direct sun exposure (applying sunscreen 30 minutes before exposure) and perhaps the use of oral and topical application of vitamins C, E, A, other antioxidants and scavengers of reactive oxygen species.

The stratum corneum, as the outermost layer, has to be kept moist since it becomes scaly and loses its elasticity when dry (Fig. 3.1). Unfortunately, moisture cannot be easily added to the skin; in fact, what moisturizers do is to help the skin to keep its own moisture. Contrary to common belief, oil-in-water emulsions may even impair the barrier function of the stratum corneum.[9] Glycerol may reverse this harmful effect on the horny layer. Glycerol-containing hand creams have proven to be effective, and facial skincare may also benefit from glycerol as an ingredient. Urea is another natural moisturizer with unique properties since it can penetrate the horny layer and keep moisture in the skin. The addition of ammonium lactate may enhance this effect.[10] However, topical preparations that contain higher urea concentrations tend to itch when applied to the dry skin of atopic individuals. Dexpanthenol is another substance that improves stratum corneum hydration (Fig. 3.2).[11]

The stratum corneum is also able to store fat-soluble substances. Many lipophilic drugs and cosmeceuticals are retained in it and slowly released. This property is used in dermatology for many creams and ointments that only require a daily application. Simple emollients provide a protective film of fat, preventing transcutaneous water loss and therefore keeping the skin moist. It is not a paradox that the higher the content of fat in the skincare product, the better it maintains skin moisture. This applies to all skin areas, from the very thin eyelid skin to the far more oily and thicker forehead skin.

It is not only the active ingredients of skincare products that are important. The art of making products that are well tolerated, easily applied, non-allergenic, non-toxic or otherwise harmful and feel comfortable on the skin must be supplemented by optimizing existing delivery systems and developing new application systems. A number of stable carrier systems have been developed that allow controlled release of the incorporated ingredients. These systems include liposomes, sphyngosomes, niosomes, multiple emulsions, microemulsions, microsponge delivery systems and thalaspheres, as well as solid lipid nanoparticles and nanostructured lipid carriers.[12] In particular, solid lipid nanoparticles have good physical long-term stability, protect incorporated labile substances against degradation, ensure controlled release

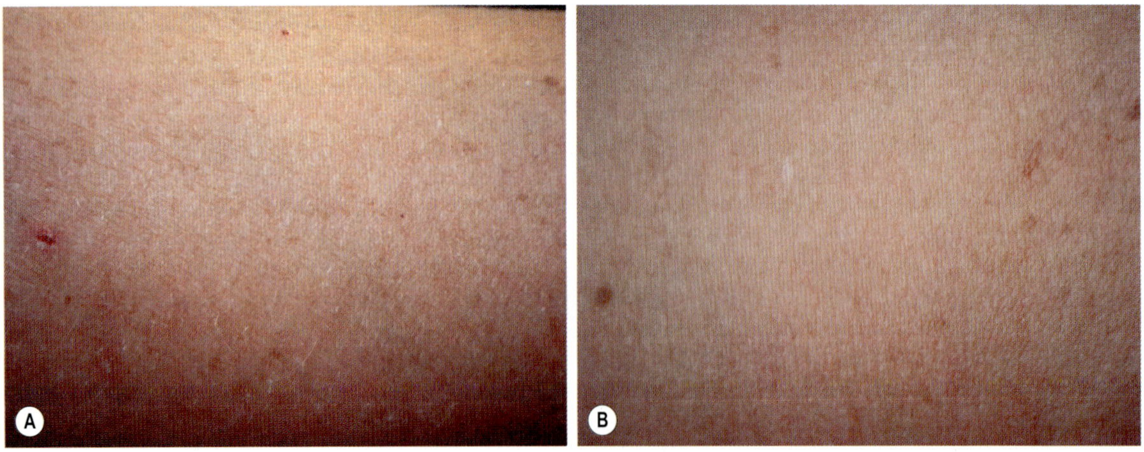

Fig. 3.1 Effect of a simple emollient on skin roughness. *A*, Before treatment; *B*, after 6 weeks of once-daily application.

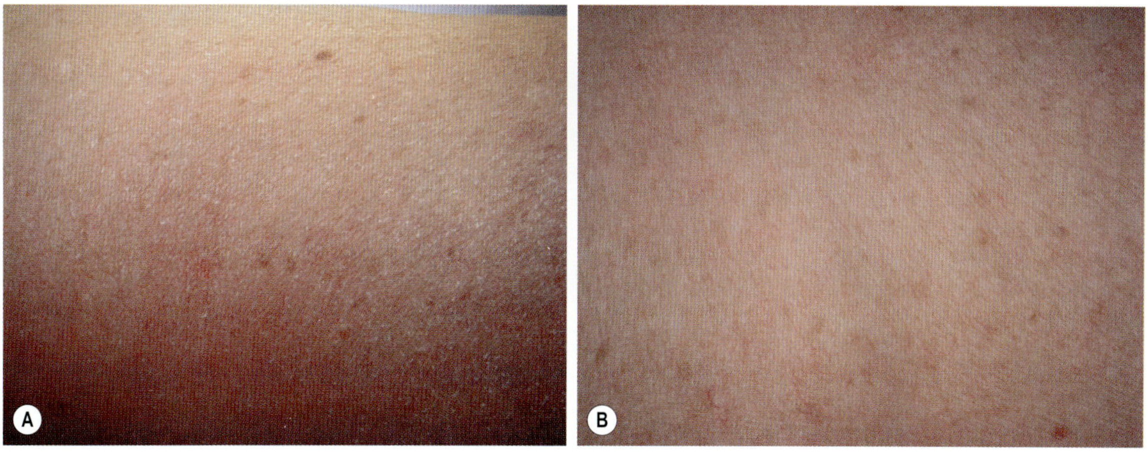

Fig. 3.2 Dex-panthenol containing cream. *A*, Before treatment; *B*, skin-smoothing effect is better than that achieved with an emollient.

of incorporated ingredients, prolong the release of perfumes and repellents, enrich active ingredients in certain skin regions, increase skin hydration and protect against UV light.

More than 80% of the visible aging of facial skin is due to UV exposure. Smoking and other exogenous influences are also important. Avoiding UV exposure and not smoking are the most important factors for beautiful skin.

Whereas UVA is relatively low in energy, it penetrates into the dermis where it causes connective tissue damage, a process erroneously called 'photoaging', although it is in fact photodamage. It causes solar elastosis, a peculiar type of connective tissue damage, blotchy hypo- and hyperpigmentation, and sun-burst vessels. On either side of the neck, a multicolored aspect, called poikiloderma of Civatte, may appear. It is therefore logical to add potent sun-protective substances to daycare products, particularly during the sunny season. High-energy UVB does not penetrate so deeply and is mainly absorbed by the DNA of the epidermis, where it is responsible for tanning, a defense mechanism of the skin against sun exposure. In the long term, however, UVB is responsible for precancerous lesions and skin carcinomas. It dries the epidermis out, causing scaling, rough hyperkeratotic areas and pigment spots. Sunscreens containing UVB-absorbing substances can be effective in preventing skin cancer development. However, sunscreens protecting against both UVA and UVB have the best spectrum of action, protecting against photoaging and also considerably reducing UV-induced immunosuppression.

Washing and cleansing of the skin are important daily skincare measures. There is no scientific proof that washing the face once daily with a mild soap is harmful and makes the skin dry. It is self-evident that the use of soaps should never be overdone and depends on the degree of soiling. Whether or not common alkaline soaps are more harmful than non-alkaline synthetic detergents and skin cleansers remains unproven since these substances are more aggressive degreasing agents than normal soaps. Many people claim that they do not tolerate perfumed soaps or detergents. It is therefore logical for these people to abandon them and not to try one soap after the other. Tolerability and cleansing properties do not depend on the price of the product.

For people who really cannot use soaps or detergents, a well-tolerated emulsion may be used instead. In fact, it is the ability of the soap or detergent to dissolve or emulsify fat that is responsible for the cleaning action. The oily part of the emulsion dissolves the debris and allows it to be removed from the skin surface.

Skin irritation is more frequent in women than in men,[13] and apparently Asian females complain more readily about skin irritation and intolerance of cosmetics than Causasians. However, skin irritability is very difficult to quantify and remains mostly a subjective impression of the individual.

COSMETIC SKINCARE

Cosmetics are defined as articles without therapeutic function (US Federal Food, Drug and Cosmetic Act, 1938). EU legislation forbids cosmetic preparations from containing active ingredients (EU 76/768). Usually, they are substances with immediate effects on skin physiology to clean, protect, maintain and regenerate the skin. Topicals with active ingredients are considered drugs.

Two major classes of cosmetics are distinguished:

- decorative cosmetics, which may also have a minor effect on skin physiology
- substitutive-regenerative cosmetics, which have a marked effect on the condition of skin, mucous membranes and their appendages, such as the hair, nails, sweat and apocrine glands, teeth and minor salivary glands.

Decorative cosmetics are effective for 'camouflage', but have no effect on photodamage. One example is the self-tanning agents that are based on dihydroxyacetone, which reacts with free amino groups of keratin to produce a decorative brown color. Although this is not harmful to the skin it has no UV-protective action.

Regenerative-substitutive cosmetics are applied to regenerate, maintain or improve good skin condition. By law, they must not have a systemic effect.

A third class of substances called cosmeceuticals has recently been introduced. These are cosmetic agents with improved and/or enhanced action, a proven benefit, but a low risk. Fruit acids, α-hydroxy acids, vitamin A and vitamin E are now considered cosmeceuticals when applied topically. They may also exhibit adverse side effects. Nutriceuticals, substances with similar actions, may be useful as absorption from the skin is often limited.

There is a great deal of advertising of products that can prevent cutaneous aging and improve photoaged skin. Many of these products have demonstrated either antioxidant or repairing activities in *in-vitro* experiments, but most have not been tested according to the stringent rules of good dermatologic practice and science. Some of the most important and effective cosmetics are sunscreens. They prevent not only sunburn, but also more harmful consequences that are not immediately seen, such as immunosuppression, DNA damage and elastotic degeneration of the connective tissue. It is important to keep in mind that even if these products are correctly used, consumers cannot remain in the sun for longer periods. The skin needs to be protected from carcinogenic UVB and the less energetic UVA. Ultraviolet light also induces release of iron into the tissues, which in turn promotes the generation of free radicals and connective tissue damage. Topical iron chelators – substances that are able to bind iron – have been shown to be protective.[14]

Oxygen radical scavengers – α-tocopherol (vitamin E), ascorbic acid (vitamin C), propyl gallate and a number of antiinflammatory agents such as ibuprofene, naproxene or hydrocortisone – prevent UV-mediated DNA damage and squamous cell carcinoma. Just as sunscreens may often contain these products, cosmetic preparations for outdoor use should also contain UV filters.

COSMOCEUTICALS

Vitamin A

Vitamin A is all-*trans*-retinol. It restores the horny layer by stimulation of keratinocyte renewal, reduces desiccation of the skin, stabilizes cell membranes and controls membrane permeability. Retinal is all-*trans*-retin aldehyde. Its action is very similar to that of vitamin A. Atmospheric oxygen oxidizes it to vitamin A acid (VAA; also known as tretinoin, *all-trans* retinoic acid or Retin A™), thus exhibiting similar, but milder, VAA effects. It is a physiological metabolite of vitamin A and is produced in the liver. Even though there is very little absorption into the blood stream, retinoic acid is a drug, not a cosmeceutical, and therefore is not allowed in cosmetic preparations. It is used topically in 0.025–0.1% concentration for acne treatment and rejuvenation, and systemically in promyelocytic leukemia. It is therefore the only substance that can turn the biological clock back. Combinations with hydroquinone or azelaic acid are potent skin depigmenting agents used for treatment of melasma. Since melasma is often provoked or exacerbated by previous inflammation, mild cortisone cream is often also added.

Vitamin A is an animal product, whereas the provitamin carotenoids occur mainly in red vegetables and fruit, such as carrots, tomatoes (containing lycopene), red berries and rose-hips.

Vitamin C

Vitamin C (L-ascorbic acid) is a very effective radical scavenger and is essential for collagen and hyaluronic acid synthesis and induction of production of other intercellular substances. It exerts a mild UV protective action and has mild antiinflammatory effects. Cosmetic preparations containing stabilized vitamin C have a positive effect on skin quality.

Vitamin C cannot be synthesized by the human body and has to be taken up with food. It is found in green vegetables and potatoes, fruit (particularly citrus fruit) and peppers. The molecule is unstable in air, light and heat, and must be promptly consumed.

Vitamin E

Vitamin E (α-tocopherol) increases the water-binding capacity of the skin and is a natural moisturizer. Its main biochemical function is to protect cell membranes against the damaging effects of UV-induced free radicals. It also inhibits the formation of peroxides, which are implicated in the aging process. It stimulates cell renewal and supports biological skin stability. Skin tension is increased, wound-healing stimulated and the final quality of the skin scar is improved. It is a strong antioxidant and after topical application for 6 to 24 hours it concentrates in the dermis, where it can exert its positive effects (Fig. 3.3).

Vitamin E is a plant product and is found in many plant oils, nuts and seeds. It stabilizes vitamin C.[15] Together, topical vitamins C and E reduce harmful UV effects (Fig. 3.4).

Some users have developed allergic contact dermatitis from vitamin E soaps and lotions. This appears to be unique to topical vitamin E preparations since systemic administration of vitamin E virtually never produces allergic reactions.

Vitamin B_3

Vitamin B3 (nicotinic acid or niacin) and its amide, nicotinamide (or niacinamide), are similarly effective since they are interconverted within the body. Niacinamide is a component of important coenzymes involved in hydrogen transfer. It is the prosthetic group of two codehydrogenases, nicotinamide adenine dinucleotide (NAD) and nicotinamide adenine dinucleotide phosphate (NADP). Topical application of niacinamide has a stabilizing effect on epidermal

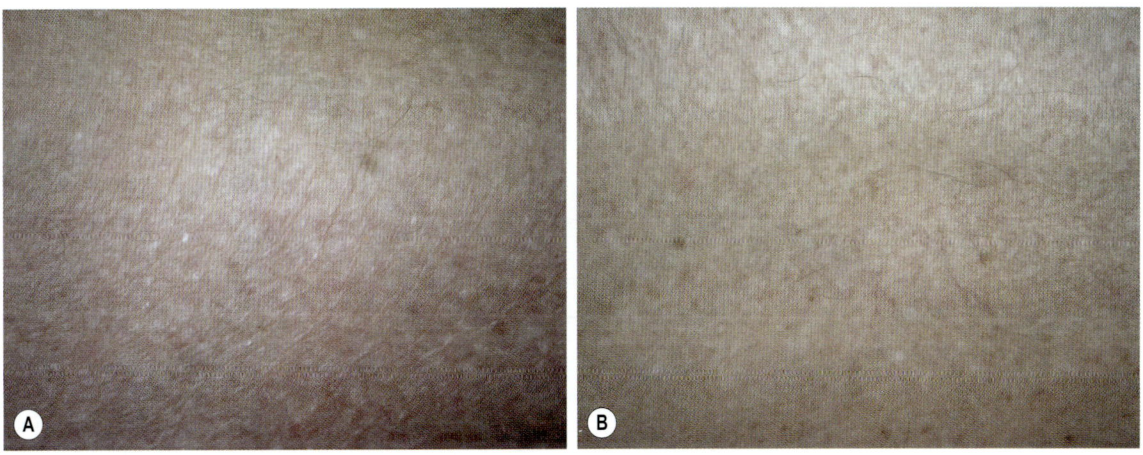

Fig. 3.3 Effect of a cream containing α tocopherol 1%. *A*, Before treatment; *B*, after 4 weeks of daily application.

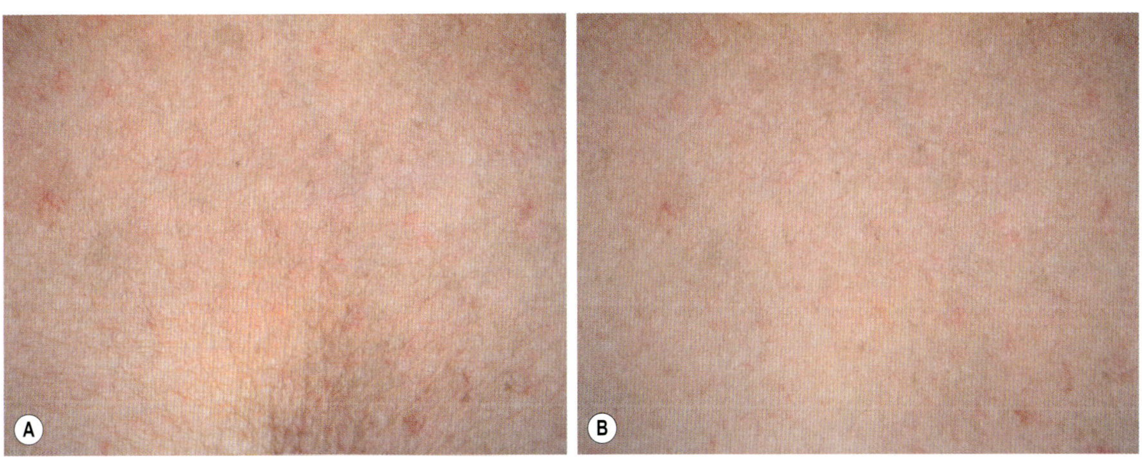

Fig. 3.4 Effect of a combined α-tocopherol 1% plus 5% vitamin C cream. *A*, Before treatment; *B*, after 8 weeks of twice-daily application.

barrier function, reducing transepidermal water loss and improving the moisture content of the horny layer. It increases protein synthesis, for instance of keratin, stimulates ceramide synthesis, speeds up the differentiation of keratinocytes and raises intracellular NADP levels. In aging skin, topical application of niacinamide improves the surface structure, smoothes out wrinkles and inhibits photocarcinogenesis. It increases the protein content of the barrier layer of the epidermis and the collagen mass in the dermis. It has antiinflammatory effects in acne, rosacea and nitrogen mustard-induced irritation. Its verifiable beneficial effects make niacinamide a suitable component in cosmetic products for epidermal barrier function disorders, for aging skin, for improving pigmentary disorders and for use on skin prone to acne and rosacea. It is well tolerated by most patients complaining of 'sensitive skin'.[16]

Vitamin K

Vitamin K (phylloquinone) has an antiedematous and antiinflammatory effect through stabilization of vessel walls, thus reducing actinic purpura and tissue iron content. The negative effect of iron overload is diminished. Its main cosmetic use is in creams to alleviate periorbital dark circles and restore facial skin color.[17]

Alpha-hydroxy Acids

Fruit acids (α-hydroxy acids (AHA)) are a group of organic acids mainly, but not exclusively, contained in fruits: glycolic, lactic, tannic, tartaric, citric, malic acid, etc. They are all radical scavengers. In addition, they are exfoliative, keratolytic, hydrating and bleaching agents. AHAs modulate the maturation of the epidermis to improve the quality of the horny layer. Their effect is related to their chemical structure and is proportional to acidity, concentration and duration of application: the lower the pH, the higher the concentration, the longer the application, the more intense the effect. In low concentrations between 2 and 10%, they can be used by the consumers themselves whereas high concentrations, which are used for skin peels, should be used by experienced persons only. Their main indications are mild acne, spotty dyspigmentation, hyperkeratoses, skin refreshing and pretreatment before chemical peeling.[18]

Beta-hydroxy Acids

Beta-hydroxy acids (β-butanoic acid, tropic acid) and polyhydroxy acids have similar actions. The latter are derived from sugars and other carbohydrates. For instance, vitamin C (ascorbic acid) is the lactone form of an AHA, but it has no effect on keratinization comparable to other AHAs. Alpha-keto acids, e.g. pyruvic acid, have similar effects, as lactic acid can be oxidized to pyruvic acid by lactate dehydrogenase. Polyhydroxy acids are also antioxidants.[19]

Dimethylaminoethanol

Dimethylaminoethanol (DMAE) has become a new 'miracle drug' in the cosmetic skincare market. Although it has been listed in the *Cosmetic, Toiletries, and Fragrance Association Dictionary* for a long time, the observation of its immediate tightening action on skin has only recently been exploited for new antiaging creams. DMAE is currently marketed as an oral nutritional supplement for memory improvement and enhancement of physical performance, but this has apparently to be separated from its action on the epidermis. The mechanism of action is thought to induce a vacuolar effect on cells of the upper skin layers, causing cell expansion and thus giving the appearance of an immediate antiwrinkle effect.[20]

Zinc

Zinc has an anti-free radical effect and is essential for many immune functions, connective tissue regeneration and wound healing. It is often used in the form of a fine white powder of zinc oxide, particularly in sunscreens. The whitish hue it gives to the skin makes these preparations cosmetically unacceptable. However, the white color can be diminished by adding brown pigments, and recently the zinc has been micronized, improving the final preparation texture.

Estrogens

Estrogens are female sex hormones that decrease considerably with the menopause. The addition of estrogen-active substances to skincare products may improve stratum corneum hydration and alleviate fine wrinkles.[21]

Soy

Soy has been known for many years to have positive nutritional and health effects. Chinese women working in the tofu industry were famous for having the most beautiful (fair, smooth, porcelain-like, fine) skin. At least one part of soy's positive action on skin is due to its relatively high content of isoflavones, phytoestrogenic substances with weak antioxidant and antiinflammatory properties. Soy phytosterols interfere with the arachidonic cascade and provide mild antiinflammatory effects. Soy beans contain the water-soluble vitamins thiamine (B_1), riboflavin (B_2), niacin, and folic and pantothenic acids, and the fat-soluble vitamins A and E. They are an important source of zinc, manganese, magnesium and calcium. Soy saponins provide active antioxidant and free-radical scavenging effects. A preparation made of the complete spectrum of soy components improved the firmness and elasticity of the skin.[22] Specific soy bean proteins interfere with melanosome transfer, resulting in more even pigmentation and pigment reduction.[22] Soy components are also used for skin conditioners and emollients (soy-bean oil), emulsifiers (soy protein hydrolysates), surfactants, emulsifiers and stabilizers (soy lecithin and phospholipids), as well as skin conditioners (soy sterol).

Green Tea

Green tea extracts improve UV-induced skin damage. Green tea polyphenols reduce UV erythema. The active substances are (−)-epigallocatechin-3-gallate and (−)-epicatechin-3-gallate, which protect against the deleterious effects of UV on immune cells such as Langerhans cells.[23] Black tea extracts, both orally and topically applied, are also able to protect against UV-induced skin damage. The active substance is theaflavin.[24]

Spearmint

Spearmint (*Mentha spicata*) can reduce the oxidizing potency of benzoyl peroxide and salvage the antioxidant properties of a variety of reducing enzymes that contain glutathione as their active component.[25]

Hamamelis

Hamamelis (witch hazel) may reduce UV-induced erythema. However, this effect depends on the way its active ingredients are distilled.[26]

Essential Fatty Acids

Essential fatty acids, particularly the n-3 type, reduce the risk of squamous cell cancer development.[27] Evening primrose oil and borage oil improve dry skin and its barrier function, especially in atopic subjects.

Beta-lipohydroxyacid

Beta-lipohydroxyacid is able to improve features of female aged skin by inducing epidermal thickening and some recipients also develop a thicker filaggrin-containing layer in the epidermis.[28]

Essential Oils

Essential oils have also been tested for their skincare effect. Lavender oil has an antiinflammatory action.[29]

Other Cosmetics

Herbs, plant oils, unsaturated fatty acids, algae, shark cartilage and so on have some – if barely detectable – skincare effect.

New Products

There are two relatively new developments in the cosmetic field: amino acids of sugar cane and kinetin.

Sugar Cane Amino Acids

Sugar cane amino acids occur in the sprouts of young sugar cane plants. They are small molecules that rapidly penetrate the skin and are the only substances known that can increase skin moisture threefold, thus improving skin tonicity. In combination with vitamin C they are highly active.

Indications of these promising new treatments are photodamage, wrinkles, pigment spots, dry skin, peeling pretreatment, acne and rosacea.

Kinetin

Kinetin (N^6-furfuryl adenine) is a plant hormone which stimulates growth. It is the substance that keeps cut leaves green but it also prevents the skin aging processes. In creams, it improves skin texture, color, pigmentation, fine wrinkles and reduces trans-epidermal water loss. It is non-irritative, non-allergenic and may be combined with other cosmeceuticals. It also alleviates reddening of facial skin.[30–32]

New Developments

There is presently a lot of research focusing on cosmetics to prevent photoaging. Some will provide modulation of DNA repair mechanisms using exogenously applied enzymes such as bacterial photolyase, while others stimulate DNA repair by exogenous UV-damaged DNA. Pretreatment with thymidine dinucleotide may interfere with the harmful effect of high-energetic UV light.

CONCLUSION

Skincare appears to be something self-evidently necessary for many women, but most men are unfamiliar with it. Two aspects of skincare have to be differentiated: basic skincare with moisturizers and treatment with cosmeceuticals. Both moisturizers and cosmeceuticals can improve the skin quality, prevent or at least diminish damage from environmental hazards, and delay signs and symptoms of aging. This is possible with minimal effort and there are excellent long-term results. However, sun protection is of paramount importance and can be derived from both basic skincare and from cosmeceuticals.

REFERENCES

1 Denda M, Koyama J, Hori J, et al. Age and sex-dependent change in stratum corneum sphingolipids. *Arch Dermatol Res.* 1993;285:415–417.

2 Green A, Martin NG. Measurement and perception of skin colour in a skin cancer survey. *Br J Dermatol.* 1990;123:77–84.

3 Seidenari S, Pagnoni A, Di Nardo A, Riannetti A. Echographic evaluation with image analysis of normal skin: variations according to age and sex. *Skin Pharmacol.* 1994;7:201–209.

4 Maheux R, Naud F, Rioux M, et al. A randomized double-blind, placebo-controlled study on the effect of conjugated estrogens on skin thickness. *Am J Obstet Gynecol.* 1994;170:642–649.

5 Fraser JK, Wulur I, Alfonso Z, Zhu M, Wheeler ES. Differences in stem and progenitor cell yield in different subcutaneous adipose tissue depots. *Cytotherapy.* 2007;9:459–467.

6 Hattori K. Okamotow. Skin fold compressibility in Japanese university students. *Okajima Folia Anat Jpn.* 1993;70:69–78.

7 Querleux B, Cornillon C, Jolivet O, Bittoun J. Anatomy and physiology of subcutaneous adipose tissue by in vivo magnetic resonance imaging and spectroscopy: Relationships with sex and presence of cellulite. *Skin Res Technol.* 2002;8:118–124.

8 McFarland RA, Kadish R. Sex differences in finger temperature response to music. *Int J Psychophysiol.* 1991;11:295–298.

9 Gloor M, Hauth A, Gehring W. O/W emulsions compromise the stratum corneum barrier and improve drug penetration. *Pharmazie.* 2003;58:709–715.

10 Gloor M, Fluhr J, Lehmann L, Gehring W, Thieroff-Ekerdt R. Do urea/ammonium lactate combinations achieve better skin protection and hydration than either component alone? *Skin Pharmacol Appl Skin Physiol.* 2002;15:35–43.

11 Gehring W, Gloor M. Effect of topically applied dexpanthenol on epidermal barrier function and stratum corneum hydration. Results of a human in vivo study. *Arzneimittelforschung.* 2000;50:659–663.

12 Müller RH, Mäder K, Gohla S. Solid lipid nanoparticles: productions, characterization and applications. *Adv Drug Deliv Rev.* 2001;47:165–196.

13 Wilhelm KP, Maibach HI, Wilson D. Irritant reactivity in males and females. *Contact Dermatitis.* 1987;17:276–280.

14 Jurkiewicz BA, Buettner GR. EPR detection of free radicals in UV-irradiated skin: mouse versus human. *Photochem Photobiol.* 1996;64:918–922.

15 Rozman B, Gasperlin M. Stability of vitamins C and E in topical microemulsions for combined antioxidant therapy. *Drug Deliv.* 2007;14:235–245.

16 Gehring W. Nicotinic acid/niacinamide and the skin. *J Cosmet Dermatol.* 2004;3:88–93.

17 Iscan Y, Wissing SA, Hekimoglu S, Müller RH. Solid lipid nanoparticles (SLN) for topical drug delivery: incorporation of the lipophilic drugs N,N-diethyl-m-toluamide and vitamin K. *Pharmazie.* 2005;60:905–909.

18 Ditre CM, Griffin TD, Murphy GF, et al. Effects of α-hydroxy acids on photoaged skin: a pilot clinical, histological and ultrastructural study. *J Am Acad Dermatol.* 1996;34:187–195.

19 Yu RJ, Van Scott EJ. α-Hydroxyacids, polyhadroxy acids, aldobionic acids and their topical actions. In: Baran R, Maibach H, eds. *Textbook of Cosmetic Dermatology.* 3rd ed. London: Taylor & Francis; 2005:77–93.

20 Morissette G, Germain L, Marceau F. The antiwrinkle effect of topical concentrated 2-dimethylaminoethanol involves a vacuolar cytopathology. *Br J Dermatol.* 2007;156:433–439.

21 Schmidt JB, Binder M, Macheiner W, et al. Treatment of skin ageing symptoms in perimenopausal females with estrogen compounds. A pilot study. *Maturitas.* 1994;20:25–30.

22 Wallo W, Nebus J, Leyden JJ. Efficacy of a soy moisturizer in photoaging: a double-blind, vehicle-controlled, 12-week study. *J Drugs Dermatol.* 2007;6:917–922.

23 Elmets C, Singh D, Tubesing K, et al. Cutaneous photoprotection from ultraviolet injury by green tea polyphenols. *J Am Acad Dermatol.* 2001;44:425–432.

24 Nomura M, Ma W-Y, Huang C, et al. Inhibition of ultraviolet B-induced AP-a activation by theaflavins from black tea. *Mol Carcinog.* 2000;28:148–155.

25 Saleem M, Alam A, Sultana S. Attenuation of benzoyl peroxide-mediated cutaneous oxidative stress and hyperproliferative response by the prophylactic treatment of mice with spearmint (*Mentha spicata*). *Food Chem Toxicol.* 2000;38:939–948.

26 Hughes-Formella B, Filbry A, Gassmueller J, et al. Anti-inflammatoryx efficacy of topical prepatations with 10% hamamelis distillate in a UV erythema test. *Skin Phamacol Appl Skin Physiol.* 2001;15:125–132.

27 Hakim I, Harris R, Ritenbaugh C. Fat intake and risk of squamous cell carcinoma of the skin. *Nutr Cancer.* 2000;36:155–162.

28 Avila-Camacho M, Montastier C, Piérard GE. Histometric assessment of the age-related skin response to 2-hydroxy-5-octanoyl benzoic acid. *Skin Pharmacol Appl Skin Physiol.* 1998;11:52–56.

29 Kim H-M, Cho S-M. Lavender oil inhibits immediate-type allergic reaction in mice and rats. *J Pharm Pharmacol.* 1999;51:221–226.

30 Rattan SJS, Clark BFC. Kinetin delays the onset of aging characteristics in human fibroblasts. *Biochem Biophys Res Commun.* 1994;201:665–673.

31 McCullough J. Furfuryl adenine – a new antiaging topical: research and clinical experience. *Skin Allergy News.* 1999;3–5.

32 Chiu PC, Chan CC, Lin HM, Chiu HC. The clinical anti-aging effects of topical kinetin and niacinamide in Asians: a randomized, double-blind, placebo-controlled, split-face comparative trial. *J Cosmet Dermatol.* 2007;6:243–249.

4 Chemical Peels

Marina Landau, Richard H Bensimon

Included on **DVD**

INTRODUCTION

Chemical peeling is a procedure used for the cosmetic improvement of skin or for the treatment of some skin disorders. Chemical exfoliating agent is applied to the skin to destruct portions of epidermis and/or dermis with subsequent regeneration and rejuvenation of the tissues. In the periorbital area, it results in improvement of the skin quality, shrinkage of redundant skin and lightening of the pigmentation.

The periorbital area is a barometer of facial aging, since it is affected by intrinsic and extrinsic factors of aging.[1] In addition, the skin in this area is tightly attached to the underlying orbicularis oculi muscle and therefore is under constant muscular movements, induced by mimetic expressions. Moreover, the periorbital skin has the thinnest epidermis and dermis. It has been shown that type I collagen content diminishes with aging in the eyelid skin due to a decrease in its synthesis.[2] All these factors contribute to the fact that the periorbital area is the first to show the signs of facial aging.

Chemical peels can be performed on the lower lid exclusively or on the whole periorbital skin. They can be a part of the full-face peeling procedure or can be performed as isolated chemical blepharoplasty. Eyelid peeling can be combined with simultaneous surgical blepharoplasty or with non-surgical procedures, such as botulinum toxin injection or tear trough deformity correction by dermal fillers.

INDICATIONS

- Periorbital wrinkling
- Upper eyelid ptosis
- Periorbital pigmentation

CONTRAINDICATIONS

- Ectropion
- Lower lid laxity (moderate to severe)
- Severe eye dryness
- Claustrophobia

INDICATIONS AND CONTRAINDICATIONS

Lower eyelid wrinkles and redundant eyelid skin are challenging for treatment. As long as the skin in this area is tight and elastic, eyelid wrinkles can be improved by infraorbital injection of small doses of botulinum toxin. If flaccid, additional relaxation will worsen the skin appearance and cause suborbital swelling. Furthermore, the lower portion of the lateral orbicularis oculi assists in elevation of the upper cheek. When it is totally paralyzed in older patients, an extra roll of skin becomes apparent at the junction of the lower eyelid and cheek skin when smiling.[3]

Lateral crow's feet in young patients are treated successfully by botulinum toxin injection. Our experience shows, however, that if these lines are not significantly worsened during animation, as happens in older individuals, the effect of muscle paralysis would not be sufficiently effective. The option of botulinum toxin injection in sub- and periorbital areas is therefore preserved for relatively young patients with tight skin. Chemical peels significantly improve this area.[4] Periorbital skin rejuvenation using medium and deep peels is achieved due to stimulation of the production of new dermal collagen and elastic tissues, with a desired overall refreshed and tightened appearance, reduction of fine wrinkles and skin tightening.[5–8]

Lower eyelid wrinkles are minimally helped by standard surgical blepharoplasty, in particular when a transconjunctival approach is used for fat removal or fat transposition. They are therefore commonly neglected during this procedure. A combination of eyelid surgery with lower eyelid peeling has been suggested as an effective and safe procedure that improves the final result of lower blepharoplasty.[9,10]

For upper eyelid blepharochalasis, surgical blepharoplasty is indicated in most cases. The results are generally good, natural and long lasting. Nevertheless, if a patient is reluctant to have surgical intervention or if full-face chemabrasion is scheduled, the periorbital procedure can be surprisingly effective on the upper eyelid as well (Fig. 4.1).[11]

Periorbital pigmentation is prevalent in 9–38% of American women under the age of 30 years.[12] This manifestation worsens with age. Histological examination of infraorbital darkening suggests that it is caused by multiple etiologic factors, including acquired dermal melanocytosis, ethnic or age-related dermal melanin deposition, postinflammatory hyperpigmentation secondary to atopic or allergic contact dermatitis, periorbital edema, skin photoaging, superficial location of the vasculature, and tear trough depression.[13,14]

Chemical peels are highly effective for the removal of melanin depositions secondary to ethnic dark circles and postinflammatory hyperpigmentation, and in skin photoaging.

Our experience shows that in ethnic dark circles, deep peels create definitive results (Fig. 4.2).

A novel use of periorbital peels is to treat younger patients who show only textural changes and who are not necessarily contemplating surgery. This approach not only opens up treatment to a much larger patient population but is also a means of keeping up with aging. The inherent improvement and tightening of the anterior lamella caused by the peel may bring enough improvement in younger patients with mild fat protrusion who may not be ready to consider surgery (Figs 4.3 and 4.4).

There are no absolute contraindications for periorbital peeling. Ectropion secondary to chemical peeling is a remote possibility and its existence is debatable.[7,15] Nevertheless, pre-existing ectropion or moderate-to-severe lower lid laxity is a relative contraindication for lower eyelid peeling, unless each is corrected surgically prior to the chemical peel.

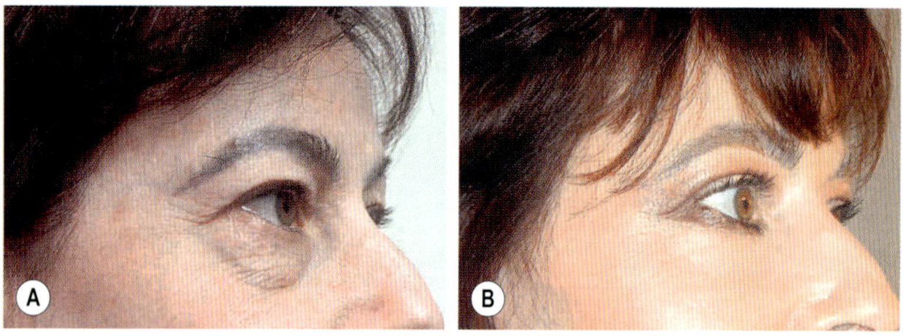

Fig. 4.1 Upper and lower eyelid: *A*, before; *B*, after full-face deep peeling.

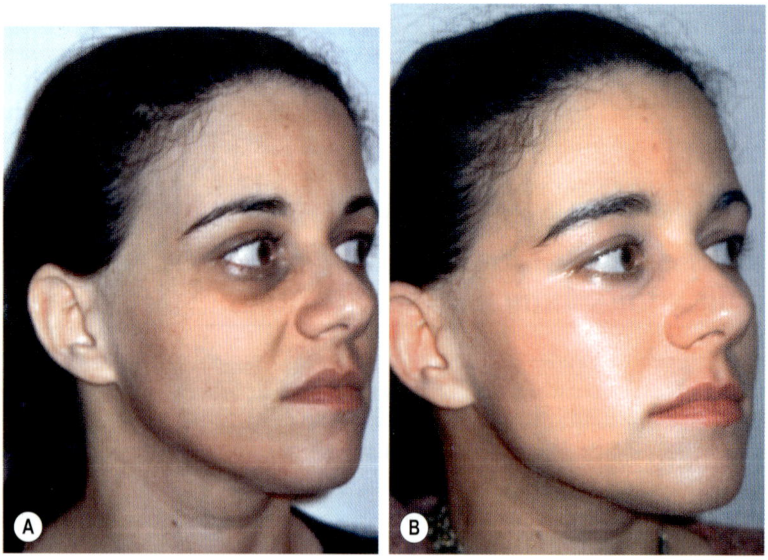

Fig. 4.2 A 28-year-old woman with periorbital pigmentation: *A*, before; *B*, after periorbital deep peeling combined with full-face medium-depth peel.

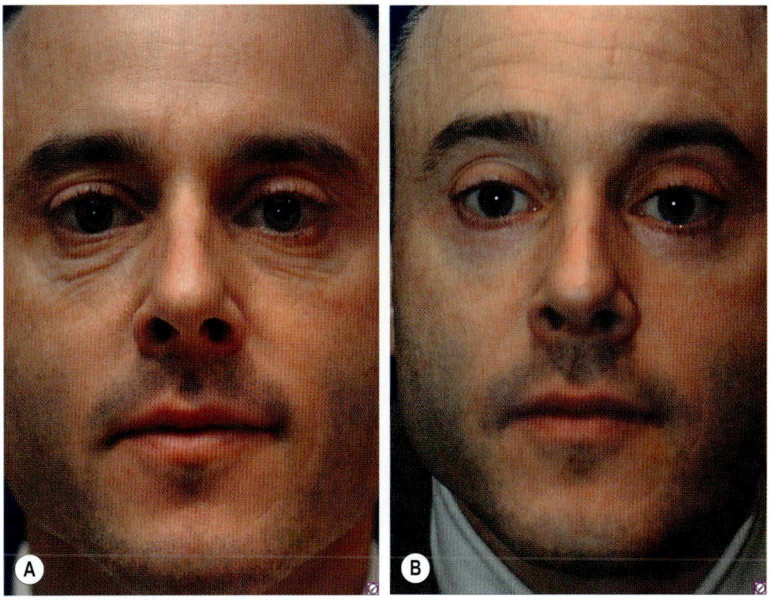

Fig. 4.3 A young man with obvious wrinkling of lower eyelid skin in sharp contrast with the rest of the face: *A*, before; *B*, after isolated deep peel of lower eyelid skin.

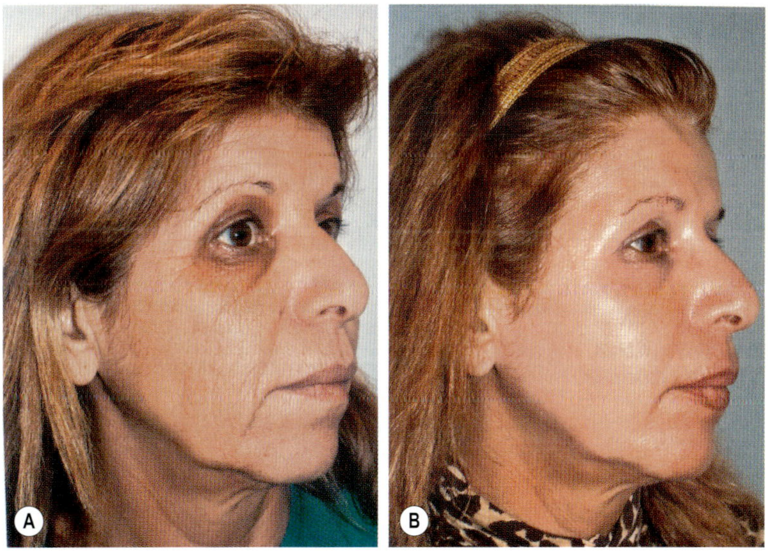

Fig. 4.4 A 56-year-old patient with evenly prematurely aged skin. Note the periorbital area: *A*, before; *B*, following full-face deep peeling.

PREOPERATIVE HISTORY AND CONSIDERATIONS

When evaluating the patient before the peel, an extensive history should be taken. The patient has to be questioned about general health status, medications such as oral isotretinoin, smoking, previous cosmetic procedures such as surgical lifts or fluid silicone injections, recurrent herpetic outbreaks, keloid formation, etc.

Skin type should be determined, based on Fitzpatrick's skin type scale. Skin preparation with bleaching creams and early reintroduction of these products in the immediate post-peel period are crucial to avoid postinflammatory hyperpigmentation in dark phenotypes.

The message of 'the deeper the peel, the more the inconvenience, the more significant the results' should be clearly conveyed and discussed with the patient.

The patient should be aware of the need to regularly apply sunscreen in the immediate post-peel period and of the possibility of using makeup to conceal post-peel redness, and advised to resume normal daily activities immediately after the procedure.

Of paramount importance is to have the patients photographed and sign the term of consent prior to the procedure.

OPERATIVE APPROACH

Chemical peels are an extremely versatile tool and are divided into three categories, depending on the depth of the wound created. Superficial peels penetrate the epidermis only, medium-depth peels damage the entire epidermis and papillary dermis, while deep peels create a wound to the level of the mid-reticular dermis.[16]

The depth of the peel is dictated by a number of factors: the chemicals that have been applied, their concentration and mode of application, and skin type and its condition. In general, the depth of the peel determines patient's inconvenience during and after the procedure, healing time, the rate of the potential side effects and the results.

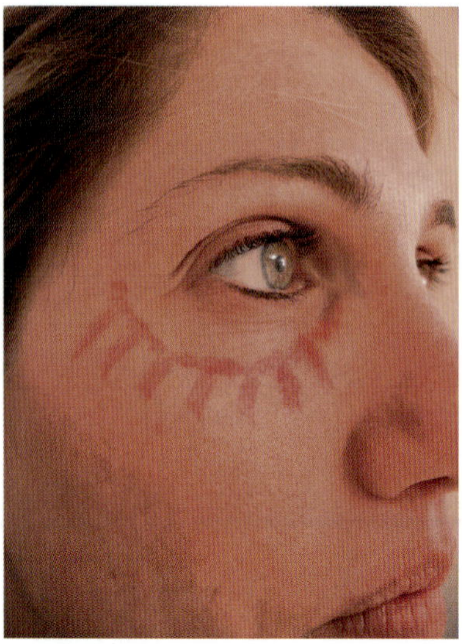

Fig. 4.5 Procedure plan: marking of the periorbital skin to be occluded and the transitional area to be peeled without occlusion.

PRE-PEEL SKIN PREPARATION

Skin can be pretreated with topical tretinoin 0.025–0.05% for 2–6 weeks, but its efficacy in periorbital skin priming is controversial.[4,6,9] Immediately before applying the chemical, the skin is thoroughly cleaned and degreased with acetone. The treatment area, particularly in the lower eyelid, is marked while the patient is in the sitting position. If an occluded deep-peel procedure is scheduled, the authors mark the area to be occluded and a marginal area in which to perform a non-occluded peel (Fig. 4.5).

To prevent any damage that might result from chemical leaking into the eye itself, the patient should be just slightly reclined, and sterile ophthalmic ointment is instilled to coat the eye globe before the procedure starts. All the extra ointment should be meticulously removed from the periorbital skin to avoid interference with the solution penetration.

CHOICE OF CHEMICAL AGENT

Various peeling solutions may be used effectively to perform periorbital peeling, including trichloroacetic acid (TCA) 35% and phenol–croton oil-based solutions. Stronger chemicals will cause a deeper wound with a greater effect on the skin.[17] The following factors must be considered when choosing chemicals: the amount of redundant skin, degree of laxity of the lower eyelid, degree of actinic damage, skin color and concomitant or previous surgical intervention.

TCA 35% is effective to remove pigmentation and fine wrinkles.[4,6,7] Nevertheless, our experience shows that for deep melanin deposits, deep peeling creates more significant and long-lasting results. The authors do not recommend higher concentrations of TCA, since the results are less predictable and the potential for scarring is higher. In order to increase the depth and efficacy of TCA peel, without increasing the concentration of the acid, the TCA can be preceded by Jessner's solution (Monheit method).[4]

TCA solution is compounded in a weight-to-volume preparation. To prepare a 35% solution, the authors dissolve 35 g of TCA crystals in a small amount of water and add water to make a total volume of 100 mL. TCA is stable in room temperature and is not light sensitive.

When attempting to treat blepharochalasis, deep peel is our first option. Deep-peeling solutions penetrate the skin to the mid-reticular dermis and create maximal effect for production of new collagen.[17] The solutions for deep peeling are composed of a combination of croton oil and phenol in various concentrations.[18] Phenol is an aromatic hydrocarbon derived originally from coal tar. Croton oil is an extract of the seed of the plant *Croton tiglium* and has been commercially prepared as croton resin since 1932. Its activity on the skin is related to free hydroxyl groups, which cause skin vesiculation even in low doses. Other chemicals in use in deep chemical peel formulas include septisol, water and vegetable oils (glycerin, olive and sesame).

The key to the peel is that the croton oil concentration is weak enough that the application technique is a main determinant of the depth reached.[19] The experienced practitioner is able to control the process in order to reach the desired depth and go no further. A thin transparent frost with a pink background denotes a peel to the papillary dermis, and this is an appropriate depth for the eyelids. Regardless of concentration used, it is always imperative to judge the depth reached by means of the visual guidelines outlined above.

A combination of different solutions can be used by an experienced physician to comply with differences in each skin area.[6] Periorbital deep peeling can be combined with medium-depth peel on the rest of the skin to prevent demarcation lines.

ANESTHESIA AND PATIENT MONITORING

The majority of patients do not require anesthesia for the peel procedure. In some cases, a combination of an oral sedative, such as lorazepam or diazepam, and an analgesic, such as tramadol, is used. Another option to be considered, especially for phenol peels, is regional block.

Periorbital TCA and phenol peels do not require any monitoring. Full-face phenol-based peel is carried out under full cardiopulmonary monitoring with intravenous hydration throughout the procedure.[20]

PEELING TECHNIQUE

BOX 4.1

1. Meticulous defatting maximizes the results of the peel
2. To avoid eye injury an almost-dry Q-tip should be employed
3. To avoid spreading of the peeling solution, an assistant holds cotton tips in the medial and lateral canthi to absorb the tears.
4. Upper eyelids are peeled while the eyes are closed.
5. For the lower eyelid procedure a patient opens the eyes wide and looks upwards
6. To blend color and textural differences a more superficial peel might be needed in the marginal area

After skin defatting with acetone, a single cotton tip is dipped in a small container containing the peeling solution and squeezed over its side to avoid dripping of the solution to other areas. The authors use commercial cotton tips and roll an additional layer of soft cotton on them to increase fluid absorption.

The upper eyelids are peeled while the eyes are closed. For the lower eyelid procedure, a patient is required to open the eyes wide and look up. At this stage, uncontrollable tearing regularly appears. It is therfore important that an assistant holds cotton tips in the medial and lateral canthi to absorb the tears and avoid spreading of the solution. For extra comfort, eyedrops of tetracaine solution can be recommended, but administration of the eyedrops has to be done very carefully since it can mask any inadvertent peel that may go into the eyes by capillarity.

As the acid encounters the skin, it coagulates and precipitates the protein, resulting in varying shades of white, called a frost (Fig. 4.6,*A*). With progressive passes, the frost becomes denser, indicating deeper penetration. Phenol peels induce immediate protein coagulation. With TCA 35%, a patient observation of the skin is needed, since this chemical creates delayed skin frosting.

Another visual clue, which is useful with deep peels on the eyelids, is epidermal sliding. This phenomenon occurs when the peel reaches the papillary dermis and the epidermis is separated from the underlying reticular dermis and slides on a thin, independent sheet. Epidermal sliding is an excellent way to judge the depth of peel in the eyelids.

POSTOPERATIVE CARE

After a phenol-based peel, the lower eyelid can be occluded for 24 hours or left unoccluded. The peripheral treatment area is left unoccluded to create a more even blending with untreated skin. If a waterproof zinc oxide non-permeable tape or a plastic mask (Neofarma® Compounding Pharmacy, Sao Paulo, Brazil) is used, after the occlusion is removed, the skin exudate is cleaned by sterile saline. The face is covered with bismuth subgalate antiseptic powder for 7 days. On the eighth day, wet soaking with tap water is used to soften the powder mask and to remove it.

If a non-occluded deep peel is employed, the skin is covered with a thin layer of petroleum ointment postoperatively. Although the recovery from a full-face peel is somewhat difficult for the patient, an isolated peel of the lower lids is easy to tolerate,

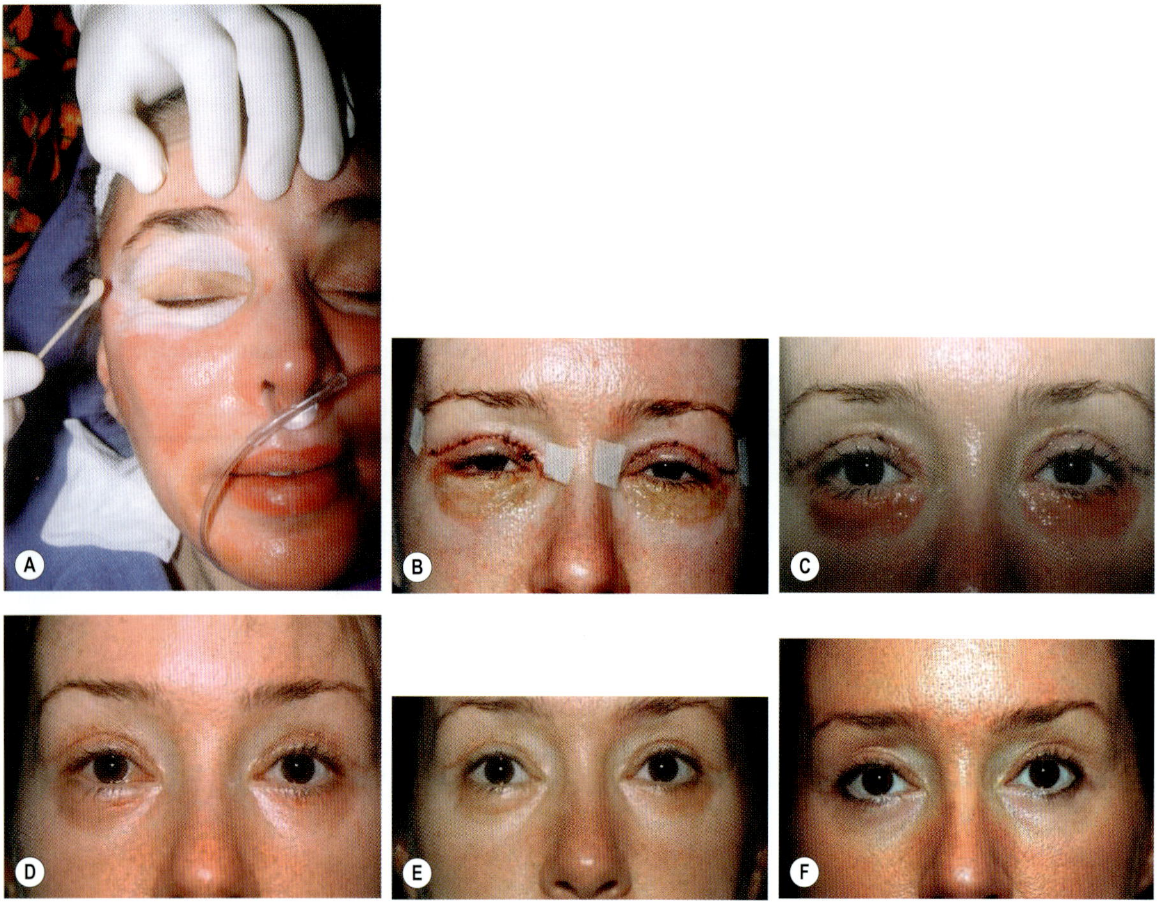

Fig. 4.6 Unoccluded lower eyelid peeling: *A*, frost forms as the acid is progressively applied on the skin; *B*, day 1 after peel; *C*, day 5 post treatment; *D*, day 10 post treatment; *E*, 3 weeks post treatment; *F*, 7 months post treatment.

with epithelialization occurring in approximately 5–7 days (Fig. 4.6,*B–F*). This is followed by about 6 weeks of redness, which is easy to camouflage with make-up or glasses.

For TCA peels, wet soakings are used immediately postoperatively. In both cases, during the next few days patients may expect to feel tightening and swelling of the skin, together with gradual darkening of the skin color. On day 3 or 5, the skin starts to crack and desquamation begins. At this stage moisturizing cream can be applied, although a few authors choose to recommend bland moisturizers (petrolatum, for instance) from day 1. Full re-epithelization is completed after 5–7 days. At this stage, the patient is advised to wear camouflage make-up and resume normal daily activities. Blunt moisturizer and high-level sun protection are recommended for the next 2–3 weeks.

SPECIAL CONSIDERATIONS FOR PERORBITAL PEELINGS

In the post-peeling period a crust is formed on the eyelid skin. The eyelids therefore become less flexible and the efficacy of the blinking mechanism, responsible for the tears dispersion, is reduced. As a result, some patients complain of ophthalmic irritation during the healing period. The authors advise all the patients to use artificial tears. Patients with severe preoperative eye dryness should be especially instructed and closely followed up.

Periorbital peeling causes extensive swelling around the eyes. In some cases, complete closure of the eyelids can occur. This possibility has to be discussed with claustrophobic patients. Some of them will benefit from antianxiety medications in the first few days after the peeling.

REPEATED PEELINGS

BOX 4.2

Repeated peelings of the lower eyelid improve the results.

Repeated peelings of the lower eyelid improve the results. Lower eyelid peel can be repeated and performed in a graded fashion. If a patient desires a quicker recovery, then a lighter peel can be done and repeated in the future with an additive effect. In this manner the lower lid skin can be peeled to the patient's satisfaction (Fig. 4.7).

Repeated sessions of TCA peel are performed 1 month apart, while phenol peels can be repeated after 3–6 months.[4,9]

COMBINATION OF PEELING WITH SURGERY

In the traditional transcutaneous lower lid blepharoplasty, the orbital fat is accessed by going through the anterior lamella and traversing the orbital septum. Once the fat has been modified, surgeons cannot seem to avoid temptation and try to improve wrinkles by pulling up on the skin and removing the excess. The contracture of the injured septum, coupled with the removal of skin, cause a vertical shortening and invariably result in rounding of the outer canthus or, worse, frank ectropion.

The author's (RHB) preference is to utilize the bi-lamellar approach – that is, access the fat in the posterior lamella through a transconjunctival approach and then manipulate the anterior lamella if necessary, be it suspension of the orbicularis oculi muscle and lateral canthi tightening and/or removal of excess skin, without invading the orbital septum. Regardless of the technique used, the last, and often very important, factor is dealing with the textural changes of aging eyelid skin.

For many patients, the combination of transconjunctival fat resection and croton oil peel is an excellent choice. If there is true excess of skin or an orbicularis oculi, and lateral canthi manipulation is deemed necessary, these can be performed after the elevation of a skin flap and a peel can be done at a later time. In this manner, both the structural and the textural changes can be dealt with appropriately while preserving the natural shape of the eye and avoiding the all-too-common 'operated' look (Fig. 4.8).

COMPLICATIONS

The list of potential complications of chemical peels includes pigmentary changes, infections, milia, acneform eruption, scarring and cardiotoxicity.

1. Pigmentary changes – Reactive hyperpigmentation can occur after chemical peels. Usually lighter complexions have lower risk for hyperpigmentation. In regional peels, especially in darker skin phenotypes or in severely sun damaged skin, a demarcation line at the margins of the peeled area can occur. If this is the case, a full-face procedure or skin camouflaging has to be considered. Hypopigmentation after phenol peels is proportional to the depth of the peel, the amount of solution used, the number of drops of croton oil in the solution, inherent skin color and post-peel sun-related behavior.
2. Infection – Bacterial and fungal complications in chemical peels are rare. Patients with a positive history of herpes simplex infection are treated prophylactically with acyclovir or valacyclovir

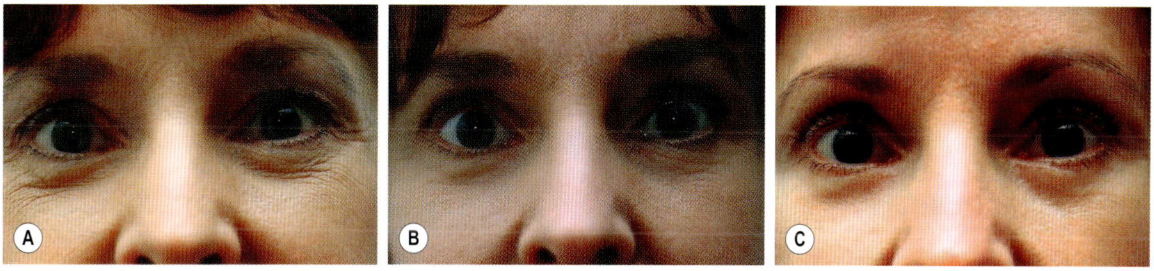

Fig. 4.7 Gradual peeling: *A*, wrinkled lower eyelid skin pretreatment; *B*, results after first peel of lower eyelid; *C*, 1 year after second peel of lower eyelid.

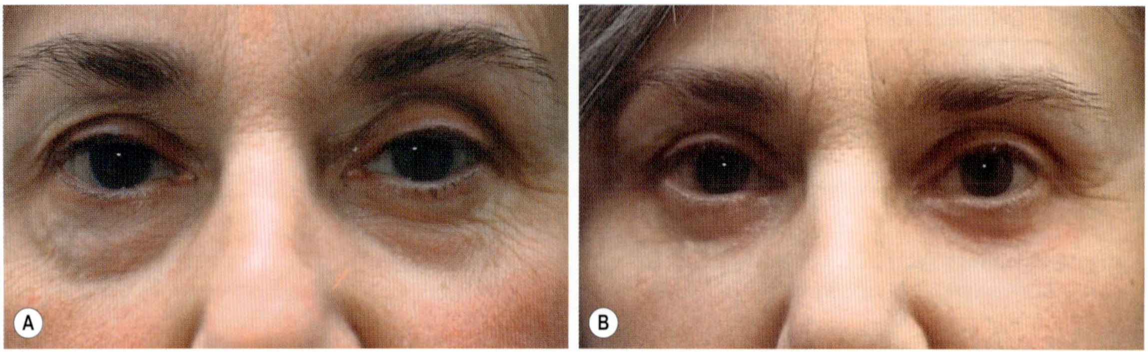

Fig. 4.8 Combination of transconjunctival blepharoplasty with lower eyelid peeling: *A*, prior to surgery; *B*, results after combination procedure.

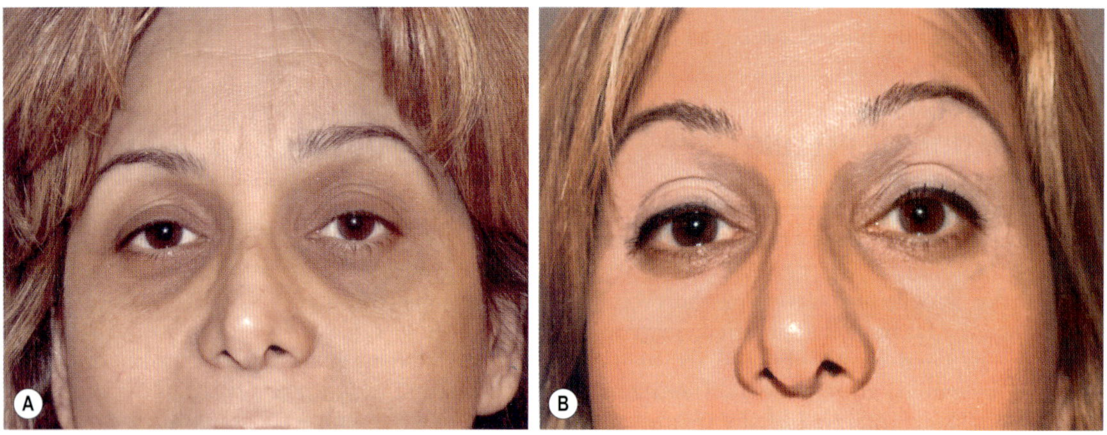

Fig. 4.9 A 44-year-old patient: *A*, before; *B*, 3 years after periorbital peeling for periorbital pigmentation.

during medium and deep peel until full re-epithelization is achieved.

3. Scarring – Scarring and cicatricial ectropion remain the most dreadful potential complications of periorbital peels. Delayed healing and persistent redness are important alarm signs for forthcoming scarring. Topical antibiotics and potent steroid preparations should be introduced as soon as this diagnosis is made. Nevertheless, this complication is extremely rare.[9,15]
4. Cardiotoxicity, milia and acneiform eruption, which can occur in full face peeling, have not been seen by the authors during the procedure in the periorbital area.

LONG-TERM RESULTS

In spite of the fact that the tightness of the eyelid skin usually seen in the first 3–6 months is not permanent, patients usually appreciated an overall improvement in their eye appearance following the peel. To prevent recurrence of mimetic periorbital wrinkles, the authors advise all patients to start periorbital botulinum toxin injections about 4 weeks postoperatively. As for patients peeled for dark circles, their satisfaction does not reduce with time (Fig. 4.9).

REFERENCES

1 Landau M. Exogenous factors in skin aging. *Curr Probl Dermatol.* 2007;35:1–13.

2 DeBacker CM, Putterman AM, Zhou L, Holck DE, Dutton JJ. Age-related changes in type-I collagen synthesis in human eyelid skin. *Ophthal Plast Reconstr Surg.* 1998;14:13–16.

3 Kane MAC. Classification of crow's feet patterns among Caucasian women: the key to individualizing treatment. *Plast Reconstr Surg.* 2003;112(suppl):33S–39S.

4 Kadhim KA, Al-Waiz M. Treatment of periorbital wrinkles by repeated medium-depth chemical peels in dark-skinned individuals. *J Cosmet Dermatol.* 2005;4:18–22.

5 Litton C, Trinidad G. Chemosurgery of the eyelids. In: Aston SJ, Hornblass MA, Meltzer MA, Rees TD, eds. *Third International Symposium of Plastic and Reconstructive Surgery.* Baltimore: Williams and Wilkins; 1982:341–345.

6 Morrow DM. Chemical peeling of the eyelids and periorbital area. *J Dermatol Surg Oncol*. 1992;18:102–110.

7 Dailey RA, Gray JF, Rubin MG, et al. Histopathological changes of the eyelid skin following trichloroacetic acid chemical peel. *Ophthalmic Plast Reconstruc Surg*. 1998;14:9–12.

8 Nelson BR, Fader DJ, Gillard M, Majmudar G, Johnson TM. Pilot histologic and ultrastructural study of the effects of medium-depth chemical facial peels on dermal collagen in patients with actinically damaged skin. *J Am Acad Dermatol*. 1995;32:472–478.

9 Gatti JE. Eyelid phenol peel. An important adjunct to blepharoplasty. *Ann Plast Surg*. 2008;60:14–18.

10 Zins JE. Invited discussion: Eyelid phenol peel. An important adjunct to blepharoplasty. *Ann Plast Surg*. 2008;60:19–20.

11 Parada MB, Yarak S, Gouvêa LG, Hassun KM, Talarico S, Bagatin E. 'Blepharopeeling' in the upper eyelids: A nonincisional procedure in periorbital rejuvenation – a pilot study. *Dermatol Surg*. 2008. [Epub ahead of print].

12 Gupta MA, Gupta AK. Dissatisfaction with skin appearance among patients with eating disorders and non-clinical controls. *Br J Dermatol*. 2001;145:110–113.

13 Yoshimura K, Sato K, Aiba-Kojima E, et al. Repeated treatment protocols for melasma and acquired dermal melanocytosis. *Dermatol Surg*. 2006;32:365–371.

14 Lowe NJ, Wieder JM, Shorr N. Infraorbital pigmented skin. Preliminary observations of laser therapy. *Dermatol Surg*. 1995;21: 767–770.

15 Wojno T, Tenzel RR. Lower eyelid ectropion following chemical face peeling. *Ophthalmic Surg.*. 1984;15:596–597.

16 Landau M. Chemical peels. *Clin Dermatol*. 2008;26:200–208.

17 Butler PE, Gonzalez S, Randolph MA, Kim J, Kollias N, Yaremchuk M. Quantitative and qualitative effects of chemical peeling on photo-aged skin: an experimental study. *Plast Reconstr Surg*. 2001;107:222–228.

18 Hetter G. An examination of the phenol-croton oil peel: Part I. Dissecting the formula. *Plast Reconstr Surg*. 2000;105: 239–248.

19 Hetter GP. An examination of the phenol-croton oil peel: part IV. Face peel results with different concentrations of phenol and croton oil. *Plast Reconstr Surg*. 2000;105:1061–1083.

20 Landau M. Cardiac complications in deep chemical peels. *Dermatol Surg*. 2007;33:190–193.

5 Lasers and Intense Light Sources

Eckart Haneke

Included on **DVD**

INTRODUCTION

The laser is a technical miracle. It was Albert Einstein who predicted the existence of laser light but it took almost another half-century until the first laser was developed. Initially, they were known as masers (microwave amplification by stimulated emission of radiation), but they were soon renamed lasers (light amplification by stimulated emission of radiation).

Laser light is unique due to its three characteristic properties. It is:

- monochromatic, which means it emits light of one specific wavelength
- coherent, which means that all light waves are in the same phase
- collimated, meaning that the light rays are all parallel.

A typical laser device consists of an optical medium, a source of excitation producing light or energy, and a set of mirrors positioned to potentiate the excitation light.

The use of lasers in selective photothermolysis was heralded in a 1980 paper by Rox Anderson, and since then lasers have found a wide range of medical applications.

'[Selective photothermolysis] relies on selective absorption of a brief radiation pulse to generate and confine heat at certain pigmented targets. An absolute requirement is that the targets have greater optical absorption at some wavelength than surrounding tissues...'

(Anderson & Parrish)

CLASSIFICATION OF LASER DEVICES (Tables 5.1–5.4)

Basic Concepts

Laser light is widely thought to penetrate the skin, where it is specifically absorbed by the target. However, this is only partially true. Firstly, the light is reflected, not only by the skin surface but also by optical grenz zones; secondly, it is transmitted through the more-or-less transparent skin; thirdly, it is scattered whenever it hits particles; fourthly, it is absorbed and its relative energy transformed into heat (Fig. 5.1). The tissue effect is caused by the absorption. The deeper the target, the more energy will be non-specifically lost by reflection and scattering, until a threshold is reached at which no tissue effects will be generated.

A laser for medical use is characterized by its wavelength (in other words its color), its mode of light emission as a continuous wave (CW) or pulsed, by the pulse width (duration of a single light pulse), by its power and by its fluence.

Wavelength

The wavelength is the color of the light used. It determines the absorption of the light energy by the pigmented target (chromophore). Many of the intended targets for treatment are beneath the skin surface and the wavelength also plays a role in determining the amount of scatter and hence the penetration depth of the light energy; penetration of visible laser light is inversely related to wavelength.

Pulse Width

Pulse width is the time interval over which the energy is delivered. For effective treatment, this pulse width should be shorter than the thermal relaxation time (TRT) of the intended target. The TRT is a measure of the time it takes for 50% of the energy absorbed by the target (i.e. heat) to diffuse into the surrounding tissue.

Fluence

Fluence is the amount of light energy per area delivered to heat a target. Sufficient energy must be provided to damage the tissues of the target. For a

Table 5.1 Laser classification by optical medium

Lasing medium	Laser type
Gas	CO_2, argon
Liquid	Dye lasers
Solid	Crystal, ruby, alexandrite, NdYag-diode

Table 5.3 Laser classification by emitted power

Low-level lasers
Medium-level lasers
Strong lasers

Table 5.2 Laser classification by emitted wavelength

Laser type	Wavelength	Color	Indications
Xenon chloride excimer	308 nm CW	UV-B	Vitiligo, psoriasis
Argon	488 nm CW	Blue	Vascular lesions
	514 nm CW	Green (secondary, weak)	Vascular lesions
KTP (frequency doubled Nd-YAG)	532 nm QS	Yellow	Telangiectasiae
Copper vapor	511 nm, 578 nm pseudo-continuous	Yellow, orange	Pigment, blood vessels
Tunable dye (argon laser pumped)	550–585 nm CW	Yellow, orange, red	Blood vessels
Pulsed dye laser (flash-lamp pumped)	585 nm pulse	Orange	Blood vessels
Q-switched ruby	694 nm QS	Red	Pigments
Alexandrite	755 nm QS, long-pulse	Near infrared	Pigments, tattoos
Diode	810 nm long-pulse	Near infrared	Hair removal
	800 nm pulse		
Nd-YAG	1060 nm CW, pulse, long-pulse, QS	Infrared	Pigments, hair removal
Nd-YAG	1360 nm	Infrared	Pigment, tattoos, coagulation, hair removal, etc.
Diode	1450 nm	Infrared	Photorejuvenation
Er-glass	1550 nm	Infrared	Photorejuvenation
Er-YAG	2940 nm pulse	Infrared	Laserablation, microablation, fractional
Carbon dioxide	10 600 nm CW, pulsed	Infrared	Resurfacing, cutting, vaporizing, fractional
Intense pulsed light	500–950 nm 600–950 580–980 nm 645–1200 nm 590–1200 nm 525–1200	Broad range visible light	Photorejuvenation, pigment lesions, telangiectasiae

CW, continuous wave; QS, Q-switch.

Table 5.4 Laser classification by delivery type of energy
Continuous wave
Pseudo-continuous (Cu vapor laser generates a train of 15 000 pulses per second, thus acting as a quasi-continuous laser)
Pulsed
Q-switched

given laser energy a smaller spot size creates a higher fluence. To calculate the fluence the equation below is used:

$$\text{fluence } (\text{J/cm}^2) = \text{energy of the beam (J)} / \text{area of the beam } (\text{cm}^2)$$

Spot Size

Spot size is the diameter of the beam at the skin surface. This parameter affects the treatment area and depth.

Repetition Rate

Repetition rate is the number of pulses per second and determines the speed of the treatment.

Energy

Energy is measured in joules and is defined as force × distance (N × m). Power is energy divided by time (J/s). Irradiance is power density, i.e. power divided by area (W/cm^2), and fluence is power × time divided by area (J/cm^2). These variables are of the utmost importance as they allow the laser parameters to be accurately determined and measured, and understanding of them makes the difference between a physician and a beautician. Lasers can be classified by power as low-level, medium-level or strong lasers.

While the specific wavelength of a laser defines its absorption spectrum and thus its principal biophysical effects, the duration of the laser emission also has a profound impact on the end result. CW lasers can be used to coagulate, cut, carbonize or vaporize tissue, or to stimulate certain cells. They usually exert important thermal effects on the tissues that absorb the energy, but there is also an effect on neighboring tissue, due to heat convection. The argon laser is a typical example of a CW laser that is used to coagulate blood vessels (port-wine stains, sun-burst vessels) and to heat up tissue (xanthelasma, small fibromas, small seborrheic keratoses).

Different techniques have been used to reduce the undesirable effect of CW lasers on adjacent tissue. The superpulse and ultrapulse techniques use

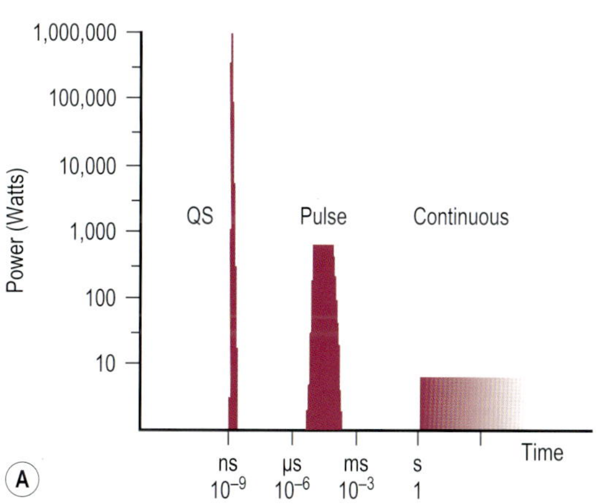

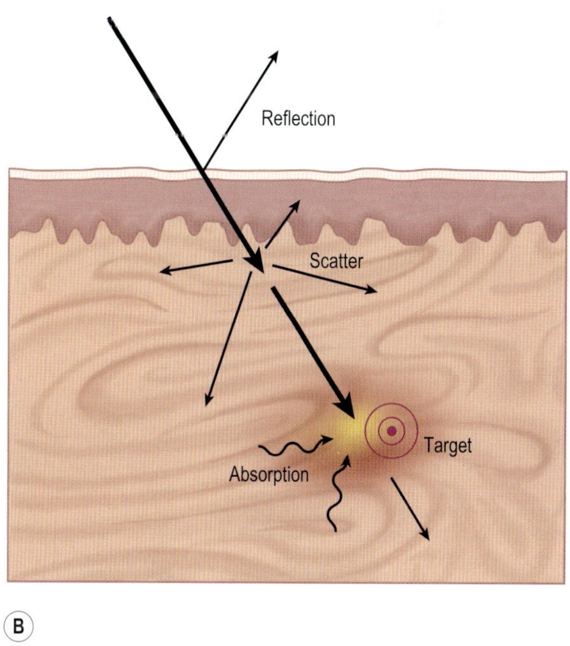

Fig. 5.1 *A*, Relationship of pulse duration and power of laser light. *B*, Light tissue interaction.

surgical carbon dioxide lasers with multiple interruptions, which give time for the tissue to cool down between pulses. Another technique is to use scanners, which reduce the possibility of inaccurate application of the laser beam by the physician.

Pulsed lasers emit short bursts of high energy light. This extreme power can lead to a number of undesirable side effects: when treating port-wine stains or telangiectasiae with a flash-lamp pumped dye laser, the power of a single pulse can be so high that the target tissues – the blood vessels and erythrocytes – explode and cause purpura, a reddish-black discoloration, which is cosmetically embarrassing. On the other hand, short pulses are shorter than the so-called thermal relaxation time, defined as half the time needed for 50% of the heat to pass to neighboring structures. When pulses remain below the thermal relaxation time of a given target no heat damage of the adjacent structures occurs.

To make a continuous wave laser into a pulsed one, a quality switch (Q-switch; QS) is necessary. This changes many of the laser properties, examples being the CW neodymium-YAG and the QS Nd-YAG lasers. Another way to modify a laser is frequency doubling, which changes the biophysical properties such as light absorption.

TYPES OF LASER

Continuous Wave Lasers for Aesthetic Enhancement

CW lasers are now rarely used in aesthetic dermatology. The three main CW lasers still used are argon, tunable dye and CO_2 lasers, now seen by many as 'historical'. Three parameters can be set by the operator: power, spot size and speed of movement (or length of shutter).

The CO_2 laser was the most important surgical laser used for cutting, vaporizing, carbonizing and, above all, for skin resurfacing. The latter procedure gives excellent results that cannot be achieved with modern non-invasive procedures. However, its main disadvantage is the long downtime period and the comparatively high risk of adverse side effects. Because its use is invasive, it will not be dealt with here. The Er-YAG laser, the light of which is absorbed 10 times more specifically by water, leaves much less thermal damage and healing is therefore faster. It may be an alternative for the treatment of prominent scars, mesh graft-like scars, excess graft tissue, some burn scars and traumatic tattoos.[1]

The argon laser, with its strong blue and weaker green emission, was the first vascular laser. Its emission wavelengths do not coincide with any of the oxyhemoglobin absorption maxima, and heat conduction from the target to neighboring structures is an additional source of tissue damage. Furthermore, before even reaching the vessels, melanin of the epidermis absorbs much of its light energy.[2] Depigmentation and epidermal necrosis are the consequences, often accompanied by scarring. Today's indications are mainly cherry angiomas, syringomas and xanthelasmata and other soft tissue lesions (Fig. 5.2 and 5.3).

The tunable dye laser, pumped by an argon laser, could be adjusted to the 577 nm oxyhemoglobin absorption maximum. It was better adapted for vascular lesions but because of its CW nature and relatively weak output its results were not really superior.

Pulsed and Q-switched Lasers

Pulsed lasers with an emission peak at 577 nm, where absorption by melanin is weaker, and with a pulse duration below the thermal relaxation time should be optimal to target superficial vessels without additional damage to surrounding structures. Q-switched lasers used in conjunction with preferentially absorbing pigments are optimal for melanotic lesions.

The flash-lamp pumped pulsed dye laser (PDL) with rhodamin G as the lasing medium emits light

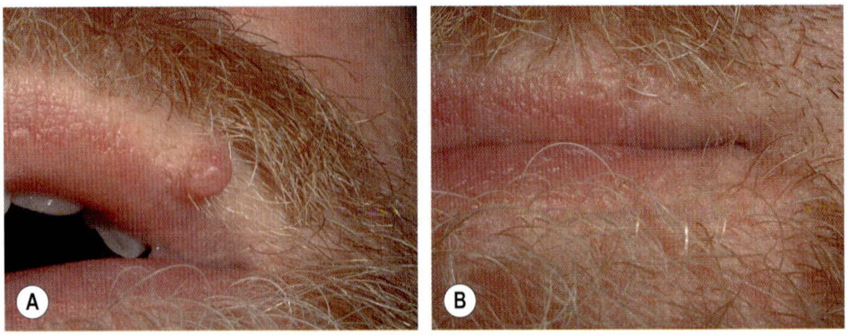

Fig. 5.2 Soft fibroma on the upper lip. *A*, Before treatment; *B*, two months after argon laser coagulation.

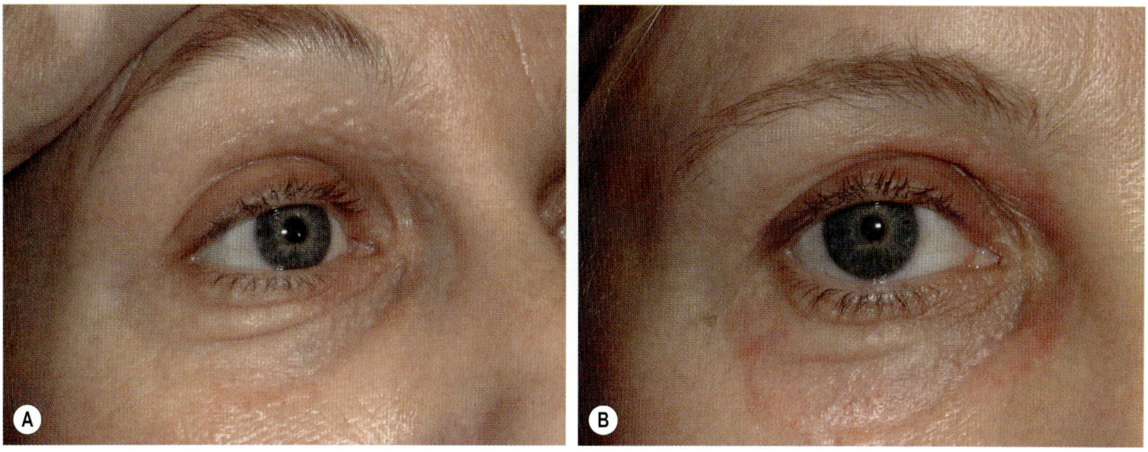

Fig. 5.3 Syringomas of the upper eye lid. *A*, Before treatment; *B*, two weeks after argon laser treatment.

between 577 and 585 nm at a pulse duration of 450 µs.[3] This is below the thermal relaxation time and thus no heat conduction occurs. Side effects are therefore rare except for transitory purpura lasting for about 2 weeks. These purpuras are due to the impact of the power being confined to a short time scale and can be prevented by using a long-pulse dye laser.[4] A comparative trial with fluence of 1 J/cm^2 below and 0.5 J/cm^2 above the purpura threshold showed that clearance of telangiectasiae is possible with both modes.[5] However, a longer pulse requires higher power densities, which are achieved with a frequency doubled Nd-YAG laser. This allows pulse widths of 1–30 ms and fluence rates of 15–20 J/cm^2.

A novel approach is the combination of a pulsed dye laser with a Nd-YAG laser. It has been shown that blood changes its absorption characteristics during subpurpuric photocoagulation, due to methemoglobin generation[6,7] increasing infrared absorption 3–5 fold.[8] This allows the energy densities of both lasers to be reduced, thus minimizing potential side effects such as scars. A study using a device with one hand-piece, delivering PDL light of 595 nm (10 J/cm^2, 10 ms pulse width, 7 mm spot size) and 100 ms later another pulse of 1064 nm Nd-YAG (70 J/cm^2, 15 ms, 7 mm) was significantly more effective than either laser alone.[9]

Pigments, both endogenous melanin as well as tattoo ink, are the main target for the so-called pigment lasers such as ruby and alexandrite. Melanin absorbs from 300–1064 nm, but minimizing interference with blood while still maintaining relatively high absorption makes a wavelength of 510 nm most suitable.[10] Although not at precisely this wavelength, the light from ruby and alexandrite lasers is absorbed at a wavelength where absorption by hemoglobin is virtually zero, allowing melanin and tattoos to be effectively treated. Although ruby laser light at 694 nm is maximally absorbed with minimal absorption by hemoglobin and water, its light pulses are too short to damage hair follicles sufficiently for it to be useful in hair removal.[11] The QS Nd-YAG laser penetrates deeper and it therefore is now also widely used for hair removal[12] as well as the removal of dermal melanin and black tattoos.[13]

Non-ablative lasers minimize the risks of temporary and permanent scarring because they leave the epidermis intact while delivering dermal irradiation with concomitant surface cooling. The absence of epidermal damage is associated with the absence of a true wound-healing response and therefore non-ablative lasers have minimal resurfacing efficacy. Because of this, multiple treatment sessions are required and there is variable and modest clinical improvement.[14–17]

Fractional (Pixellated) Lasers

Fractional lasers are novel devices the use of which is grounded in the theory of selective photothermolysis. Their use involves creation of microscopic treatment zones (MTZs) of controlled width, depth and densities, which are surrounded by viable skin.

While ablative lasers produce excellent skin rejuvenation but with considerable downtime, non-ablative photorejuvenation is much less efficacious but has the advantage that there is no downtime. Ablative and non-ablative lasers both create large macroscopic zones of thermal damage, which are defined by the laser spot size. A new type of laser light delivery with patterns of 100 to over 1500 microscopic treatment zones/cm^2 was developed both with non-ablative lasers[18,19] and with CO_2 and Er-YAG lasers. Small channels of controlled width, depth and densities of connective tissue damage are produced that are less than 200 μm wide. Within 1 hour of non-ablative laser irradiation, well-defined columns of both epidermal and dermal thermal damage are seen, with an intact overlying stratum corneum. Within 24 hours, viable cells migrate from the periphery toward the MTZs and microscopic epidermal necrotic debris (MEND) is formed. MEND comprises epidermal and dermal thermally damaged cells as well as melanin and elastin.[20] It is extruded transepidermally within 3–7 days. Cellular markers of dermal wound healing and neocollagenesis are expressed within the treatment areas.

Fractional ablative lasers produce tiny holes reaching into the epidermis and upper dermis which are surrounded by normal skin. They increase in depth and width with increasing pulse energies.[21] Channels up to 1600 μm deep can be safely made with the CO_2 or Er-YAG fractional lasers. The effect of ablative fractional lasers is much more pronounced, but healing takes at least a week.

Hair Removal Lasers

Hair density and distribution are important factors in psychosocial relations. Both too little and too much hair can be extremely embarrassing.

Hair removal with lasers is one of the most popular cosmetic treatment methods. Depending on hair color – the darker the better – and skin complexion – the lighter the better – long-lasting results are usually achieved after 5–10 sessions.

Long-lasting to almost permanent removal of unwanted hair has become possible with new laser devices. They are mainly based on long-pulsed alexandrite, diode and Nd-YAG lasers or intense pulsed light (IPL) sources, and by 2004 more than 22 different types of machine were available. It has been shown that photoepilation is much more efficacious than needle epilation, hurts less, is about 60 times faster and the results are aesthetically better.[22] However, skillful photoepilation requires a great deal of experience.[23,24]

The basis of photoepilation is the interaction of light and its target. About 5% of light is reflected by the stratum corneum. Light scatter on tissue inhomogeneities is the most important cause of energy loss because the laser beam loses its collimation and coherence (see Fig. 5.1). This loss can be reduced by choosing a greater spot size. Laser wavelength is another important variable: the longer the wavelength the deeper the penetration, up to about 1050 nm, when absorption by tissue water begins to increase. Choosing the right wavelength allows the target structure to be specifically heated without damaging the neighboring structures; this phenomenon is called selective photothermolysis. Follicular melanosomes are believed to be the targets of laser and IPL epilation,[25] and dendritic melanocytes have also been found in the bulge, the region of the follicular stem cells. In the hair bulb, most melanin is present in anagen phases III–VI and this is the phase to be chosen for the treatment. Since only about 50–70% of facial hair is in anagen, multiple treatment sessions are necessary for a good result.

Intense Pulsed Light Sources

IPL has a broad spectrum of wavelengths potentially targeting several skin structures. It is used for vascular and pigment lesions as well as hair removal and photorejuvenation.

While the first IPL device was a very complex machine, demanding expert skills in order to achieve good results, the newer units are simpler to operate. They usually have at least two different treatment windows in order to either target hemoglobin or melanin. For hair removal and induction of collagen neosynthesis, longer wavelengths in the near infrared are preferred. The light pulses are commonly divided into two or three portions that are temporally spaced so that the surrounding tissue can cool down while the target remains hot, thus adding heat to the target with each subpulse.

IPL has, until now, been associated with minor and only transient side effects. Pain, erythema, hypo- or hyperpigmentation, and superficial crust or vesicle formation have been the most commonly reported adverse effects in applications for both photorejuvenation and depilation.[26] The potential for ocular side effects has been alluded to, with previously reported cases of facial treatments deliberately avoiding direct application of IPL to the upper lids and protecting them from exposure by small external plastic shields.

USE OF LASERS

Preoperative History and Considerations

As with all cosmetic procedures, patient selection and preparation are of utmost importance.

Skin type, according to Fitzpatrick, is an important factor as it determines the risk of post-laser hyper- and hypopigmentation. Light skin is easier to treat and has far fewer complications. In many conditions the laser light has to go through the epidermis and its absorption by melanin is an unwanted effect, not only reducing the energy that reaches the sub-epidermal target but also causing the heating of the epidermis, leading to necrosis, slough, pigment disturbance and a risk of scarring. Tanning before laser treatment is therefore strongly discouraged. Lifestyle, current medications, supplementations and skincare, previous cosmetic treatments including surgery, and a good psychological status with realistic expectations have to be considered. As all laser treatments, ablative as well as non-ablative, can reactivate herpes simplex, antiviral prophylaxis is indicated when there is a previous history of this condition. Special concern is necessary in patients taking photosensitizing drugs or gold medications. It is the laser physician's task to explain that cooperation and compliance with the recommended post-laser regimen ensures normal healing and helps to avoid complications (Table 5.5). A patient who is likely to be noncompliant or unable to avoid sun exposure is not a good candidate for most laser procedures. Generally, men are better candidates for ablative laser therapies because their skin is often thicker. However, men are often negligent in using sunblockers to prevent pigmentary disturbances.

The potential dangers accompanying laser and IPL treatments have been well documented.[27] Several major areas in which 'professional error' can occur are deficient training, incorrect operation of the laser or light source, failure to perform test treatments, and misdiagnosis. The training of staff to suitable standards and ensuring that only clinicians who have been trained in dermatology are allowed to operate lasers and other light sources are important steps in minimizing this kind of error. Test treatments, knowledge of appropriate laser and light settings and probe handling, as well as use of cooling media and appropriate shields/blocks are important factors in minimizing skin damage and further sequelae.

There are some absolute prerequisites for rational laser treatment:

- correct diagnosis and indication
- patient history, including prior treatments with lasers, light, peels, dermabrasion and other cosmetic surgeries
- standardized informed consent; an informed consent form should be available and explained to the patient (Table 5.6).
- standardized clinical photography
- a suitable laser test field – it should be similar to the treatment area but preferably less visible
- treatment
- adequate follow-up and control photography
- avoidance of treatment of unclear or suspicious pigmented lesions.

Both the physician and the patient have to understand these facts so that the most appropriate laser can be chosen for the treatment based on the particular needs and desires of the patient. Non-ablative photorejuvenation (subepidermal resurfacing) causes almost no downtime but gives only weak-to-moderate improvement; fractional lasers give better results but with some days of redness and crusting, particularly

Table 5.5 Comparison of laser and intense pulsed light

	Laser	IPL
Light	Monochromatic, coherent, collimated	Polychromatic, non-coherent, non-collimated
Pulses	Usually one depending on wavelength	Multiple stacked
Target	Single	Several, depending on spectral range used
Handpiece	Small, light	Large, bulky
Treatment time	Longer	Shorter
Cooling	Various systems: direct contact, gel, cold air, cryogen spray	Contact gel and cooling handpiece

Table 5.6 Consent form for laser treatment (adapted from M Cantisano-Zilkha, *Understanding Chemical Peels*)

A laser treatment is not a 'cure all' treatment. It can give marked improvement for appropriate conditions. It is important that you have a thorough understanding of what the laser can and cannot do for your particular condition.

I, ____________________________________, give my consent for Dr_______________________to perform a laser treatment on my face or other area of my body_____________________to treat the following conditions:

____

I understand that this is a program of treatments and that I may need several sessions to achieve my best results.

_________I understand that the degree of improvement I can expect to see depends on many variables and therefore cannot be guaranteed. Additionally, I understand that strict adherence to the physician's instructions is necessary to ensure my best results.

_________I understand that Dr_____________________has the right to discontinue my treatment at any stage if he or she thinks that I am not following instructions, or if he or she believes that no further improvement is possible.

_________I understand that the laser treatment is an outpatient procedure done in the office. I also understand that I can expect to have some minutes of stinging or burning sensations during and after the procedure, but this will stop.

_________I understand that during healing from the laser therapy, my skin may look red and darker, depending on the laser used and the condition treated and that I may be unable to work. My particular laser treatment and its relationship to my ability to work have been discussed with me by Dr___________________.

_________I consent to have my photographs taken before, during and after my treatment. These may be used for educating future patients and in possible publications and promotions. My name will not be used.

_________Although complications are rare, they occur. Prompt recognition and treatment of any complication is necessary to decrease its potential danger. It is extremely important that I follow doctor's instructions exactly and that I notify the office if I have any of the following complications:

- ☐ Skin infections, usually appearing as a red tender area, often with a scab
- ☐ Cold sore on my lips or face
- ☐ Allergic reaction to any medications I am using
- ☐ Any medication taken, including food supplements and 'natural' drugs
- ☐ Appearance of thick scars or keloids in the areas of my laser therapy
- ☐ Prolonged sensitivity to the sun and harsh climate
- ☐ Persistent areas of increased or decreased pigmentation
- ☐ Eye problems

Read and understood:

___________________________ ____________

Patient signature Date

___________________________ ____________

Witness signature Date

with the ablative pixellated lasers; ablative lasers, meanwhile, yield by far the best results but lead to considerable patient downtime. Even a series of non-ablative laser treatments will scarcely produce the same results as a single CO_2 or Er-YAG resurfacing. On the other hand, a series of very superficial Er-YAG peels may also be performed and these will give the patient very limited downtime.[28] These options have to be discussed with the patient beforehand.

Immediately before the laser treatment, the skin is cleansed as small foreign particles may take up laser energy, be heated and be 'burned into' the skin. Hair should be shaved 2–3 days prior to hair removal, and for other procedures immediately before the start of treatment.

Treatment

It is wise to treat a test area before performing a full-face treatment. This may also be treated as a test of whether or not the patient will require anesthesia or whether cooling will be sufficient. Preauricular skin is the optimal laser test area. After the laser test, the skin is cooled with a cool pad for about 30 minutes. Where there is good tolerance, light-skinned persons may be treated immediately, while individuals with Fitzpatrick type III and above are better treated the next day. Moles should not be included in the treatment zone. Before each new session, the clinician should discuss with the patient how well the previous session was tolerated, in order to determine if the laser/IPL parameters should be adjusted.

Patients should be reminded to stay out of the sun. Protective goggles must be worn and the eyes must be shut during therapy. When treating the eyelids directly, protective shields should be applied. Before starting the treatment a contact gel is usually applied, which couples the handpiece to the skin to minimize energy loss and also cools the skin surface. Use of a gel depends on the particular laser device, as some have built-in contact cooling. In other types the epidermis can be given a short spray of a cooling gas immediately before emission of the light beam. Cooling reduces the discomfort of the treatment and protects the epidermis from undue heat.[29] Each laser/IPL shot is felt like a sting or short burn, and when working near the eyes the patient will notice a light flash. Any swelling is trea ted by the cooling, but care has to be taken not to freeze the skin as this again will damage the skin. Depending on reaction to the treatment, the appointment for the next treatment session should be fixed before the departure of the patient to ensure that they remember that non-ablative laser treatments require a series of sessions.

Optimizing Outcomes

There are a number of areas that can be addressed in order to optimize treatment outcomes. These are:

- select skin type
- select target chromophore
- assure sun avoidance between sessions
- offer herpes simplex prophylaxis if requested
- select the right wavelength
- use cooling (pre and/or post-treatment)
- train staff
- increase energy by 10–20% each session
- promise less than you can give.

Immediate Post-treatment Care

The laser/IPL causes a certain degree of irritation of the skin, which is normal and usually lasts for about 24 to 48 hours. Blistering is – in most cases – a sign that the fluence was too high or surface cooling was not sufficient. The resulting scab must not be removed by the patient, and he/she has to be advised that this will result in temporary hypopigmentation, sometimes followed by postinflammatory hyperpigmentation. In patients with a tendency to develop melasma a consistent antimelasma treatment should be started even before the first session and should be continued until about 6 months after completion of the laser/IPL treatment.

The skin reaction is more intense after a treatment with a fractional laser, and crusting may last for several days after an ablative fractional laser therapy.

Encouraging the use of mild moisturizers, soap-free cleansers and sunscreen in the post-operative period is of paramount importance.

Side Effects

Non-ablative treatments using the principle of selective photothermolysis are usually free of serious adverse side effects. As mentioned above, local swelling, which often becomes less intense in subsequent sessions,[30] responds to cooling, which also reduces the development of blisters. A slight discoloration after treatment is common and resolves by itself; hyperpigmented spots will look darker after treatment, indicating that the target was actually hit. Purpura may be seen when a PDL with short pulses is used; these take about 2 weeks to disappear. Pigmentary disturbances may develop when the laser/IPL-treated skin is exposed to the sun too early.

Most recently, bilateral anterior uveitis with permanent ocular damage has been reported. This occurred in a beauty therapy salon after IPL treatment for periocular dyspigmentation was given without the use of eye shields.[31]

INDICATIONS

The main indications for laser and IPL treatment are:

- port-wine stains
- telangiectasiae
- pigmentary disturbances
- photodamage
- hypertrichosis
- scars.

Port-wine Stains

Port-wine stains can be treated with a variety of lasers and IPL sources. The ideal wavelength is 577 nm, but because laser light is completely absorbed at this wavelength the laser beam would not penetrate to the undersurface of the vessel and complete obliteration of the vessels would therefore be hard to achieve.[32] This is why a wavelength of 585 nm with a flash-lamp pulsed dye laser is usually chosen; 595 nm PDL are now also available.[30,33,34] As outlined above, very short pulses do not damage surrounding cells but have the disadvantage of producing post-treatment purpura. Long pulses in the millisecond range are commonly used to avoid this complication. Another possibility is the use of compression.[35]

Preparation of the skin for port-wine stain treatment depends on the requirements of the particular laser used. After preparation it is cooled. The pattern with which a port-wine stain is treated depends on the user, but as several sessions are almost always required overlapping is commonly avoided. The full therapeutic benefit of each session can be seen after 2–3 months, thus treatment for a large port-wine stain may be a long procedure.

Argon, argon-pumped CW tunable dye and copper vapor lasers are no longer recommended for the treatment of port-wine stains. However, they are still very useful for senile angiomas. The Nd-YAG laser, with its deeper penetration, is sometimes used to treat nodular angiomatous lesions.

The use of lasers in infantile hemangiomas is still disputed although a proactive approach is generally recommended for large hemangiomas with functional impairment, risk of ulceration and dramatic cosmetic disfigurement.[36]

Acquired Vascular Lesions

Acquired vascular lesions of the face are mainly telangiectasiae, rosacea-associated erythema, spider nevi, poikiloderma of Civatte, venous lakes and cherry angiomas.

Telangiectasiae are usually treated in a tracking mode[37] (Fig. 5.4). Many lasers are suitable for their treatment, the light of which is sufficiently absorbed by blood. As described above for port-wine stains, thin vessels can be effectively treated with the flash-lamp pumped dye laser. Thicker vessels have been shown to benefit from a combined treatment with a PDL and Nd-YAG laser[9] or with stacked pulses (multiple pulses superimposed on one another on the same area) of an IPL[38] (Figs 5.4 and 5.5). Where individual vessels cannot be seen, as in rosacea-associated erythema and Civatte's poikiloderma, large spot-size devices, particularly IPLs, are advantageous. They are used with a 25 to 35% overlap in order to avoid visible treatment fields. However, the bulky handpiece decreases its maneuverability in concave areas such as around the nose. The treatment area is not immediately visible due to direct contact between the handpiece and the skin.

Pigmentary Disturbances

Pigmentary disturbances may be treated with a variety of lasers and IPL machines according to the specific wavelengths emitted. The thermal relaxation

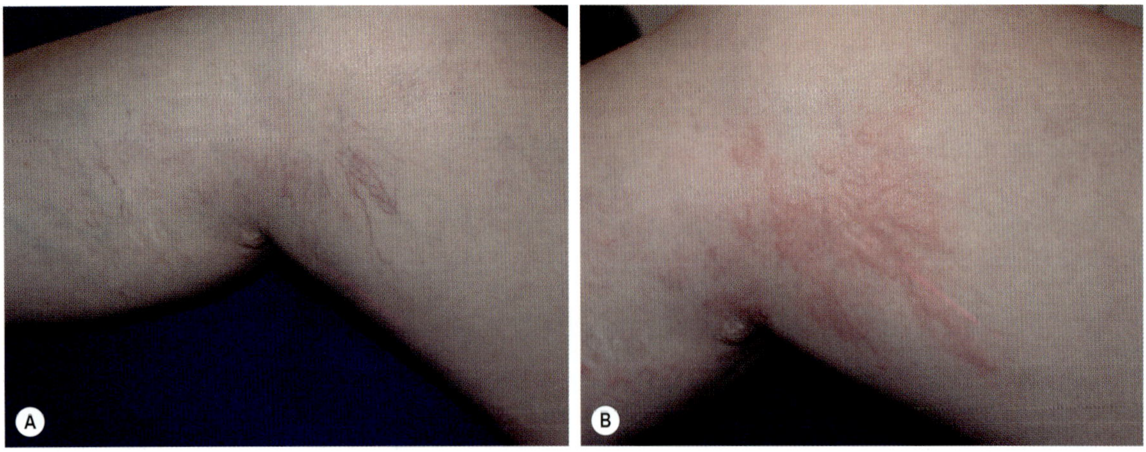

Fig. 5.4 Large caliper telangiectasiae. *A*, Before laser treatment; *B*, immediately after treatment with the frequency-doubled Nd-YAG laser with contact cooling, showing redness and edema.

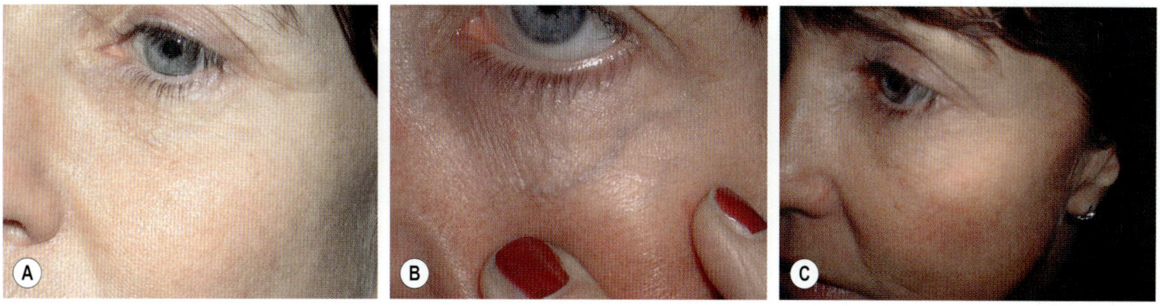

Fig. 5.5 Periocular vein. *A*, Before treatment; *B*, the vein is more visible upon stretching the overlying skin; *C*, after three sessions with an IPL device.

time of the melanosomes, which are about 0.5 μm in diameter, is about 250 ns. Laser light with sufficient absorption by melanin and with very short pulses should theoretically be optimal for treatment. The QS ruby laser, with its wavelength of 694 nm and pulse duration of 25 to 40 ns, can selectively target melanosomes without damaging the surrounding tissue.[39] However, there are many other lasers targeting melanin because it has a very broad spectrum of absorption. Both wavelengths (488 and 514 nm, CW) of the argon laser, the frequency doubled Nd-YAG (KTP) laser (532 nm, 5–10 ns, fluence 2–2.5 J/cm^2 at 10 Hz, spot size 1–3 mm) (Fig. 5.6), QS alexandrite (755 nm, 50–100 ns, fluence 6–7 J/cm^2) and the QS Nd-YAG (1064 nm, 10 ns, fluence 8 J/cm^2, spot size 3 mm for nevus of Ota) all target melanin. Although the longer wavelengths are not so well absorbed by the melanin this light penetrates deeper and can thus also remove dermal pigment.[40]

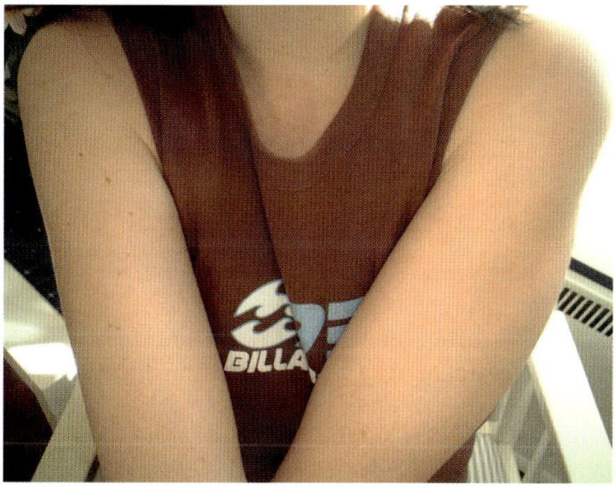

Fig. 5.6 Pigment spots on the arms. *Right*, untreated; *left*, after two sessions with the 532 nm QS Nd-YAG laser.

Dermatitis papulosa nigra, a frequent condition in skin types V and VI in black Africans and Afro-americans as well as Orientals, responds well to the Nd-YAG laser.[41]

Tattoos

Tattoos are due to exogenous pigments like black ink, but also exist in a variety of other colors. While the removal of black tattoos does not usually pose problems, colored tattoos are more difficult to target (Figs 5.7 to 5.9). Another problem is the depth of the tattoo: lay tattoos are usually much deeper and less regular than professional ones. Their removal is therefore more difficult. Furthermore, most lasers also target the overlying melanin, leading to (temporary) depigmentation. This is the reason why tanned individuals should not be treated with lasers that preferentially target melanin, but with the QS 1064 Nd-YAG. Transient hyperpigmentation can also occur and prelaser hydroquinone treatment may be advisable in those tending to develop postinflammatory hyperpigmentation or melasma. It is still not known exactly what happens to the tattoo particles, particularly with multicolored tattoos of organic permanent dyes. Some relatively light colors, such as white, flesh-tone and red, may undergo immediate darkening.[42,43] The alexandrite laser is good for black, blue and most green colored particles. The QS ruby laser is effective in removing black, green and blue inks, but relatively ineffective for red and yellow colors. The QS KTP laser with its 532 nm wavelength is used to remove red and orange tattoos. All treatments have to be repeated until sufficient blanching or complete removal is achieved. It is important to stress this in advance as many patients expect a single treatment.

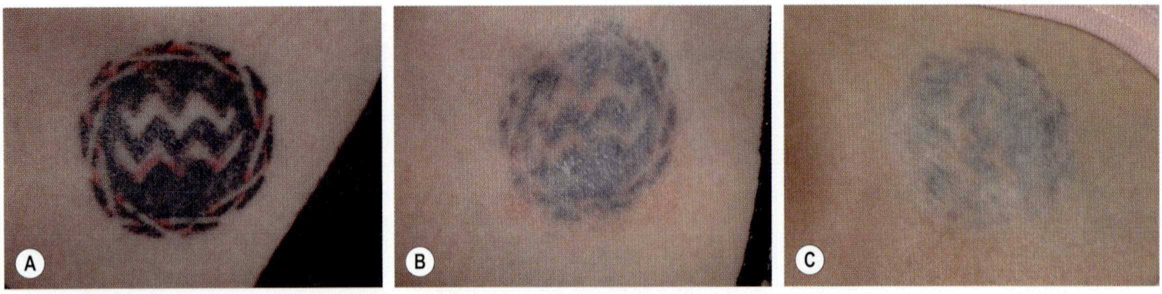

Fig. 5.7 Mainly black tattoo with small red portion. *A*, Before treatment; *B*, 4 months after first QS alexandrite laser session; *C*, 2 months after third treatment session showing residual bluish-black pigment.

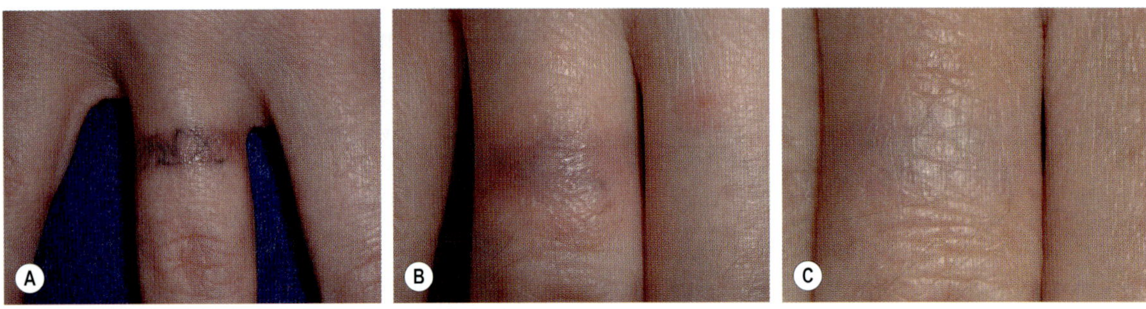

Fig. 5.8 Tattoo in shape of a ring. *A*, After two sessions with a QS Nd-YAG laser; *B*, 2 weeks after a final alexandrite laser session; *C*, 3 months after the last laser treatment.

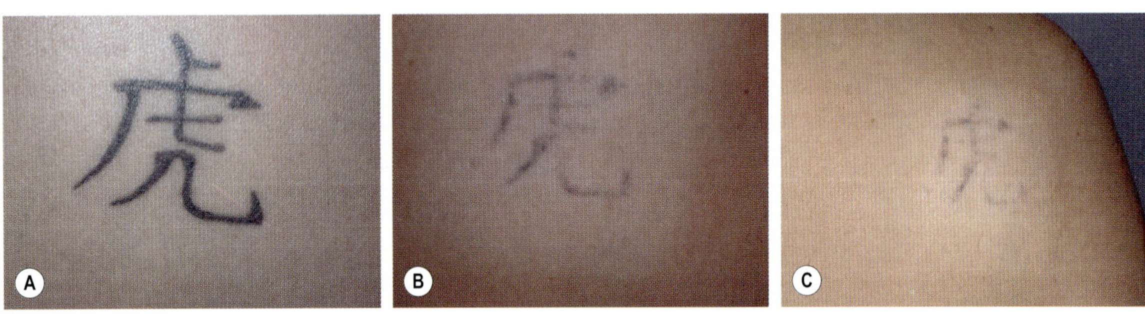

Fig. 5.9 Ornamental black tattoo. *A*, Before treatment; *B*, 3 weeks after QS alexandrite laser; *C*, laser treatment also reduced normal melanin pigment.

Photorejuvenation

Photorejuvenation, also called subepidermal resurfacing, is a non-ablative or fractional laser treatment which removes telangiectasiae, pigment spots, other skin irregularities, solar elastosis and superficial wrinkles, improves skin texture and reduces skin laxity. A wide variety of lasers and IPL devices can be used, which not only vary in wavelength emitted, but also in pulse width, spot size, repetition rate, pulse stacking, compression and cooling systems. Cooling systems have a profound influence on the fluence to be administered to achieve the result required. General treatment recommendations concerning most of the parameters mentioned therefore cannot be given here but depend on the particular device being used. As mentioned above, a test treatment in a relatively inconspicuous area is always recommended, although with experience and familiarity with the particular laser used the need for tests prior to full-face treatments will diminish. Moreover, the parameters used will also depend on the particular treatment plan, i.e. when pigment lesions are more important they will be treated first and either another laser or different treatment parameters will be chosen for consecutive sessions. Skin type is important too, as types I and II are best suited to treatment with shorter wavelengths than types III and IV. Asian skin reacts differently and requires extra experience. Most devices are used with two to three passes per session and several sessions some 3 to 6 weeks apart. The combination with botulinum toxin A injections was reported to give significantly better results on fine lines and small wrinkles.[44]

Hair Removal

Hair removal has become a very popular cosmetic procedure in the last decade.[45] Since its introduction, the technology has changed considerably: from waxing to thermolysis, electrolysis and now laser-assisted techniques based on selective photothermolysis. In order to have a long-term effect on hair growth both the bulb (hair matrix) as well as the bulge (stem cell region) have to be damaged with the laser. Hitting the hair bulb requires the hair to be in the growth (anagen) phase. The hair bulb is located deep in the dermis, or even in the superficial hypodermis, requiring relatively long wavelengths, which are able to penetrate that deep. The laser pulses have to be of sufficient duration to bring enough energy to the required depth, but need to do so without damaging the overlying epidermis. The thermal relaxation time of the follicle is roughly 10 times that of the epidermis. Optimal pulse width would therefore be 40–100 ms.[45] To make the laser light penetrate deeper a larger spot size is used.

Nd-YAG light of 1064 nm penetrates deeply, but is poorly absorbed by melanin. To overcome this disadvantage a mineral oil–carbon solution is used.[46,47] It is applied to the shaved or waxed skin surface and massaged into the follicular openings. Excess material is wiped away about 10 minutes prior to starting treatment. The laser treatment is delivered at a fluence of 2–3 J/cm^2, pulse width 10–20 ns, repetition rate of 10 Hz and spot size of 7 mm. It is thought that the effect is produced both by the thermal effect of the carbon particles being heated by absorption of the laser light and by the kinetic energy of the carbon particles which are hit by the light and propelled into the surrounding follicular cells. Treatment is performed in scanning movement until all carbon particles have disappeared. This procedure achieves a subjective and objective reduction of hair density, which was apparently not permanent.

A long-pulsed Nd-YAG laser was able to remove between 20 and 40% of the unwanted hair per session with almost complete hair removal after 4–6 sessions.[48]

The ruby laser emits light at a wavelength of 694 nm, which can be used to specifically target melanin. There is apparently enough melanin in the follicle to act as a chromophore for hair removal, although the epidermis also contains melanin that absorbs ruby laser light. It has been observed that the pulse width of the QS ruby laser beam is too short to damage the hair follicle sufficiently and because of this a 3 ms, 10–75 J/cm^2 normal mode ruby laser with a repetition rate of 0.5 Hz, a 10–12 mm spot size and a cooling handpiece was developed (Epilaser®). Fifteen to twenty per cent of its energy penetrates through the entire dermis to damage the hair follicle.[49] The handpiece is firmly pressed against the epidermis to minimize epidermal damage and to allow for deeper light penetration. Topical hydroquinone treatment is advised in darkly pigmented or tanned patients prior to laser treatment. The fluence in skin types III and IV is around 10 J/cm^2, and in fair skinned people up to 75 J/cm^2. However, the ideal treatment parameters have to be adapted to each single patient and session. This procedure gives longer-lasting hair reduction than the Nd-YAG carbon particle method. When the hair regrows it is usually thinner and lighter in color. Staged multiple retreatments are now generally recommended. Another ruby laser, with a 0.8 ms pulse width, 1.2 Hz and 4–6 mm spot size, has also been used.

Alexandrite lasers that are used in QS mode for pigmented lesions and tattoos are now also available in a long pulse mode with pulse widths between 2 and 20 ms.[50] Alexandrite laser light is less well absorbed by epidermal melanin than that of the ruby laser, and hence more darkly pigmented skin types may be treated with alexandrite lasers. Skin cooling is, however, a prerequisite to reduce potential epidermal damage from the high energy and relatively long pulses. Its large spot size and repetition rate of 1–5 Hz allow large skin areas to be treated in a reasonable time. Clearance rates observed are between 33 and 80%.[22,51–54] A pneumatic skin flattening device has been shown to considerably reduce the pain felt during laser treatment as compared to a dynamic cooling device.[55]

Diode lasers emitting light at either 800 or 810 nm have a pulse width of 5–100 ms. This allows skin types up to III to be treated with fluences of up to 60 J/cm^2; darker skin requires lower levels. A rectangular tip of 9 × 9 mm and a repetition rate of 2 Hz permits the treatment of large hairy areas in a relatively short time. Clearance rates are between 25 and 60%, depending on the time of follow-up and the number of sessions.[56–58] Skin cooling is necessary and usually achieved with a chilled tip built into the handpiece. However, the sapphire lens has to be cleaned after every few laser shots in order to remove burnt hair remnants that may reduce the laser intensity but also heat the epidermis when heated by the laser beam.

IPL systems have a broad spectrum of incoherent light with wavelengths from 500 nm to 1200 nm. These systems allow not only hypertrichosis to be treated but also benign pigmented and vascular lesions.[59] IPL devices have a range of selection parameters for the laser physician to choose from and these usually make IPL treatment more demanding than when using lasers. Wavelength range and fluence are chosen according to skin type – the darker the skin, the longer the wavelength. The pulses can be stacked and applied as a single, double or up to a 7-fold pulse, with intervals between 1 and 300 ms. These variables can be chosen individually or programs pre-defined by the manufacturer of the device can be used. The spot size is usually rectangular and very large compared to that of most lasers, which makes up for one of their major disadvantages: the slow repetition rate of approximately 0.3 Hz. Apparently, actual fluences are often not precisely what is indicated by the manufacturers.[60] Clearance rates range from 60% to over 80%.[61–64]

Scars

Scars can be treated with a variety of lasers. The rationale behind their use is either to inhibit deposition of excess collagen to avoid hypertrophic scars and keloids, or to reduce scar vascularization and redness and to debulk scars.[65,66] Observation has shown that the microvasculature is not the sole target of the pulsed dye laser: it also makes scars more pliable as well as less erythematous, hypertrophic and itchy (Figs 5.10 and 5.11).

Microscopic examination of scars after laser treatment showed finer and more fibrillar collagen. For hypertrophic scars, two to four treatments with the PDL, 585 nm, at fluences of 6–7 J/cm^2, a 5 or 7 mm spot size and adjacent, non-overlapping pulses were used whereas keloids required two to six treatments.

Fractional photothermolysis has intensively been studied in acne, surgical and traumatic scars. Even though CO_2 and Er-YAG ablative resurfacing remain unsurpassed for the treatment of facial rhytides, both methods have yielded lesser improvements for scarring, with keloids usually recurring soon after treatment. This is probably due to the fact that the depth of tissue ablation is limited. Fractional lasers achieve significant depth of penetration, leading to improvements in scars similar to those-achieved with the ablative lasers. Another advantage of fractional lasers is that the risk of pigmentary disturbance, even in higher skin pigmentation types, is greatly reduced. High energies, with deep tissue coagulation, are apparently associated with the best clinical improvement. In a large series of

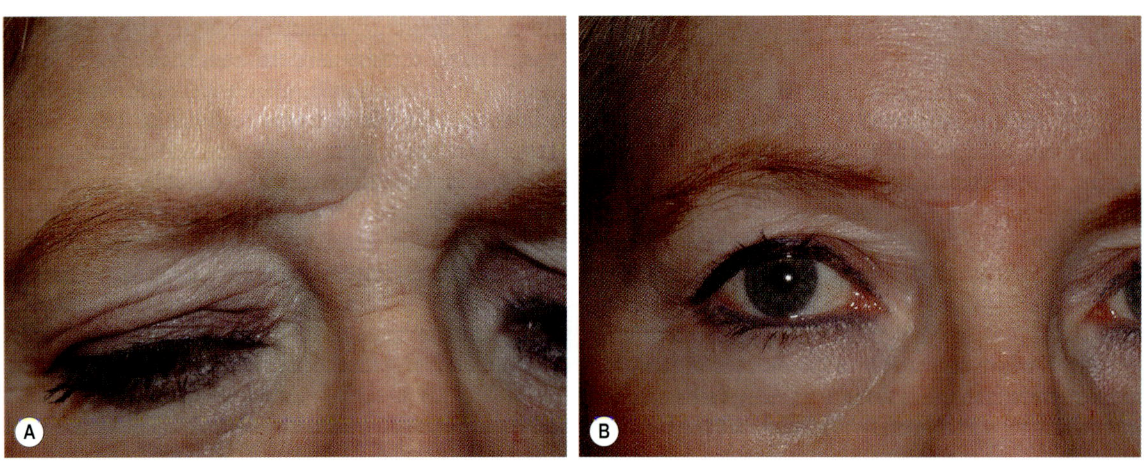

Fig. 5.10 Scar from car accident. *A*, before treatment; *B*, after three laser sessions.

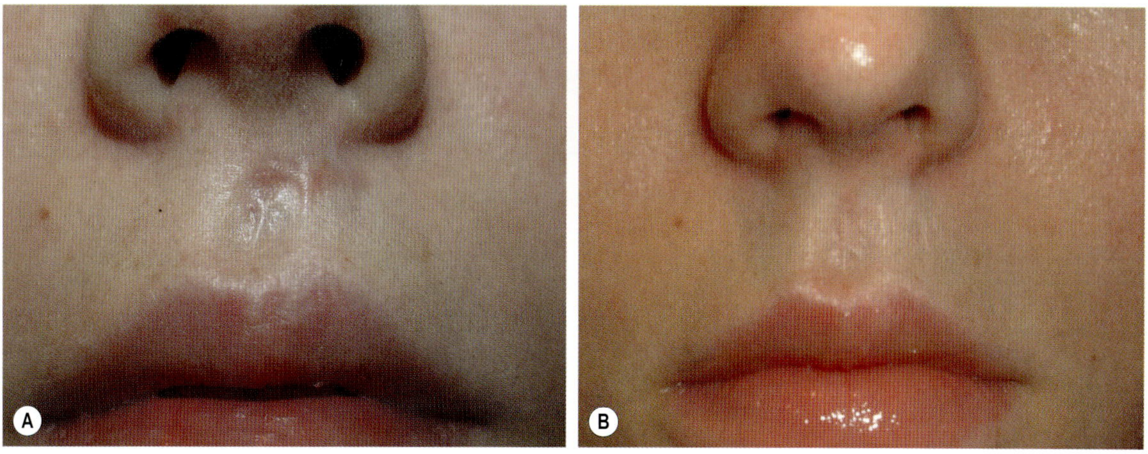

Fig. 5.11 Partly hypertrophic scar from bike accident. *A*, Before treatment; *B*, after three sessions with the long-pulsed Nd-YAG laser.

181 patients with skin types I–III and 176 patients with skin types IV–VI and acne scarring, one to five treatments with the Fraxel (SR750) laser at a pulse energy of 25 mJ, 125 MTZ/cm^2 and eight non-overlapping passes, with additional treatment at 25–35 mJ and 125 MTZ/cm^2 for another four to ten passes produced greater than 75% improvement in 12% of the patients and 50–75% improvement in 73% of patients. Only one patient developed postinflammatory hyperpigmentation, and there was one case of localized scarring that resolved with intralesional corticosteroid injection.[67] Clinical improvement of 51–75% in nearly 90% of treated patients up to 6 months after two to five treatments was shown in another study of 53 patients.[68] Yet another study of 29 patients yielded moderate-to-marked improvements in acne scarring after three to five treatments with the newer Fraxel SR1500 (Fraxel *re:store*™) laser at 40 mJ/MTZ and treatment levels of 7–10, and advanced level 1, corresponding to 23–35% of skin area treated.[69]

It is particularly interesting that erythematous and specifically hypopigmented scars have shown improvements lasting up to 6 months[70,71] whereas repigmentation of hypopigmented scars by excimer laser treatment diminished relatively soon and required re-treatments at 1–4 months.[72] Neither ablative nor non-ablative lasers have managed the improvement in hypopigmentation achieved by treatment with the Fraxel laser. Long-term follow-up will be required to determine the longevity of repigmentation from fractional resurfacing. The mechanisms of action are still unclear, although epidermal injury stimulates melanocyte proliferation and migration from the wound periphery.[73,74] The formation of microscopic areas of epidermal and dermal injury from fractional resurfacing probably stimulates both melanocyte proliferation and migration. It is possible that hypopigmented scars as well as vitiligo contain dormant melanocytes that are stimulated by controlled wounding.[75] Fractional lasers have also been used successfully in the treatment of striae rubrae and albae. Although striae rubrae responded to pulsed dye laser treatment, striae albae were largely unresponsive. Patients with striae rubrae and albae received one to four fractional resurfacing sessions at energies of 16–20 mJ and 125 MTZ/cm^2 per pass for final densities of 1000–1500 MTZ/cm^2. Improvements were greater than 50%.[76]

Finally, CO_2 and Er-YAG fractional ablative lasers are now on the market that give better skin-tightening results than the non-ablative ones but also require approximately 2 days for healing of the oozing and crusting. With the fractional CO_2 laser, 400–1600 MTZ/cm^2 at 10–20 mJ was given for photodamage, skin laxity[77] and acne scars.[78] With the Er-YAG laser, fluences of 2.5–25 mJ/cm^2 were used.[79]

Laser-assisted liposuction is a combination of liposuction with Nd-YAG laser treatment which leads to considerable skin tightening due to the tissue shrinking brought about by the heat of the laser.[80] This treatment is discussed in Chapter 12.

CONCLUSION

Lasers are powerful instruments for many different indications. They are technical miracles requiring basic biophysical and biooptical knowledge in order to use them adequately. In principle, lasers are excellent tools to treat multiple skin disorders with safety and efficacy but a training course is necessary to obtain maximum benefits while reducing risks.

REFERENCES

1 Eberlein A, Schepler H, Spilker G, et al. Erbium:YAG laser treatment of post-burn scars: potentials and limitations. *Burns* 2005;31:15–24.

2 Neumann R, Knobler R, Leonhartsberger H, et al. Comparative histochemistry of port-wine stains after copper vapor laser (578 nm) and argon laser treatment. *J Invest Dermatol.* 1992;99:160–167.

3 Tan OT, Murray S, Kurban AK. Action spectrum of vascular specific injury using pulsed irradiation. *J Invest Dermatol.* 1989;92:868–871.

4 Dierickx CC, Casparian JM, Venugopalan V, et al. Thermal relaxation of port-wine stain vessels probed in vivo: the need for 1–10 millisecond laser pulse treatment. *J Invest Dermatol.* 1995;105:709–714.

5 Alam M, Dover JS, Arndt KA. Treatment fo facial telangiectasia with variable-pulse high fluence pulses dye laser: comparison of efficacy with fluences immediately above and below the purpura threshold. *Dermatol Surg.* 2003;29:681–685.

6 Alves OC, Wainberg E. Heat denaturation of metHb and HbNO: e.p.r. Evidence of a new hemichrome. *Int J Biol Macromol.* 1993;15:273–279.

7 Barton JK, Loui S, Black JF. Optical and magnetic resonance changes in photothermally coagulating blood. *Proc SPIE.* 2002;4609:10–19.

8 Black JF, Barton JK. Time-domain optical and thermal analysis of blood undergoing laser photocoagulation. *Proc SPIE.* 2001;4257:341–354.

9 Karsai S, Raulin C. News in the treatment of vascular skin lesions. In: Plewig G, Thomas P, eds. *Fortschritte der praktischen Dermatologie and Venerologie.* Berlin: Springer; 2007:575–576.

10 Sherwood KA, Murray S, Kurban AK, et al. Effect of wavelength on cutaneous pigment using pulsed irradiation. *J Invest Dermatol.* 1989;92:717–720.

11 Goldberg DJ. Laser- and light-based hair removal: an update. *Expert Rev Med Devices.* 2007;4:253–260.

12 Tanzi EL, Alster TS. Long-pulsed 1064 nm Nd:YAG laser-assisted hair removal in all skin types. *Dermatol Surg.* 2004;30:13–17.

13 Kilmer SL, Anderson RR. Clinical use of the Q-switched ruby and the Q-switched Nd:YAG (1064 nm and 532 nm) lasers for treatment of tattoos. *J Dermatol Surg Oncol.* 1993;19:330–338.

14 Ross EV, Sajben FP, Hsia J, et al. Nonablative skin remodeling: Selective dermal heating with a mid-infrared laser and contact cooling combination. *Lasers Surg Med.* 2000;26:186–195.

15 Goldberg DJ. Full-face nonablative dermal remodeling with a 1320 nm Nd:YAG laser. *Dermatol Surg.* 2000;26:915–918.

16 Lupton JR, Williams CM, Alster TS. Nonablative laser skin resurfacing using a 1540 nm erbium glass laser: a clinical and histologic analysis. *Dermatol Surg.* 2002;28:833–835.

17 Fournier N, Dahan S, Barneon G, et al. Nonablative remodeling: a 14-month clinical ultrasound imaging and profilometric evaluation of a 1540 nm Er:Glass laser. *Dermatol Surg.* 2002;28:926–931.

18 Manstein D, Herron GC, Sink RK, et al. Fractional phothermolysis: A new concept for cutaneous remodeling using microscopic patterns of thermal injury. *Lasers Surg Med.* 2004;34:426–438.

19 Laubach H-J, Tannous Z, Anderson RR, et al. Skin responses to fractional photothermolysis. *Lasers Surg Med.* 2006;38:142–149.

20 Hantash BM, Bedi VP, Sudireddy V, et al. Laser-induced transepidermal elimination of dermal content by fractional photothermolysis. *J Biomed Opt.* 2006;11:041115.

21 Hantash BM, Bedi VP, Kapadia B, et al. In vivo histological evaluation of a novel ablative fractional resurfacing device. *Lasers Surg Med.* 2007;39:96–107.

22 Görgü M, Aslan G, Akoz T, Erdogan B. Comparison of alexandrite laser and electrolysis for hair removal. *Dermatol Surg.* 2000;26:37–41.

23 Lanigan SW. Incidence of side effects after laser hair removal. *J Am Acad Dermatol.* 2003;49:882–886.

24 Kautz G, Rick K, Sandhofer M, eds. *Photoepilation.* Darmstadt: Steinkopff; 2007.

25 Ziering CL. Laser assisted hair removal: a review of current technology. *In J Cosmet Surg.* 1998;6:71–75.

26 Moreno-Arias GA, Castelo-Branco C, Ferrando J. Side effects after IPL photodepilation. *Dermatol Surg.* 2002;28:1131–1134.

27 Greve B, Raulin C. Professional errors caused by lasers and intense pulsed light technology in dermatology and aesthetic medicine: preventive strategies and case studies. *Dermatol Surg.* 2002;28:156–161.

28 Tay YK, Kwok C. Minimally ablative erbium:YAG laser resurfacing of facial atrophic acne scars in Asian skin: a pilot study. *Dermatol Surg.* 2008;34:681–685.

29 Bodendorf MO, Grunewald S, Simon JC, Paasch U. Efficacy and cosmetic results of contact gel cooling of the skin during non-ablative laser procedures. *J Dtsch Dermatol Ges.* 2008;6:647–652.

30 Galeckas KJ, Ross EV, Uebelhoer NS. A pulsed dye laser with a 10-mm beam diameter and a pigmented lesion window for purpura-free photorejuvenation. *Dermatol Surg.* 2008;34:308–313.

31 Pang ALY, Wells K. Bilateral anterior uveitis after intense pulsed light therapy for pigmented eyelid lesions. *Dermatol Surg.* 2008;34:1276–1279.

32 Huldsbergen-Henning JP, van Gemert MJC, Lahaye CTW. Clinical and histological evaluation of port-wine stain treatment with a microsecond-pulsed dye-laser at 577 nm. *Laser Surg Med.* 1984;5:375.

33 Ross EV, Uebelhoer N, Domankevitz Y. Use of a novel pulse dye laser for rapid single pass purpura-free treatment of telangectasias. *Dermatol Surg.* 2007;33:1466–1469.

34 Yoon HJ, Lee DH, Kim SO, Park KC, Youn SW. Acne erythema improvement by long-pulsed 595-nm pulsed-dye laser treatment: a pilot study. *J Dermatolog Treat.* 2008;19:38–44.

35 Kauvar A, Rosen N, Khrom T. A newly modified 595-nm pulsed dye laser with compression handpiece for the treatment of photodamaged skin. *Lasers Surg Med.* 2006;38:808–813.

36 Willenberg T, Baumgartner I. Vascular birthmarks. *Vasa.* 2008;37:5–17.

37 Bernstein EF, Kligman A. Rosacea treatment using the new-generation, high-energy, 595 nm, long pulse-duration pulsed-dye laser. *Lasers Surg Med.* 2008;40:233–239.

38 Ross BS, Levine VJ, Ashinoff R. Laser treatment of acquired vascular lesions. *Dermatol Clin.* 1997;15:385–396.

39 Herd RM, Dover JS, Arndt KA. Basic laser principles. *Dermatol Clin.* 1997;15:355–372.

40 Goldberg DJ. Laser treatment of pigmented lesions. *Dermatol Clin.* 1997;15:397–407.

41 Schweiger ES, Kwasniak L, Aires DJ. Treatment of dermatosis papulosa nigra with a 1064 nm Nd:YAG laser: Report of two cases. *J Cosmet Laser Ther.* 2008;10:120–122.

42 Kilmer SL. Laser treatment of tattoos. *Dermatol Clin.* 1997;15:409–417.

43 Anderson RR, Geronemus R, Kilmer SL, et al. Cosmetic tattoo ink darkening. A complication of Q-switched and pulsed laser treatment. *Arch Dermatol.* 1993;129:1010.

44 Khoury JG, Saluja R, Goldman MP. The effect of botulinum toxin type A on full-face intense pulsed light treatment: a randomized, double-blind, split-face study. *Dermatol Surg.* 2008;34:1062–1069.

45 Wheeland RG. Laser-assisted hair removal. *Dermatol Clin.* 1997;15:469–477.

46 Goldberg DJ. Topical solution-assisted laser hair removal. *Lasers Surg Med.* 1995;7S:47.

47 Nanni CA, Alster TS. Optimizing treatment parameters for hair removal using a topical carbon-based solution and 1064-nm Q-switched neodymium:YAG laser energy. *Arch Dermatol.* 1997;133:1546–1549.

48 Bencini PL, Luci A, Galimberti M, Ferranti G. Longterm epilation with long-pulsed neodymium:YAG laser. *Dermatol Surg.* 1999;25:175–178.

49 Grossman MC, Dierickx C, Farinelli BS, Flotte T, Anderson RR. Damage to hair follicles by normal-mode ruby laser pulses. *J Am Acad Dermatol.* 1996;35:889–894.

50 Boss WK, Usal H, Thompson RC, Fiorillo MA. A comparison of the long-pulse alexandrite laser hair removal system. *Ann Plast Surg.* 1999;42:381–384.

51 Goldberg DJ, Ahkami R. Evaluation comparing multiple treatments with a 2-msec and 10-msec alexandrite laser for hair removal. *Lasers Surg Med.* 1999;25:223–228.

52 Lloyd JR, Mirkov M. Long-term evaluation of the long-pulsed alexandrite laser for the removal of bikini hair at shortened treatment intervals. *Dermatol Surg.* 2000;26:633–637.

53 McDaniel DH, Lord J, Ash K, Newman J, Zukowski M. Laser hair removal: a review and report on the use of the long-pulsed alexandrite laser for hair reduction of the upper lip, leg, back, and bikini region. *Dermatol Surg.* 1999;25:425–430.

54 Nanni C, Alster TS. Long-pulsed alexandrite laser-assisted hair removal at 5, 10, and 20 millisecond pulse durations. *Lasers Surg Med.* 1999;24:332–337.

55 Bernstein EF. Pneumatic skin flattening reduces pain during laser hair reduction. *Lasers Surg Med.* 2008;40:183–187.

56 Williams RM, Gladstone HB, Moy RL. Hair removal using an 810 nm gallium aluminum arsenide semiconductor diode laser. A preliminary study. *Dermatol Surg.* 1999;25:935–937.

57 Campos VB, Dierickx CC, Farinelli WA, Lin TY, Manuskiatti W, Anderson RR. Hair removal with an 800 nm pulsed diode laser. *J Am Acad Dermatol.* 2000;43:442–447.

58 Lou WW, Quintana AT, Geronemus RG, Grossman MC. Propsective study of hair reduction by diode laser (800 nm) with long-term follow-up. *Dermatol Surg.* 2000;26:428–432.

59 Greve B, Raulin C. Medizinische dermatologische Lasertherapie. *Hautarzt.* 2003;54:594–602.

60 Ash C, Town G, Bjerring P. Relevance of the structure of time-resolved spectral output to light-tissue interaction using intense pulsed light (IPL). *Lasers Surg Med.* 2008;40:83–92.

61 Schroeter CA, Raulin C, Hürlimann W, Reineke T, De Potter C, Neumann M. Hair loss in 40 hirsute women with an intense light source, the Photoderm VL. *Eur J Dermatol.* 1999;9:374–379.

62 Troilius A, Troilius C. Hair removal with a second-generation broad spectrum intense pulsed light source – long-term follow-up. *J Cutan Laser Ther.* 1999;1:173–178.

63 Weiss RA, Weiss MA, Marwaha S, Harrington AC. Hair removal with a non-coherent filtered flash-lamp intense pulsed light source. *Lasers Surg Med.* 1999;24:128–132.

64 Sadick NS, Weiss RA, Shea CR, Nagel H, Nicholson J, Prieto VG. Long-term photoepilation using a broad-spectrum insense pulsed light source. *Arch Dermatol.* 2000;136:1336–1340.

65 Alster TS. Improvement of erythematous and hypertrophic scars by the 585 nm pulsed dye laser. *Ann Plast Surg.* 1994;32:186.

66 Alster TS. Laser treatment of erythematous/hypertrophic pigmented scars in 26 patients. *Plast Reconstr Surg.* 1995;95:91.

67 Weinstein C, Bosnich R. High energy fractional resurfacing for acne scarring (abstr). *Lasers Surg Med.* 2007;S19:34.

68 Alster TS, Tanzi EL, Lazarus M. The use of fractional laser photothermolysis for the treatment of atrophic scars. *Dermatol Surg.* 2007;33:295–299.

69 Chrastil B, Glaich A, Goldberg LH, et al. Fraxel SR1500 for the treatment of acne scars (abstr). *Lasers Surg Med.* 2007; S19:34.

70 Glaich AS, Chrastil B, Rahman Z, et al. Fractional photothermolysis for treatment of hypopigmented scars (abstr). *Lasers Surg Med.* 2007;S19:59.

71 Glaich AS, Chrastil B, Goldberg LH, et al. Fractional photothermolysis for the treatment of post-inflammatory erythema resulting from acne vulgaris (abstr). *Lasers Surg Med.* 2007;S19:60.

72 Alexiades-Armenakas MR, Bernstein LJ, Friedman PM, et al. The safety and efficacy of the 308-nm excimer laser for pigment correction of hypopigmented scars and striae albae. *Arch Dermatol.* 2004;140:955–960.

73 Hirobe T. Proliferation of epidermal melanocytes during the healing of skin wounds in newborn mice. *J Exp Zool* 1983;227:423–431.

74 Bergamaschi O, Kon S, Doine A, et al. Melanin repigmentation after gingivectomy: A 5-year clinical and transmission electron microscopic study in humans. *Int J Periodontics Restorative Dent.* 1993;13:85–92.

75 Fulton JE, Rahimi AD, Mansoor S, et al. The treatment of hypopigmenation after skin resurfacing. *Dermatol Surg.* 2004;30:95–101.

76 Kawashita MY, Niwa ABM, Alves EV, et al. Treatment of stretch marks with Fraxel laser (abstr). *Lasers Surg Med.* 2007; S19:72.

77 Rahman Z, Tanner H, Tounas J, et al. Ablative fractional resurfacing for the treatment of photodamage and skin laxity (abstr). *Lasers Surg Med.* 2007;S19:15.

78 Levy JL, Fournier N, Mordon S. CO_2 fractional resurfacing combined with air cooling: histologic investigation and optimal parameters determination (abstr). *Lasers Surg Med.* 2007;S19:17.

79 Pozner JN, Goldberg DJ, Glanz S. Fractional erbium resurfacing: histologic and early clinical experience (abstr). *Lasers Surg Med.* 2007;S19:73.

80 Katz B, McBean J. Liposuction. The new laser liposuction for men. *Dermatol Ther.* 2007;20:448–451.

6 Photodynamic Treatment

Eckart Haneke

Included on **DVD**

INTRODUCTION

Photodynamic treatment (PDT) was first described more than a century ago, but due to lack of appropriate photosensitizers it was virtually forgotten for over 50 years. General photosensitization brought about by the systemic nature of the drugs that were available at the time prevented its general use. With the development of a range of new drugs, PDT is now readily available as a new therapeutic option in various fields of medicine, particularly dermatology.

DEFINITION OF PDT

PDT is defined as the selective destruction of malignant or fast-growing cells by light activation of a photosensitizing substance in the presence of oxygen. However, new research has now broadened its indications.[1] Of the many modern photosensitizers, the most commonly used in dermatology are the prodrugs 5-aminolevulinic acid (ALA) and its methyl ester (Me-ALA).

Living cells are capable of heme biosynthesis. This is, however, quantitatively restricted by the activity of intracellular ALA synthase, which limits the endogenous synthesis of ALA and thus all further steps of the heme synthesis. Heme itself, by means of a negative feedback, inhibits ALA synthase.

There is little ALA synthase activity in the normal cell nucleus, which makes ALA from the aminoacid glycine and succinyl coenzyme A. Normally, ALA is transferred from the mitochondrion into the cytosol where it is synthesized to coproporphyrinogen via porphobilinogen and uroporphyrinogen. The coproporphyrine is again transferred into the mitochondrion and protoporphyrinogen is synthesized. This then undergoes molecular transformation to protoporphyrin IX (PpIX). This is the origin of heme, which is made by adding Fe^{++} via ferrochelatase. Heme has a strong negative feedback on the mitochondrial ALA synthase. Since the amount of intracellular iron is limited, PpIX – the photosensitizer – accumulates, rendering the cell susceptible to light of the appropriate wavelength.

Adding exogenous ALA bypasses the limiting step of endogenous ALA synthesis and leads to a significant increase in the intracellular quantity of porphyrins (Fig. 6.1). Since heme synthesis depends on the cell's activity, malignant cells, which are highly active, take up relatively more exogenous ALA and produce more PpIX, rendering them more sensitive to light irradiation. Neither ALA nor Me-ALA – the substances currently approved for the treatment of superficial skin cancer – are by themselves active, but they are precursors of the light-sensitizing compound PpIX.

ALA selectivity for malignant cells is about 1.5 times that for normal ones, while that of Me-ALA is over 8 times.[2] This allows shorter application times for Me-ALA cream compared to ALA cream. Furthermore, most non-malignant cells are virtually left intact. Absorption of ALA and Me-ALA through normal skin is minimal and there is no increase in light sensitivity.[3] Thus, in contrast to injectable photosensitizers, the topical application of the precursor of a physiological porphyrin has nearly zero systemic risk and general photosensitivity does not develop.

The preferential uptake of the completely innocuous precursor and subsequent endogenous synthesis of protoporphyrin by the target cells is the major advantage of using ALA or Me-ALA, thereby restricting the phototoxic effect to the application site. Irradiation with light, which induces an active state in the photosensitizer,[3] stimulates it to generate reactive oxygen species (ROS). These then kill those target cells that preferentially synthesized or took up the photosensitizer (Table 6.1). ROS induces cellular damage, causing in turn cytotoxicity and immunomodulation, and finally apoptosis, necrosis and vessel occlusion (Fig. 6.2).[3,4] The damage

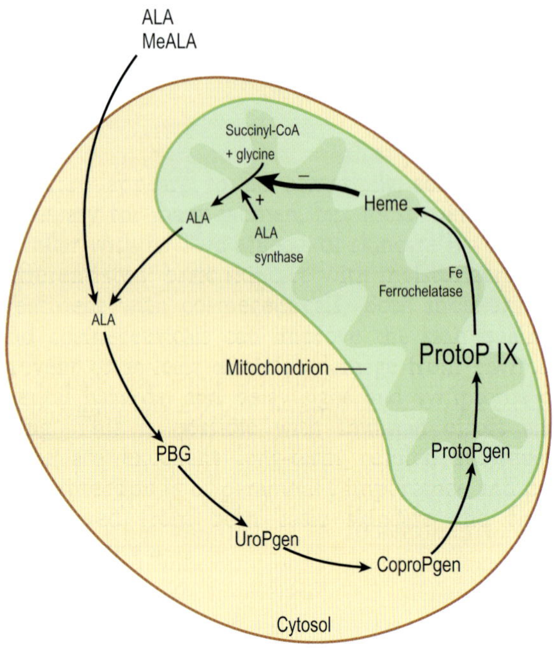

Fig. 6.1 Protoporphyrin synthesis in the cell after exogenous application of ALA or MeALA, respectively.

Table 6.1 Requirements for effectiveness of photodynamic treatment
• Tissue affinity to the photosensitizer
• Incubation time of photosensitizer on the skin (time of application)
• Light source
• Tissue oxygenation
• Type of target cell

resulting from PDT needs to overwhelm cellular repair mechanisms, a level that is reached at what is referred to as the minimum photodynamic dose. The role of heat during light irradiation is not yet entirely clear.[5] The photosensitizer is activated by light, which elevates electrons to a higher energy level causing fluorescence. Upon return of the photosensitizer to its normal state, electrons are donated to the oxygen, turning it into reactive oxygen species. These in turn cause direct cellular damage with immunomodulation and cytotoxicity, leading to apoptosis, cell death and vascular effects (Fig. 6.2).

DRUGS USED FOR PHOTODYNAMIC TREATMENT IN DERMATOLOGY

In dermatology two prodrugs are used that are taken up by the cells and converted into the potent photosensitizer protoporphyrin IX: ALA and MeALA.[6] Other drugs that are used in ophthalmology, urology, cancer treatment and internal medicine (for example systemic ALA, verteporphin, ethyl etiopurpurin and mesotetraphenylporphine sulfonate) do not play an important role in dermatology.

5-Aminolevulinic Acid

In the USA, the Food and Drug Administration (FDA) approved ALA as the first topical photosensitizing agent for the treatment of actinic keratoses. Because it is a small hydrophilic molecule, ALA is readily absorbed through abnormal keratin while normal keratin protects healthy surrounding skin.[7] ALA is converted to PpIX, which, as described above, is a potent photosensitizer, and cannot be further converted to the non-photosensitizing heme because of limited supplies of iron. Application times of up to

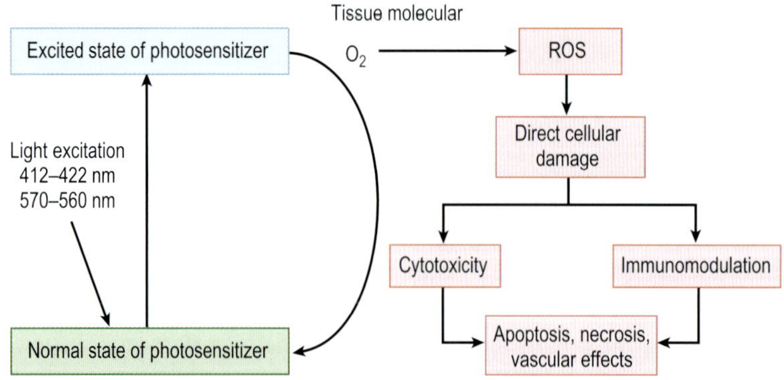

Fig. 6.2 Principle of photodynamic treatment.

4 hours confine PpIX production mainly to the target site. Longer application may lead to a larger reaction area.[8] Since PpIX is readily degraded by the absorbed light – a process called photobleaching or photodecomposition – photosensitization typically resolves within 24 hours of application, but patients should be advised not to expose the treatment area to (sun) light immediately after treatment. The maximal light absorption peak is at 409 nm, but smaller peaks occur at 509, 544, 584 and 635 nm. The FDA approval is based on a 14- to 18-hour application period even though efficacy has been demonstrated with shorter incubation periods (1 hour), which is more convenient for both patients and physicians.[9]

Recently, a low-concentration, liposome-encapsulated ALA cream has become available for use in light-induced skin rejuvenation. Measurements of skin fluorescence distribution patterns by fluorescent photography after topical application of low concentrations of ALA (0.5 and 1% preparations encapsulated in liposomes) were compared to those obtained after treatment with 20% ALA in moisturizing cream. These showed that skin fluorescence intensity with the low-concentration, liposome-encapsulated ALA reached saturation level after approximately 2 hours. The fluorescence decayed linearly within 15 minutes of the end of the application and was back to baseline within 8 hours. In contrast, the fluorescence of areas treated for more than 1 hour with the more concentrated ALA preparation in moisturizing cream was very uniform, with a linear relationship to incubation time (0–3 hours). The fluorescent intensity (15.2–57.9%) continued to increase after the end of the treatment application, eventually reaching a fluorescence of 1.6 9 times that at the end of the application, 8 hours afterwards. Thus, by changing the ALA vehicle from a moisturizing cream to liposome encapsulation, the ALA concentration can be lowered by a factor of 40 and still induce the same skin fluorescence. This also eliminates the need for occlusion, and the low post-treatment fluorescence suggests a significantly reduced risk of post-treatment phototoxicity.[10]

Aminolevulinic Acid Methyl Ester

Me-ALA was approved by the FDA in 2004 for the treatment of actinic keratoses. Me-ALA is provided as a 160 mg/g cream to be applied under occlusion for 3 hours followed by red light activation (570–670 nm with a total dose of 75 J/cm^2, or by red LED light at a light dose of 37.5 J/cm^2), after which complete photobleaching should have occurred. Me-ALA is more lipophilic and has better specificity for tumors and diseased skin than ALA.[2,3,11] However, Me-ALA and ALA were recently suggested to exhibit similar levels of efficacy.[12]

LIGHT SOURCES FOR PDT

Red light activation generates heat, which makes PDT for tumors almost unbearable without cold air cooling; local anesthesia is an alternative. Red LED light causes much less discomfort.

ALA and Me-ALA are converted to PpIX, the main absorption peak of which is in the blue light spectrum at 409 nm. The use of this wavelength is limited, however, by its maximal penetration of only 1.5–2 mm. In the USA, Blu-U® (DUSA Pharmaceuticals, Wilmington, MA) and Omnilux Blue™ (Photo Therapeautics Inc., Carlsbad, CA) are available as blue light sources. Red light (>600 nm) is absorbed much less and higher energy levels are necessary to get the same effect as blue light, but red light has the advantage that it penetrates approximately 8–10 mm. This deeper penetration can, however, be limited by melanin.[13] Red LED light sources are widely used in Europe, while intense pulsed light (IPL) is used in both the USA and Europe, particularly for photorejuvenation.

A great number of indications have been investigated in the last 20 years (Table 6.2), but not all have proven to be of value.

Table 6.2 Indications of PDT described in the literature[1]

Premalignant and malignant lesions	Actinic keratoses, Bowen's disease (squamous cell carcinoma in situ), superficial basal cell carcinoma, other non-melanotic skin cancers*, cutaneous T cell lymphoma, extramammary Paget's disease*
Inflammatory conditions	Acne vulgaris, psoriasis*
Infections	Dermatophytosis, onychomycosis, leishmaniasis, warts*, molluscum contagiosum
Benign conditions	Sebaceous hyperplasia, sebaceous nevus
Cosmetic indications	Photorejuvenation

*We, personally, do not consider these diagnoses to be good indications for PDT

PHOTODYNAMIC DIAGNOSIS

PDT is also useful for diagnosis (photodynamic diagnosis, PDD) of malignant skin lesions and their precursors, since dysplastic cells, which selectively take up more ALA or Me-ALA than normal ones, exhibit a characteristic purple-red fluorescence upon irradiation with violet-blue light (Wood's light), thus outlining the extent of superficial skin cancers and/or differentiating them from inflammatory lesions.[14]

Blue light treatment of acne is most probably a kind of endogenous PDT as *Propionibacterium acnes* produces porphyrins that act as endogenous photosensitizers. *Propionibacterium acnes*-inhabited follicles also show the characteristic porphyrin fluorescence.

CONTRAINDICATIONS AND RESTRICTIONS

Contraindications are rare, and limited to some specific photodermatoses as well as allergies to ALA and Me-ALA. Pigmented lesions are not indicated for PDT, as melanin is a fluorescence quencher and may also inhibit light penetration[4] (Table 6.3).

PDT of precancerous lesions and superficial skin cancers has some restrictions:[4]

- PDT is a blind method, i.e. a biopsy is needed to make or confirm the diagnosis and the therapeutic result.
- Drug penetration cannot be measured exactly in routine practice.
- Light penetration cannot be measured and may not only depend on the depth of tumor invasion but also on skin type and pigmentation.
- The ideal light for treatment would be blue light at around the absorption and excitation wavelength of PpIX, but this penetrates only 1–1.5 mm, which may be sufficient for actinic keratoses, but not for lesions deeper than the level of the dermo–epidermal junction. Red light is an alternative as it penetrates much deeper, but higher energy is needed. Fortunately, it is no problem to administer enough light energy in the red color range to treatment sites. However, treating the superficial part of an early invasive lesion and leaving the deeper parts behind, thus burying it, is probably one of the main reasons for recurrences.

Table 6.3 Photosensitizing drugs contraindicated in PDT
• Griseofulvin
• Thiazidics
• Tetracycline
• Sulfonylurea
• Sulfonamides
• Phenothiazine

THERAPEUTIC ALTERNATIVES

There are a variety of therapeutic alternatives, both for medical and cosmetic indications. Imiquimod, a biological response modifier, is also indicated for precancerous lesions and superficial skin cancers and has shown a rejuvenation potential when used for field cancer treatment.[15] Chemical peels, alone and in combination with cryotherapy, are effective in eradicating superficial actinic keratoses and considerably improving skin quality. Even topical 5-fluorouracil can be used for single and multiple actinic keratoses and superficial basal cell carcinomas, and gives some skin improvement.

PATIENT SELECTION

Patients are selected according to their skin condition. Those with serious photodamage, exhibiting multiple actinic keratoses and/or superficial basal cell carcinomas (BCCs), are particularly good candidates for PDT as this is one of the ideal methods for field cancer treatment. When ALA or Me-ALA are applied over a larger area and irradiated, even subclinical lesions become obvious, their extent shown by post-treatment redness.

LESION PREPARATION AND TREATMENT

Before starting PDT a precise diagnosis is made. Hyperkeratotic, invasive and pigmented lesions should not be treated using PDT. Most benign lesions, except for sebaceous glands, which do take up ALA and Me-ALA, also fail to respond.

Depending on the type of treatment intended, patients have to be prepared in different ways. The most common indication, actinic keratoses (Fig. 6.3), requires removal of hyperkeratoses, either by light curettage or salicylic acid ointment, because they protect the lesions from drug and light penetration. Superficial BCCs are treated with two sessions, 4 to 6 weeks apart (Fig. 6.4). Nodular BCCs are not a good

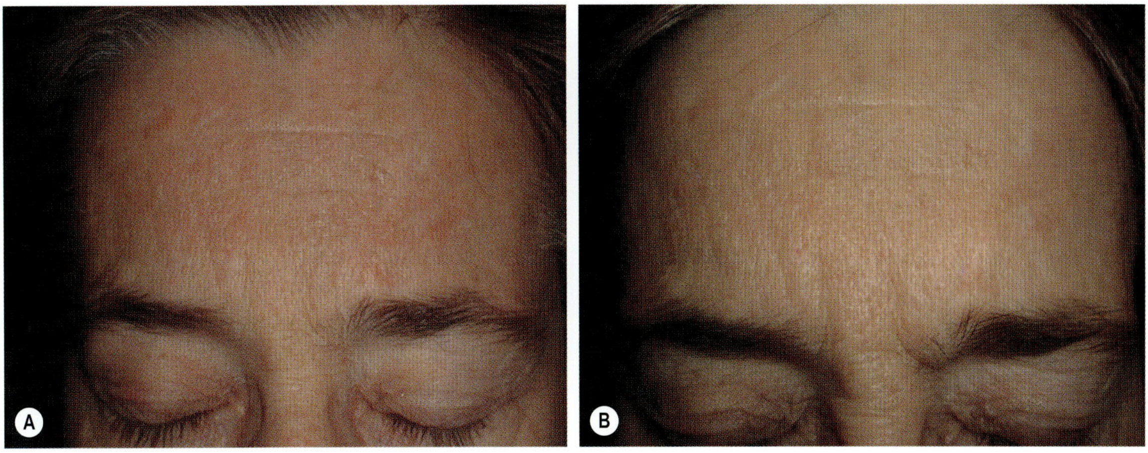

Fig. 6.3 Actinic keratoses on the left side of the forehead in a 63-year-old female patient with skin type II. *A*, Before treatment. *B*, 6 weeks after Me-ALA PDT.

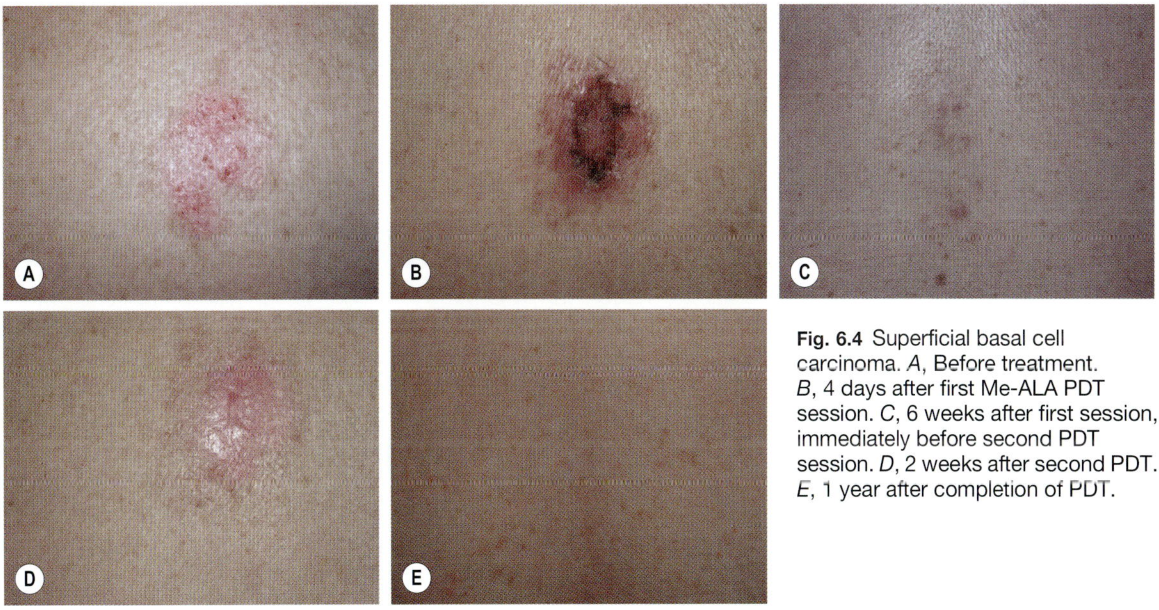

Fig. 6.4 Superficial basal cell carcinoma. *A*, Before treatment. *B*, 4 days after first Me-ALA PDT session. *C*, 6 weeks after first session, immediately before second PDT session. *D*, 2 weeks after second PDT. *E*, 1 year after completion of PDT.

indication, but they may be treated after debulking, for example by curettage. Blood, however, should not be allowed to remain on the bottom of the lesion. Each single lesion is marked and painted with the ALA solution (or covered with the Me-ALA cream), which is then occluded with a non-transparent tape. Light irradiation is applied for the duration required for the drug used. For field therapy, the entire face or cosmetic unit is treated with the ALA solution or Me-ALA cream and is usually irradiated after a shorter application time. The eyes are protected with goggles. Blue light is used for ALA, and both red LED or IPL light may be used for Me-ALA. Cold-air cooling reduces the pain from the hot red light, and gel cooled by the handpiece diminishes pain during IPL treatment. When treating the eyelids or other areas near the eyes corneal shields should be used.

For sebaceous hyperplasias, deepithelialization prior to ALA/Me-ALA application is useful; this can be achieved with one or two pulses with the Er-YAG or CO_2 laser or by superficial shaving. No anesthesia is necessary. This allows better penetration of the drug and gives fewer recurrences. We have also successfully used a similar approach for treatment of a sebaceous nevus which was planed with a #23 scalpel blade. After re-epithelialization,

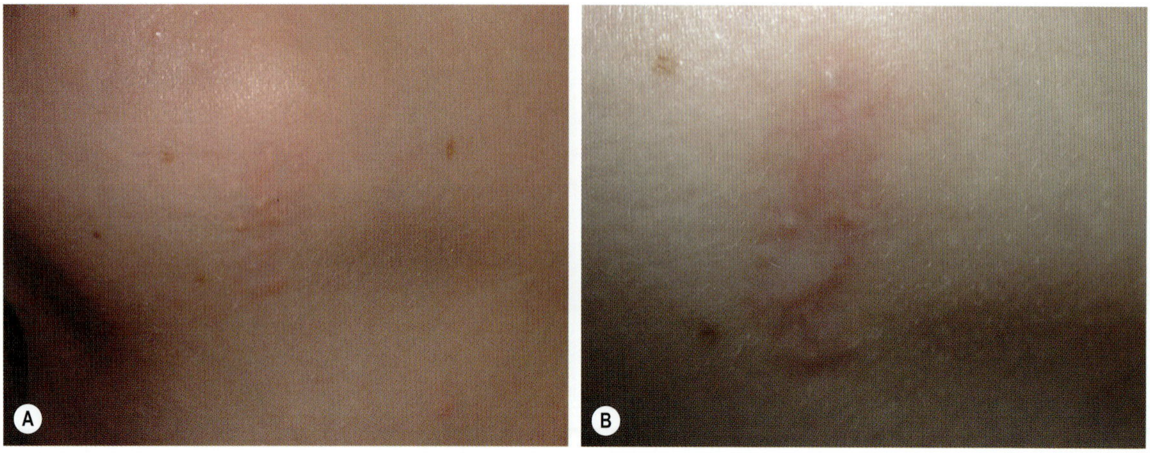

Fig. 6.5 Sebaceous nevus. *A*, After superficial shaving. *B*, 6 weeks after Me-ALA PDT.

the remaining, deeper-seated glands were then irradiated with red light after Me-ALA application for 3 hours under occlusion (Fig. 6.5) (unpublished observation).

After treatment of actinic keratoses, a red area is usually visible for 1 to 3 days, but some patients develop intense erythema and crusting, which can last for more than a week (Fig. 6.6). We have seen this particularly in red haired and blond people. Post-treatment care involves applying emollients and cooling in case of edema. Topical steroids are rarely needed.

Bowen's disease and BCC require a second session of PDT after approximately 6 weeks (Fig. 6.7), which is also performed when an actinic keratosis does not completely disappear. An attempt has been made to overcome the problem of incomplete drug and light penetration by debulking nodular BCCs, applying fractionated irradiation to reduce photobleaching of the PpIX, giving intralesional injections of ALA and applying interstitial light irradiation. However, we feel that complete excision combined with histologic margin control should be the first option for high-risk tumors. Invasive squamous cell carcinoma is not a PDT indication.

When using PDT for photorejuvenation, red spots may occur as a sign that subclinical actinic keratoses were in the treatment field. With telangietasias being the major problem, a cut-off filter at around 500 nm is used, while for blotchy skin wavelengths from 560 nm are preferred with the use of an IPL. However, the latter treatment relies more on the IPL light power than on the PDT action.

Cure and improvement rates are summarized in Table 6.4.

PDT FOR PHOTOREJUVENATION

Improvement of photodamage after PDT with 20% ALA solution applied for 15–20 hours was observed in patients who were irradiated with blue light. Of 32 patients, 72% were observed to have an

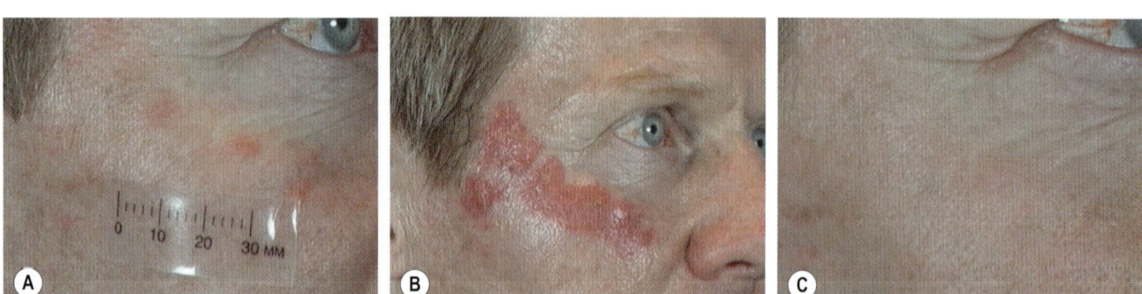

Fig. 6.6 Multiple actinic keratoses in a 45-year-old man with skin type I, freckles and red hair. *A*, Before PDT. *B*, 1 week after MeALA PDT. *C*, Completely normal skin a year after PDT.

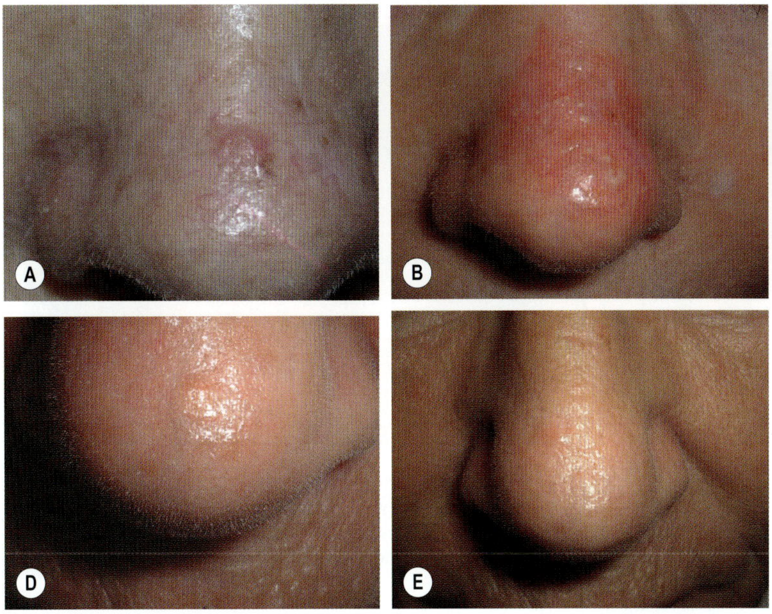

Fig. 6.7 BCC recurrence after cryosurgery. *A*, Before PDT. *B*, 2 days after Me-ALA PDT. *C*, 6 weeks after first PDT. *D*, Immediately after second PDT. *E*, 1 year after second PDT.

Table 6.4 Cure and improvement rates of various skin conditions with PDT

Diagnosis	Cure rate/improvement	Recurrence rate
Actinic keratosis	Single treatment: 65% (25–100%)	~20%
	Repeated treatments: 85% (70–90%)	
Bowen's disease (squamous cell carcinoma in situ)	80% (60–100%)	
Superficial basal cell carcinoma	50–100%	44%*/18%**
Other basal cell carcinoma	10–100%	57%
Cutaneous T cell lymphoma, extramammary Paget's disease		
Acne	Improvement:	
Comedones	45% red/58% blue + red, no ALA	
Inflammatory lesions	63% red/76% blue + ered, no ALA	
Photorejuvenation	Improvement in:	
	photoaging 80%	
	dyspigmentation 95%	
	fine lines 55%	

*ALA
**Me-ALA

improvement in skin texture. Application of ALA for short periods (1–3 hours) followed by blue light exposure was also seen to decrease sallowness and fine skin wrinkling as well as to improve mottled hyperpigmentation.[9] Nowadays, most authors use IPL as the activating light source (Fig. 6.8), as it has a therapeutic effect even without the use of ALA (see Chapter 5). A split-face study compared two treatments 1 month apart of either IPL alone or IPL plus ALA. An enhanced cosmetic effect was observed in the group with the combination of IPL plus ALA.[16] Another study designed to measure

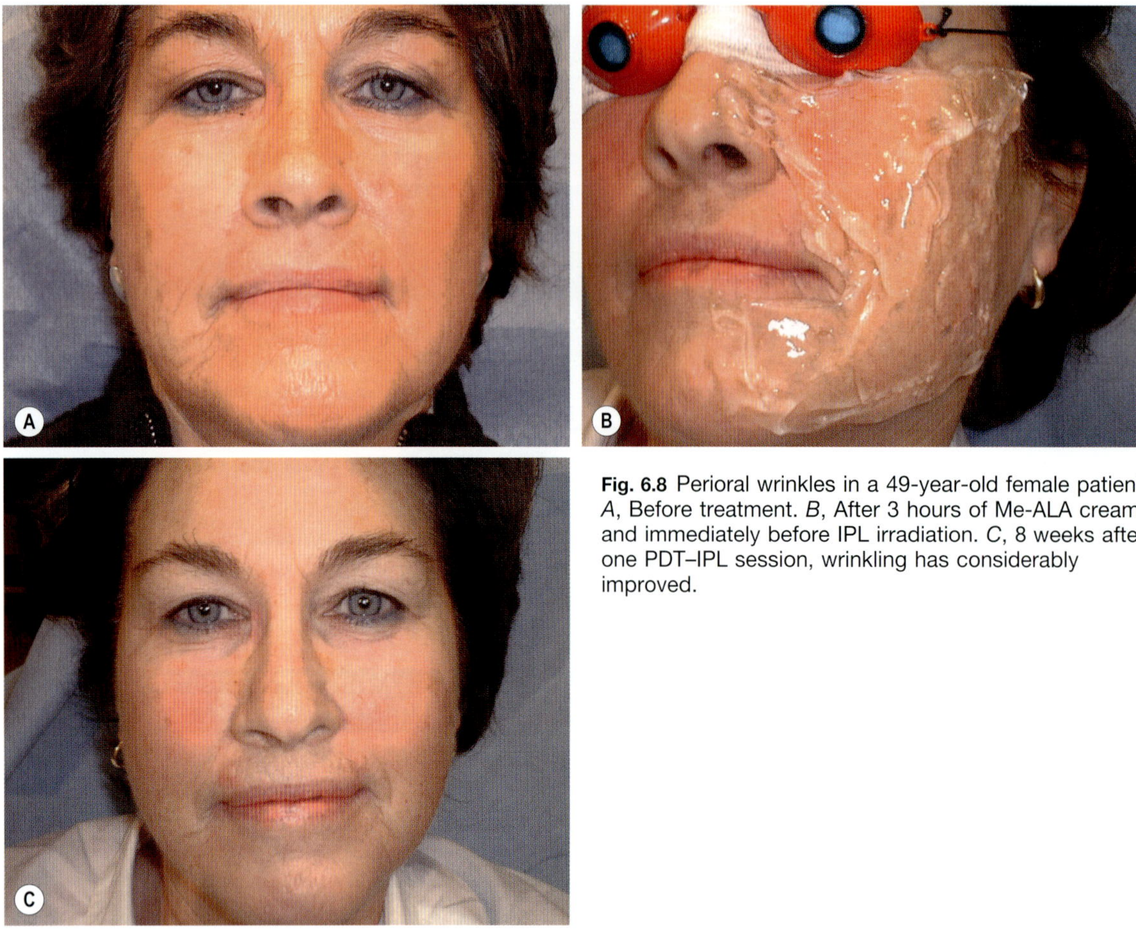

Fig. 6.8 Perioral wrinkles in a 49-year-old female patient. *A*, Before treatment. *B*, After 3 hours of Me-ALA cream and immediately before IPL irradiation. *C*, 8 weeks after one PDT–IPL session, wrinkling has considerably improved.

the effects of treatment with combined ALA and IPL and with IPL alone, compared two groups of patients, both of whom received three treatments, 3 weeks apart. It was found that the combined treatment produced greater improvement for the effects of photoaging (80% versus 50%), mottled pigmentation (95% versus 65%), and fine lines (55% versus 20%).[17] While in the first study there were more adverse effects in the combination treatment group (erythema, edema and peeling, for example), there was no difference in adverse side effects between the two groups in the latter study.[17–19] Post-procedure treatment usually does not require more than normal skincare, although immediately afterwards a cool pack may reduce any hot or burning feelings. On the other hand, the inflammation that may be induced by the treatment probably also adds to the positive rejuvenation effect.

A small study evaluated the effect of fractionated laser treatment plus Me-ALA-PDT. Four women with Fitzpatrick skin types II or III, mild to moderate rhytides and no actinic keratosis in the perioral area were treated. The perioral area was treated with two sessions of fractional resurfacing with the Fraxel SR laser, 3 weeks apart. Immediately after each fractional treatment Me-ALA was applied on one half of the perioral area and 3 hours later the area was illuminated with red light in a dose of 37 J/cm^2. There was more improvement in superficial wrinkles in three out of four patients on the combined treatment side. In one patient, the investigator found no significant difference when comparing the two sides whereas all patients noted greater improvement in the combined fractional and PDT-treated side compared to the side treated only with fractional surfacing.[20]

Guidelines for PDT photorejuvenation using IPL devices and ALA have recently been described.[21]

Long-term results from photodynamic rejuvenation are comparable to other rejuvenation techniques. For tumor PDT, consistent follow-up is necessary in order to detect potential recurrences as early as possible and in order to decide whether further PDT or an alternative treatment may be necessary.

Adverse effects include photosensitivity, which depends on the amount and duration of ALA or Me-ALA applied, skin necrosis of tumor cells with consecutive scarring as well as hypopigmentation and hyperpigmentation.[20] The degree of scarring, however, is entirely dependent on the amount of tissue destruction by the treated tumor.

CONCLUSIONS

In conclusion, PDT is a relatively new therapeutic method with the potential for scarless removal of cutaneous precancers and superficial cancers, as well as improvement of photodamaged skin. Its main advantage in the treatment of malignancy is the ability to perform field therapy. In acne, its advantage is to reduce the need for antibiotics.

REFERENCES

1 MacCormack MA. Photodynamic therapy in dermatology: An update on applications and outcomes. *Sem Cut Med Surg*. 2008;27:52–62.
2 Peng Q, Warloe T, Berg K, et al. 5-aminolevulinic acid based photodynamic therapy. *Cancer*. 1997;79:2282–2308.
3 Braathen LR. Photodynamic therapy: when and why? *J Eur Acad Dermatol Venereol*. 2002;16:227.
4 Hancke E. Photodynamic therapy for scarless removal of facial precancer and superficial carcinomas. In: Bosniak S, Cantisano-Zilkha M, eds. *Minimally Invasive Techniques of Oculofacial Rejuvenation*. New York: Thieme; 2005:151–157.
5 Orenstein A, Kostenich G, Tsur H, Kogan L, Malik Z. Temperature monitoring during photodynamic therapy of skin tumours with topical 5-aminolevulinic acid application. *Cancer Lett*. 1995;95:227–232.
6 Wolf P, Rieger E, Kerl H. Topical photodynamic therapy with endogenous porphyrins after application of 5-aminolevulinic acid: an alternative modality for solar keratosis, superficial squamous cell carcinomas, and basal cell carcinoma? *J Am Acad Dermatol*. 1993;23:17–21.
7 Kennedy JC, Pottier RH. Prossdc. Photodynamic therapy with endogenous protoporphyrin IX: basic principles and present clinical experience. *J Photochem Photobiol B*. 1990;6:143–148.
8 Jeffes EW, McCullough JL, Weinstein GD, et al. Photodynamic therapy of actinic keratoses with topical aminolevulinic acid hydrochloride and fluorescent blue light. *J Am Acad Dermatol*. 2001;45:96–104.
9 Touma D, Yaar M, Whitehead S, et al. A trial of short incubation, broad-area photodynamic therapy for facial actinic keratoses and diffuse photodamage. *Arch Dermatol*. 2004;140:33–40.
10 Christiansen K, Bjerring P, Troilius A. ALA for photodynamic photorejuvenation – optimization of treatment regime based on normal-skin fluorescence measurements. *Lasers Surg Med*. 2007;39:302–310.
11 Fritsch C, Homey B, Stahl W, et al. Preferential relative porphyrin enrichment in solar keratoses upon topical application of delta-aminolevulinic acid methylester. *Photochem Photobiol*. 1998;68:218–221.
12 Kuijpers DI, Thissen MR, Thissen CA, et al. Similar effectiveness of methyl aminolevulinate and 5-aminolevulinate in topical photodynamic therapy for nodular basal cell carcinoma. *J Drugs Dermatol*. 2006;5:642–645.
13 Ceburkov O, Gollnick H. Photodynamic therapy in dermatology. *Eur J Dermatol*. 2000;10:568–575.
14 Fritsch C, Goerz G, Ruzicka T. Photodynamic therapy in dermatology. *Arch Dermatol*. 1998;134:207–214.
15 Metcalf S, Crowson AN, Naylor M, et al. Imiquimod as an anti-aging agent. *J Am Acad Dermatol*. 2007;56:422–425.
16 Goldman MP, Atkin D, Kincaid S. PDT/ALA in the treatment of actinic damage. Real world experience. *Lasers Surg Med*. 2002;14S:79.
17 Alster TS, Tanzi EL, Welsh EC. Photorejuvenation of facial skin with topical 20% 5-aminolevulinic acid and intense pulsed light treatment: a split-face comparison study. *J Drugs Dermatol*. 2005;4:35–38.
18 Dover JS, Bhatia AC, Stewart B, et al. Topical 5-aminolevulinic acid combined with intense pulsed light in the treatment of photoaging. *Arch Dermatol*. 2005;141:1247–1252.
19 Gold MH, Bradshaw VL, Boring MM, et al. A: Split-face comparison of photodynamic therapy with 5-aminolevulinic acid and intense pulsed light versus intense pulsed light alone for photodamage. *Dermatol Surg*. 2006;32:795–801.
20 Ruiz-Rodriguez R, López L, Candelas D, Zelickson B. Enhanced efficacy of photodynamic therapy after fractional resurfacing: fractional photodynamic rejuvenation. *J Drugs Dermatol*. 2007;6:818–820.
21 Nootheti PK, Goldman MP. Aminolevulinic acid-photodynamic therapy for photorejuvenation. *Dermatol Clin*. 2007;25:35–45.

7 Skin-Tightening Devices

Included on **DVD**

Radiofrequency and infrared technologies

Alessandra Haddad, Marian Cantisano-Zilkha

BASIC CONCEPTS

Improvement in skin laxity following laser treatments was first observed in the early 1990s during ablative resurfacing treatments with a CO_2 laser.[1,2] While it was initially assumed that the benefits of these treatments were due to the removal (ablation) of tissue, cosmetic improvements were often more significant than could be explained by ablation of tissue alone.[3] Ablation typically removed 20 μm of tissue, but a residual thermal zone of 60–120 μm depth was also created.[3] The temperature rise and duration of this heating were sufficient to denature collagen, leading to a visible contraction of the skin during treatment. This led to a tighter, fresher look as a component of the ablative laser treatment. Results seen after a long-term follow-up showed histologically that resurfacing techniques are an effective alternative to deep phenol peels. On the negative side, prolonged recovery time, long training and learning curves for the practitioner, added to the high incidence of complications (scarring, dischromias, infections and pain), caused the decline of resurfacing procedures.

That has led to a question: Is it possible to get the benefits of tissue tightening non-ablatively?

The answer is yes, and non-ablative tissue tightening is one of the newest and most exciting procedures in the aesthetic marketplace today (Table 7.1).

Grekin and colleagues published the first large prospective study evaluating a radiofrequency (RF) resurfacing system (Visage®) for treating wrinkles.[4] The results of this study, involving 95 individuals with mild to severe photodamage in the periorbital or perioral regions, showed positive improvement in the Fitzpatrick Wrinkle Score. The degree of improvement was linked with the severity of wrinkles at baseline. Primary adverse effects were transient postinflammatory hyperpigmentation (26%) and hypertrophic scarring (4%). They concluded that the efficacy of RF resurfacing may be comparable with that of laser resurfacing. In addition, RF resurfacing may provide more rapid healing and less pain and erythema than CO_2 lasers. Similar results are possible with non-ablative skin-tightening devices.[4,6]

The goal of this chapter is to provide an understanding of non-ablative skin tightening. We will examine what is required for tissue tightening, as well as the different approaches available today. As it is common, there are many conflicting and confusing claims made by manufacturers, and hopefully this chapter will allow readers to make an

Table 7.1
Ablative rejuvenation.
• CO_2 and erbium YAG devices • YSGL device (Pearl)
Semi-ablative rejuvenation
• Fractional CO_2 or erbium
Non-ablative
• Radiofrequency • Infrared

informed analysis in their decision to use non-ablative technologies.

DEFINITIONS AND TERMINOLOGY

Collagen

Before going further, it is worthwhile to give some definitions. Collagen is a family of structural proteins, providing strength and resilience to the skin and other tissues.[5] Collagen is produced by fibroblasts in an early-stage form called procollagen. It is composed of a triple helix of protein chains, with interchain bonds creating a crystalline structure for the collagen.

Type I collagen is the most common form of collagen found in the dermis and provides the tensile strength of the skin. This form of collagen is also believed to be a key component in skin aging, since the quantity has been shown to be lower in photodamaged skin and to increase after some skin rejuvenation treatments.[3,4] Type III collagen is the second most common form of collagen found in the skin and forms thinner diameter fibers than type I collagen. Both procollagen and type III collagen are formed initially in the wound-healing process, with type I collagen being produced later.[6]

Skin Laxity

As part of the aging process, the skin reduces its production of elastin and collagen, the main structural proteins in the dermis. With less support structure in the skin, areas can sag due to gravity. Common areas for this to occur are the neck, jowls, underarms, and the abdomen, particularly postpartum (Fig. 7.1).

As part of the treatment of skin laxity, it is important to differentiate skin that is sagging due to laxity from skin that is sagging due to excess fat. As a general rule, thin skin without underlying excess fat can be treated most effectively.

Collagen Contraction

The goal in treating skin laxity is to create a bulk change in the support structure of the skin to counteract the skin laxity caused by aging. If sufficient heat is delivered to the collagen, the structure of the collagen will change, causing the fibers to contract and thicken. An extreme example of collagen denaturation is cooking: we have all seen how a slice of bacon shrinks as it is heated.

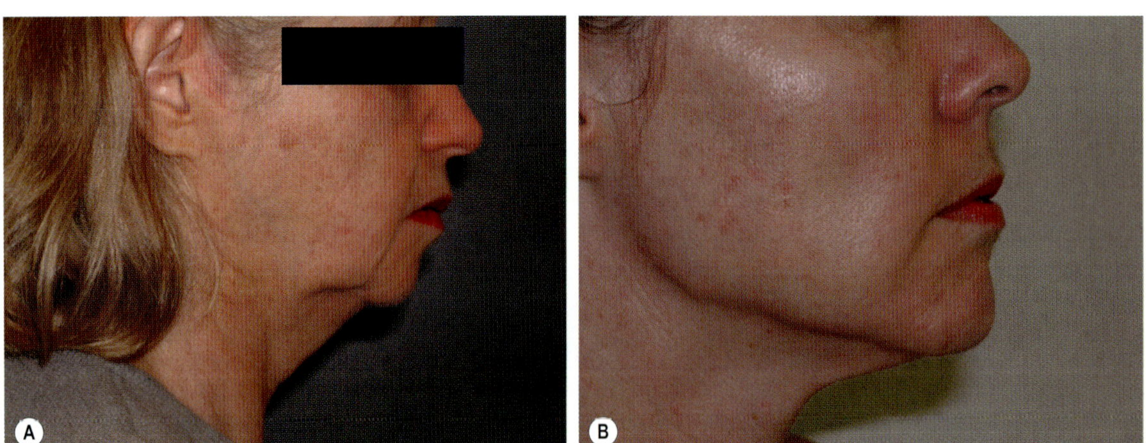

Fig. 7.1 These photographs show examples of skin laxity due to aging. Common areas in which skin laxity occurs are the lower half of the face, underarms and abdomen. (Photographs courtesy of Alessandra Haddad, MD).

While most of the laboratory studies on collagen shrinkage or denaturation have been performed ex vivo, these studies have shown that heated collagen transforms from the crystalline triple-helical structure to an amorphous, random-coil structure through breakage of the hydrogen bonds linking the protein strands of the triple helix.[7] This creates a thickening and shortening of the collagen fibers as the chains fold and assume a more stable configuration, as shown schematically in Figure 7.2. This immediate collagen contraction can be used for cosmetic treatments to treat skin laxity or other signs of aging on the face or body.

It should be noted that this immediate tissue tightening is different from the long-term collagen stimulation caused by a thermally induced wound response. These immediate changes can be observed both during treatment and through electron micrograph studies.

Sustained Volumetric Heating

As noted, temperature is a key component in collagen contraction or denaturation but it is not the only factor. While some people refer to a 'magic temperature' for collagen contraction, this is actually a misleading statement. Knowing only the temperature achieved in the dermis is not sufficient to understand if collagen denaturation will occur. Collagen contraction will occur only through a combination of time and temperature – or sustained volumetric heating. The collagen must be heated to a temperature and kept there for a sufficient length of time. This combination varies; similar collagen contraction can be achieved at a lower temperature if the duration of the heating is increased, but the heat must be delivered uniformly over the treatment area.

Studies have shown that, for a 5°C decrease in temperature, the duration of the heating must be increased by an order of magnitude (10 times) to achieve a similar degree of collagen contraction.[3] So while millisecond pulses are sufficient for collagen contraction at the temperatures achieved during CO_2 treatments, significantly longer pulse times are required for the treatment temperatures used in non-ablative treatments. All the protocols for the proven non-ablative treatments of skin laxity include multisecond treatment times.

The target depth for skin laxity treatments is the dermis. This will require a balance: providing the heat at a superficial level will not create the volume changes that are desired, while heating too deeply might affect the subcutaneous fat. To achieve this balance, the heat should be targeted at a depth of a couple of millimeters (Table 7.2).[8]

Cooling

While the temperature required in the dermis for collagen contraction with multisecond exposure times is above 55–60°C, a blister will form if the epidermal temperature is above 50°C. It is obvious

Table 7.2 Requirements for a skin laxity device
• Sustained volumetric heating
• Heat at the appropriate depth
• Uniform heating to obtain the maximum contraction
• Cooling system to protect epidermis
• Histological and scientific evidence of the results
• Cost per procedure reasonable (no or few consumables)

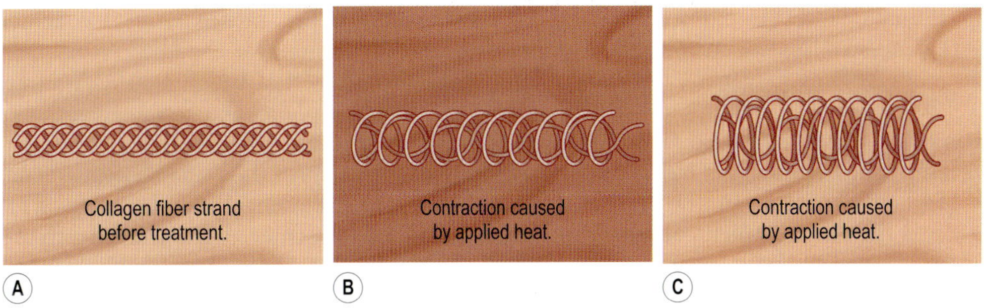

Fig. 7.2 Collagen response to uniform controlled heat. *A*, Schematic diagram demonstrating structured triple helix molecule of collagen. *B*, Initial response of collagen from a structured triple helix to a random coil structure. *C*, Long-term collagen rebuilding continues for 3–12 weeks after treatment.

that cooling will play a major role in any non-ablative approach to the treatment of skin laxity. In fact, with the heat that is deposited to contract the collagen, aggressive cooling before, during and even after the heating pulse is required. Postcooling helps protect the epidermis, as the intense heat from the dermis diffuses to the surrounding tissue. Forms of cooling can include parallel cooling through a sapphire window or cryogen cooling.

Neocollagenesis

It is important to differentiate between immediate collagen contraction and longer-term collagen production. Neocollagenesis is simply the formation of new collagen, for example as occurs during a wound response. This longer-term production of new collagen was the goal of the early laser-based non-ablative skin rejuvenation treatments. In this process, laser treatments trigger a thermally induced wound response. This response can be triggered at a temperature much lower than is required for immediate collagen contraction. Also, most of the demonstrated procedures for new collagen production require multiple treatments to obtain the desired results. In addition to evidence from before and after photographs, these results can be observed histologically by examining the collagen fibers prior to and a few months after the treatment.

APPROACHES TO THE TREATMENT OF SKIN LAXITY

To the best of the authors' knowledge at the time of publication, only a few approaches to the treatment of skin laxity have published histological evidence of immediate collagen contraction. Some of these approaches are the Titan™ by Cutera, the ThermaCool® device by Thermage®,[9,10] Visage™ by Arthrocare Corp (Sunnyvale, CA), and Accent XL® by Alma Lasers (Caesarea, Israel). While this does not mean that other devices may not effectively treat skin laxity, the reader should look for scientific evidence and medical papers before making a decision.

Various lasers, such as the Nd:YAG 1450 nm and Nd:YAG 1540 nm, emitting in the mid-infrared, have been used for the treatment of fine wrinkles and acne scars. However, these lasers need multiple treatments with a delayed and relatively minimal clinical softening of the wrinkles. They do not produce deep dermal tightening or lifting since they affect only the superficial parts of the dermis.

New devices have emerged to treat skin laxity and wrinkles in a non-ablative way, regardless of skin type and color. These devices are of three types:

1. devices using only RF[11,12]
2. devices using RF combined with infrared energy
3. devices using near- and mid-infrared pulsed light, the so-called infrared skin-tightening devices.

All these devices use different frequencies. The choice of energy and appropriate frequency that will be selectively concentrated in the dermis is of cardinal importance.

Optical energy (intense pulsed light and lasers) is absorbed by melanin chromophores in the epidermis and hair shafts, and hemoglobin in vessels. This kind of energy cannot treat wrinkles because collagen fibers, which are involved in the pathophysiology of wrinkling, do not contain chromophores.

To satisfy the need for energy, which acts on the dermis without affecting the epidermis, RF and infrared radiation were found to be the most appropriate tools. The main difference between lasers and RF is that lasers affect collagen in the upper dermis, improving fine lines, wrinkles and skin texture, while RF energy is able to penetrate deeper into the skin and affect the deeper dermis and subcutaneous layers, causing tightening and improvement to the underlying tissue structure, but with little change in skin texture.

RF is considered more selective to the depth of the dermis targeted than infrared frequencies. In the past, it has been used mainly in surgery, but now it is also considered to be the newest alternative in skin-tightening procedures and will be further discussed later in this chapter.

Infrared Technology

The general goal of tissue tightening is to provide enough heat to the dermis while protecting the epidermis. We will describe the Titan™ in more detail, since one of the authors (AH) has achieved very consistent results over the last 2 years.

In the Titan™ (Cutera, Inc., CA), water is the target chromophore and a wavelength is selected based on the absorption characteristics of water.

Figure 7.3 shows the water absorption curve. Based on this curve, wavelengths in the range of 1100–1800 nm are used to achieve heating at a depth of 1–2 mm. This depth is chosen to heat the dermis, but without any risk of heating the subcutaneous fat. There is a strong water absorption peak in the 1400–1500 nm range, and this wavelength is filtered from the Titan™ output to further optimize the treatment.

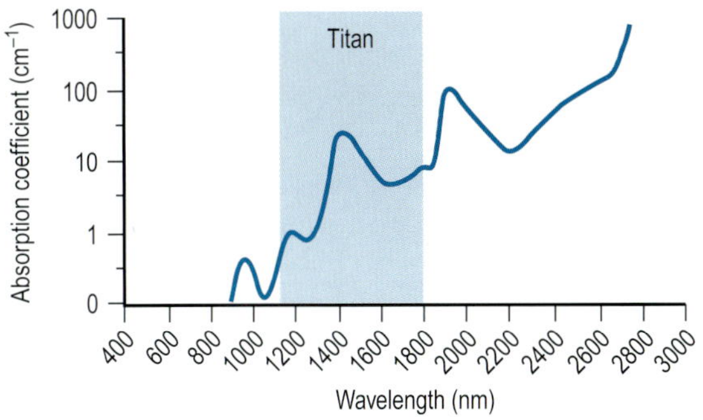

Fig. 7.3 Absorption curve of water. The range 1100–1800 nm provides the moderate absorption needed for heating at a depth of 1–2 mm.

Each Titan™ treatment pulse consists of a multi-second exposure. The temperature profile in the dermis can be measured through animal studies. Figure 7.4 shows a cross-section with a maximum temperature rise of approximately 25°C. This maximum temperature occurs at a depth of approximately 1–2 mm, whereas the epidermis is protected through contact cooling with a sapphire window.

The heating provided by the Titan™ has been shown histologically to provide immediate changes to the collagen.[9–12] The denaturing of the collagen fiber can be seen in Figure 7.5.

This immediate collagen contraction can also be seen clinically. Many physicians will treat one side of the face before moving to the other side. In the middle of the procedure, the physician lets the patients sit up and confirm that they can see the difference in the treated and untreated sides. This is not simply edema since, in most of the area treated, edema would create a swelling that would make the area look worse, not tighter.

To demonstrate that these results can be consistently reproduced, a retrospective study of over 1000 patients was performed. In this study, covering results from four different practices, physicians reported a satisfaction level above 80% with the Titan™.[13,14] The safety of the Titan™ device was also examined as part of this retrospective study. Only two side effects were reported in over 1000 treatments. Both of these side effects healed without complication.

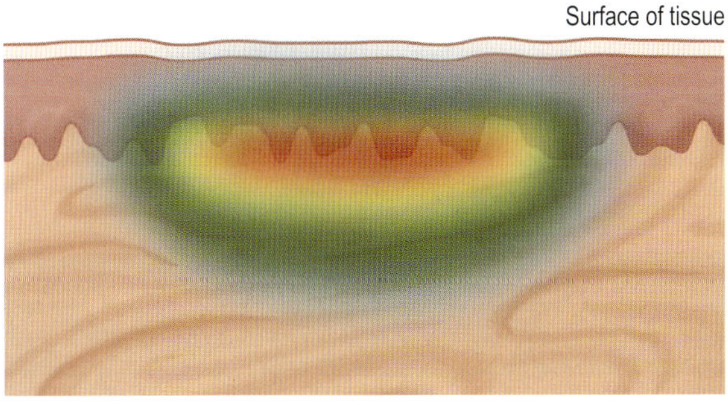

Fig. 7.4 Thermal camera measurement of a cross-section of animal tissue following a Titan™ pulse. The maximum heating is shown in red and occurs approximately 1–2 mm below the surface.

Since the Titan™ uses an infrared light source (lamp), each handpiece has a finite lifetime, either 10 000 or 15 000 pulses. Based on the replacement cost and the number of pulses per treatment, the cost per procedure is roughly $90. With typical procedure fees in the range of $800–2500 per procedure based on a survey of Titan™ users across the USA and Brazil, this per procedure cost is acceptable.

PREPARATION AND INFRARED SKIN-TIGHTENING TECHNIQUE

Preoperative Considerations

- Conduct a patient consultation complete with medical history prior to treatment.
- Clean the skin, including removal of all make-up and other skincare products. Any creams or products left on the skin can interact with the light and increase the risk of unwanted side effects.
- Shave any hair in the area to be treated. Hair in the treatment area may not allow full contact of the handpiece with the skin.
- Preoperative photographs should be taken with consistent technique (patient positioning, camera settings and room lighting).
- These treatments can be tolerated without anesthesia. The use of sedation, nerve blocks or local injectable anesthetics is not recommended for these treatments as patient feedback is very important and, with the proper technique, is not required. Topical anesthesia can be used if desired. It must be completely removed prior to treatment.

Optimizing Outcomes

- When treating near the mouth, rolled-up gauze can be placed between the lips and teeth to protect the teeth from discomfort.
- Some physicians make this treatment part of an overall skincare regimen along with topical retinoids, topical vitamin C, sun protection and/or microdermabrasion.
- Do not treat over areas with tattoos.

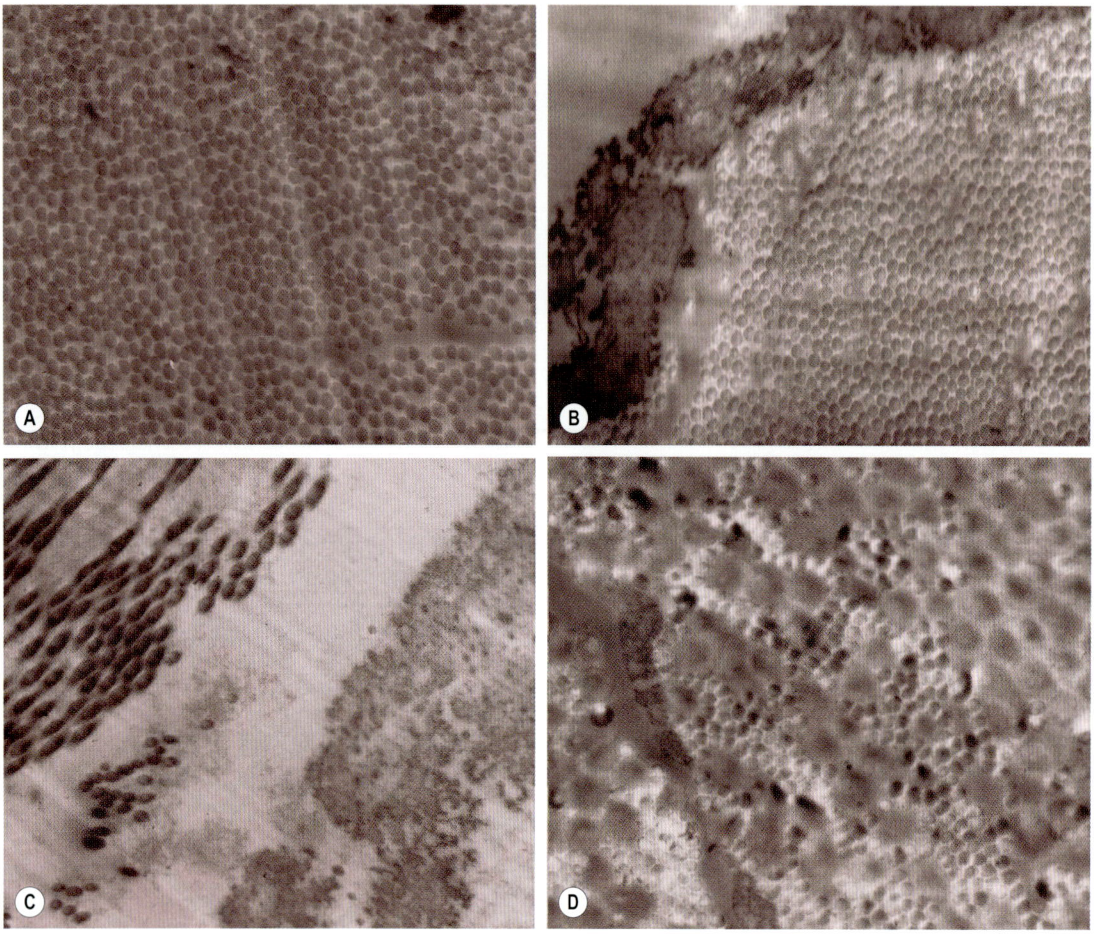

Fig. 7.5 Transmission electron microscopy of collagen fibers at the 0 to 1 mm depth. *A*, Control showing typical cross sectioned collagen fibers. *B*, Collagen fibers after four passes at 30 J/cm^2. The left-hand side shows normal morphology while the right demonstrates a transition to contracted collagen. *C*, Collagen fibers after four passes at 45 J/cm^2. The entire field shows contracted collagen. *D*, Collagen fibers after four passes at 65 J/cm^2. Many fibers are contracted to several times their normal size. Original magnification × 4320. (Brian Zelickson, M.D.)

- Extreme caution should be used when treating near the eye, taking care to avoid ocular damage from the light. Patient eye protection appropriate for the given treatment should be used. The light should always be pointed away from the eye and only applied to the skin outside of the orbital rim. Skin at the edge of the orbital rim can be treated by pulling it away from the eye while simultaneously holding the goggles in place, so treatment is kept outside of the orbital rim.

Titan™ Treatment Parameters

- Fluency should be adjusted as low as 28 J/cm^2 and raised to as high as 46 J/cm^2 based on patient tolerance and the area being treated (Table 7.3).
- Sensitive areas and bony areas may require lower fluences for some patients.
- It is common to feel a sensation at the end of the heat cycle, depending on the area that is treated. This should resolve as the handpiece is moved to the next treatment spot. If the patient still feels this sensation, or heat, stop the treatment and cool the area with the handpiece and/or ice pack.

Table 7.3 Typical starting fluence in a treatment area

Skin type	Fluence (face, neck, and chest)	Fluence (body)
I–VI (including tanned skin)	34–38 J/cm^2	36–46 J/cm^2

Recommended Technique

- When the face is being treated, it is typically divided into three regions (forehead and both cheeks), as shown in Figure 7.3. Similar-size areas can be treated when treating the neck, generally divided into two or three regions. One section at a time is treated, completing all passes in that area before moving to the next.
- Apply a layer of clear gel (such as ultrasound gel), approximately 3 mm thick, to the treatment area. For patient comfort, reapplication of cooled gel as the treatment progresses may be helpful.
- Hold the handpiece to ensure complete contact of the window with the surface of the skin to be treated. Activate the exposure with the foot pedal. Do not lift the handpiece until the audible tone and the blue light have ended: losing contact with the skin during a pulse can result in blistering and increased risk of side effects.
- Instruct the patient to alert you if the discomfort level becomes intolerable.
- Place the next pulse adjacent to the previous one without overlapping.
- Always observe the epidermis during the treatment, watching for signs of damage (epidermal separation or gray coloration). If damage is seen, stop the treatment, cool the skin and reduce the fluence before continuing.
- Apply all passes (usually three to four) in one area before beginning treatment in the next area. This allows for sustained heating. As the skin temperature increases with each pass, it may be necessary to lower the fluence by a small amount on the latter passes for patient comfort.
- Extreme caution should be used when treating near the eye, taking care to avoid ocular damage from the light. Patient eye protection appropriate for the given treatment should be used. The light should always be pointed away from the eye and only applied to the skin outside of the orbital rim. Skin at the edge of the orbital rim can be treated by pulling it away from the eye while simultaneously holding the goggles in place, so treatment is kept outside of the orbital rim.
- Erythema is a common immediate reaction seen from this treatment. This typically resolves within 2 hours but can last longer.

Postoperative Care

- Localized erythema may also be present and typically resolves within 24–48 hours. If prolonged erythema occurs, future treatments should be performed at a lower fluence.

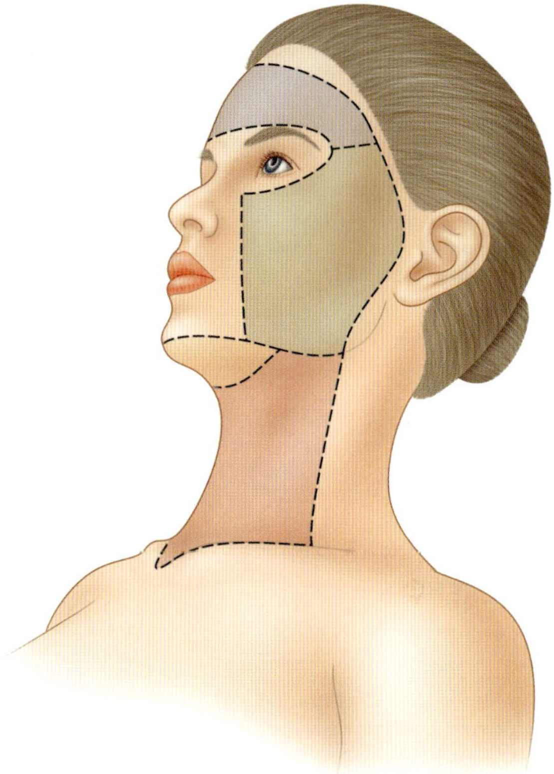

Fig. 7.6 Example segmentation of the face/neck for Titan™ procedure.

- If a wound develops, an antibiotic ointment may be recommended.
- Treatment intervals of 4 weeks are commonly used, with an average of two to four treatments.

See Figures 7.6 and 7.7.

CONCLUSION

There are multiple criteria as you evaluate the different approaches to skin tightening. Collagen contraction can only be obtained through sustained volumetric heating, often requiring multisecond pulses for the non-ablative approaches discussed in this book. With the significant heat that is delivered during treatment, cooling will be a critical element for safety. Any manufacturer should also be able to support their marketing claims with both histological and clinical evidence. A good skin laxity device should also offer consistent results, leading to a high level of patient satisfaction. Finally, the operating cost of the device should be reasonable to allow you to offer a fair procedure cost while obtaining a good return on your investment. Only when all these criteria are met should you consider purchasing and working with a skin laxity device.

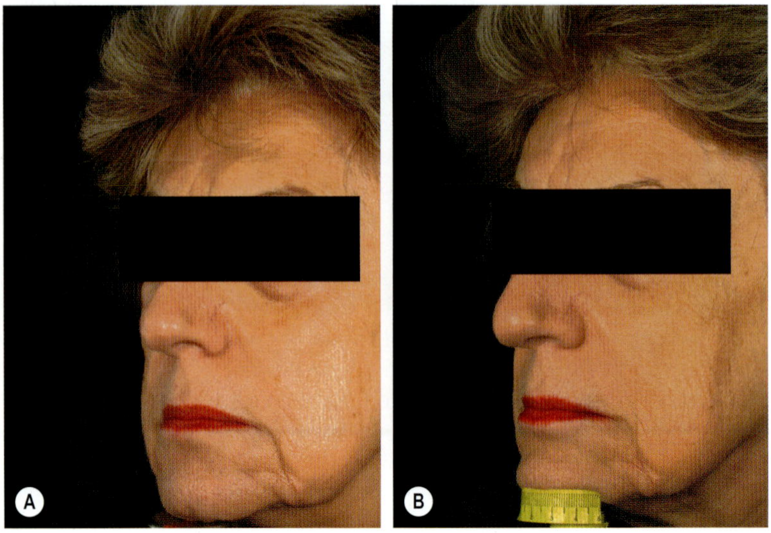

Fig. 7.7 Pre- and post- two treatments of Titan™ - 38-41J: 200 shots each session.

REFERENCES

1 Kirsch KM, Zelickson BD, Zachary CB, et al. *Ultrastructure of collagen thermally denatured by microsecond domain pulsed CO_2 laser. Paper presented at the 17th Annual Meeting of the American Society of Lasers in Medicine and Surgery, Phoenix*; April 1997.
2 Fitzpatrick RE, Rostan EF, Marchell N. Collagen tighetening induced by carbon dioxide laser versus erbium:YAG laser. *Lasers Surg Med*. 2000;27(5):395–403.
3 Ross VE, McKinlay JR, Anderson RR. Why does carbon dioxide resurfacing work? *A review, Arch Dermatol*. 1999;135(4):444–454.
4 *American Society for Aesthetic Plastic Surgery. Cosmetic Plastic Surgery National Data Bank Statistics*. http://www.surgery.org/download/2005stats.pdf.
5 Grekin RC, Tope WD, Yarborough Jr JM, et al. Electrosurgical facial resurfacing: a prospective multicenter study of efficacy and safety. *Arch Dermatol*. 2000;136(11):1309–1316.
6 Schmults CD, Phelps R, Goldberg DJ. Nonablative facial remodeling. *Arch Dermatol*. 2004;140:1373–1376.
7 Lennox FG. Shrinkage of collagen. *Biochim Biophys Acta*. 1949;3:170–187.
8 Narins RS, Tope WD, Pope K, Ross EV. Effects associated with a radiofrequency tissue tightening device: rare, preventable, and correctable with subcision and autologous fat transfer. *Dermatol Surg*. 2006;32:115–124.
9 Zelickson B, Ross V, Kist D, Counters J, Davenport S, Spooner G. Ultrastructural effect of an infrared handpiece on forehead and abdominal skin. *Dermatol Surg*. 2006;32:897–901.
10 Zelickson BD, Kist D, Bernstein E, et al. Histological and ultrastructural evaluation of the effects of a radiofrequency-based nonablative dermal remodeling device. *Arch Dermatol*. 2004;140:204–209.
11 Ruiz-Esparza J. Noninvasive skin tightening induced by radiofrequency and infrared light devices. In: Goldman MP, ed. *Cutaneous and Cosmetic Laser Surgery*. Elsevier; 2006.
12 Dierickx C. The role of deep heating for noninvasive skin rejuvenation. *Lasers Surg Med*. 2006;38:799–807.
13 Taub AF, Battle Jr EF, Nikolaidis G. Multicenter clinical perspectives on a broadband infrared light device for skin tightening. *J Drugs Dermatol*. 2006;5:771–778.
14 Battle Jr EF, Fincher EF, Moy RL, Nikolaidis G, Taub AF. Multicenter clinical perspectives on Titan. *Journal of Drus Dermatology*. 2006;5:771–778.

Radiofrequency technology

Reynaldo M Javate, Nikolaos Trakos, Raul T Cruz Jr

INTRODUCTION

Redundant facial, neck or body laxity is a major feature of aging. Just a few years ago, the only choice for the treatment of skin laxity was surgery or ablative lasers. As previously discussed in this chapter, technology continues to evolve, and procedures that once required major surgical intervention are gradually being replaced by minimally invasive treatments. Recently, monopolar radiofrequency (MRF), bipolar radiofrequency (BRF) and infrared light sources have been introduced for non-ablative tissue tightening by volumetric heating of the deep dermis.

RF energy is different from optical energy because it depends on the electrical properties of the skin, rather than on the levels of pigmentation, for the selective thermal destruction of targeted areas, which is known as electrothermolysis. Systems using RF current alone have achieved good results for skin resurfacing, with comparable efficacy to laser resurfacing and potentially more rapid healing.

Two typical configurations of electrodes are used in RF devices: the unipolar and the bipolar. In a unipolar system, electric energy is emitted through the metallic tip of the electrode and transmitted to the target tissue in a depth, which can be estimated as half the electrode size (Fig. 7.8). In the face, therefore, a 5 or 10 mm tip can be used with a penetration depth of 2.5 mm. In a bipolar system, the penetration depth is estimated as half the distance between electrodes (Fig. 7.9). Although they differ in the way the RF current is controlled and directed at the target tissue, there is no difference in the final tissue effect at the same RF. The bipolar handpiece creates local, superficial dermal heating on delicate areas, such as the face. The unipolar and larger handpieces provide deep dermal and subdermal heating of larger areas.

MONOPOLAR SYSTEMS

Monopolar systems deliver energy through one electrode. A relatively small contact point is applied to the treatment area, while a larger ground electrode is placed on the body in a location far from the active electrode. A cylindrical electrode is applied to the skin surface, concentrating the electrical

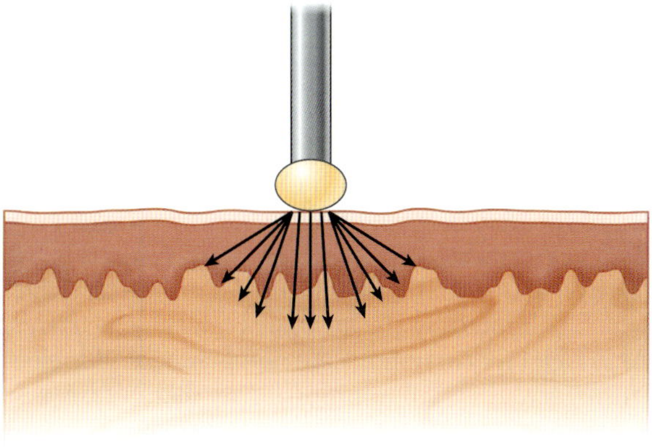

Fig. 7.8 Schematic representation of a unipolar system.

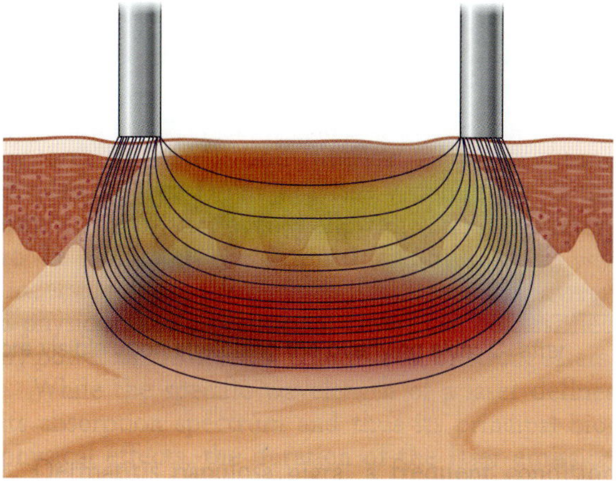

Fig. 7.9 Schematic representation of a bipolar system.

energy near the tip of the electrode, decreasing rapidly with distance. The depth of penetration is approximately half the electrode size. For example, the penetration depth of a 10 mm electrode is about 5 mm, which is deep enough to reach muscles. Monopolar systems are popular in electrosurgery where a small electrode is used because it is able to create a high power density on the surface of the electrode. The primary disadvantage of a monopolar system is that its behavior as the current passes through the body to the grounding electrode is unpredictable. Monopolar systems commonly used in aesthetic medicine include Visage®, Thermacool® (Thermage), Radiage® (now renamed Pellevè™) (Ellman Int. Inc.) (Table 7.4), and others previously described.

Radiofrequency serves as the primary principle employed in the Ellman Dual RF Surgitron Unit[1] and Ellman Surgitron Dual RF S5 device (Fig. 7.10) (Ellman International Inc, New York), used in the procedure Radiage (now renamed Pellevè™) which has been utilized in oculofacial plastic surgery to date.[2] One of the authors (RMJ), had conducted studies on Radiage which was one of the studies submitted to the Food and Drug Administration (FDA) and had given lectures worldwide on the topic Nonablative 4 MHz Dual Radiofrequency Treatment for Periorbital Rhytides and Midface Laxity. Last May 18, 2009, the FDA had granted clearance to Pellevè™, for the non-ablative treatment of mild to moderate facial wrinkles and rhytides for skin phototypes I–IV.

The latest monopolar application, currently in the final 544 Investigational Protocol of the US Food and Drug Administration (FDA) process, is able to penetrate to a depth of 100 mm. This device, the

Table 7.4 A brief comparison between two non-ablative RF technologies

Thermage system	Ellman (Pellevè™) system
1. Very high 6 MHz RF with high leakage current	1. Optimum 4 MHz RF with low leakage current
2. External cryo cooling of skin surface	2. Monoclysmic thermal gels for external cooling
3. Capacitive coupling of RF to skin	3. Patented capacitive coupling for RF energy device
4. Non-standard special electrode with essentially flat broad area contact surface	4. Ball or spherical proprietary composition alloy electrode to provide a uniform electric field and optimum transfer of non-ablative energy
5. Deeply penetrating RF heating	5. Primarily surface RF heating and energy transfer to optimally re-orient charged particles
6. High-power RF for deep penetration	6. Low power RF is sufficient
7. Minimizes skin burning by cryocooling	7. Minimizes skin burning by low power, constant electrode movement and efficient energy transfer
8. Copper/steel electrodes	8. Highly conductive proprietary composition alloy electrodes for inherent electrode cooling effect

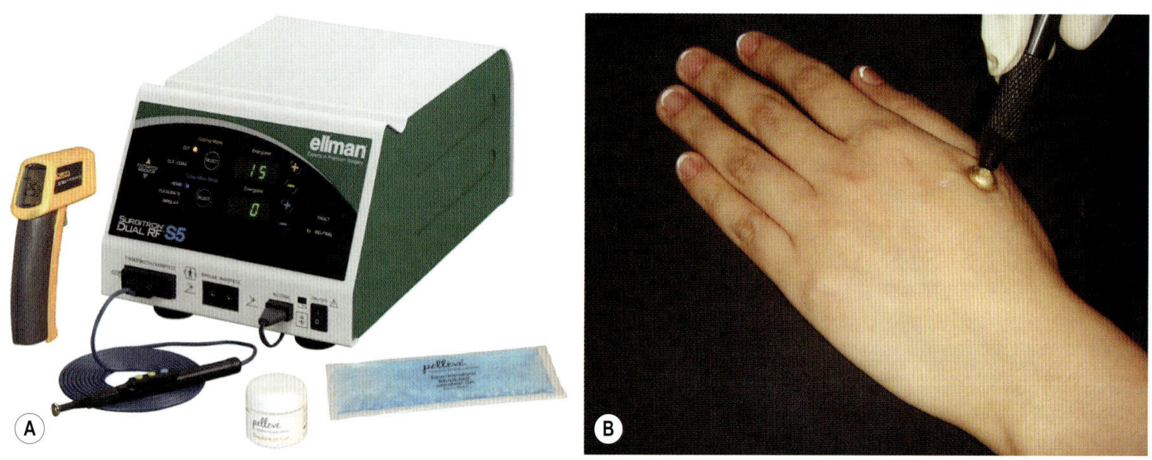

Fig. 7.10 A, Ellman Surgitron Dual RF S5 device, Wrinkle Treatment Handpiece and RF Cool Gel. **B,** A 10 mm Wrinkle Treatment Handpiece is moved in a circular motion on top of the hand of the patient.

Lipotron® (RevecoMED International, Anaheim, CA), unlike its predecessors, will be used not only for wrinkle reduction, rejuvenation of the face, and cellulite smoothing, but also for body contouring. The most significant feature of the Lipotron® (Fig. 7.11), with its depth of heat penetration, is that it affects the visceral fat as well as the subcutaneous fat. It operates at 0.5 MHz and feels like a warm massage to the patient.

BIPOLAR SYSTEMS

Bipolar systems pass an electrical current between two electrodes separated by a fixed distance. Both electrodes are applied to the treated area, and electrical current flows only in the area between the electrodes. The penetration depth of the electric current is approximately half the distance between the electrodes. The primary advantage of bipolar systems is the controlled distribution of RF current inside the tissue, which is limited by the area between the electrodes. Although bipolar systems are not as suitable for electrosurgery, they are appropriate for hemostasis and controlled vessel contraction using an intravascular catheter. There are certain bipolar devices used in aesthetic medicine that combine the action of infrared diode laser and RFs (Polaris™) and the action of

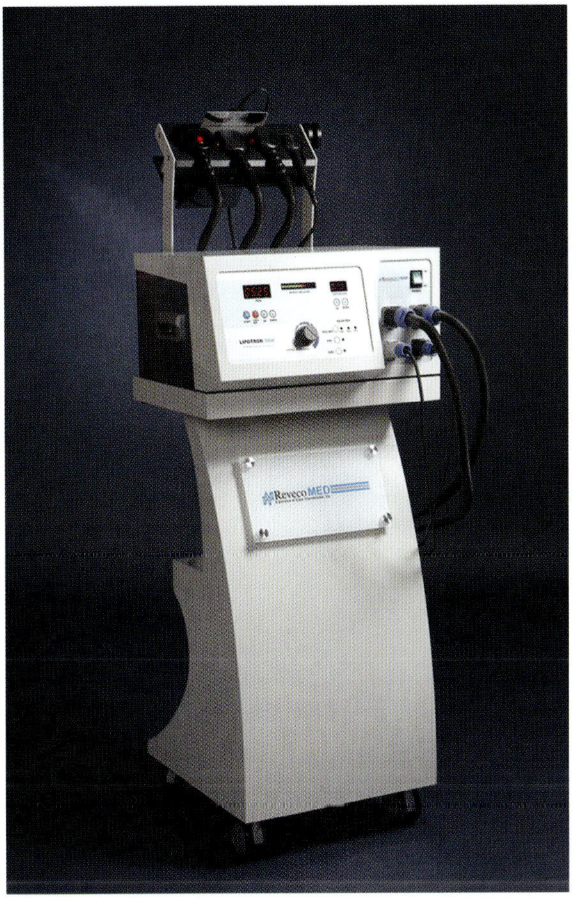

Fig. 7.11 Lipotronic device.

pulsed light and RFs (Aurora™). Both (Syneron Medical Ltd, Yokneam, Israel) use the BRF system. Polaris™ combines RF with infrared energy of 900 nm diode laser and Aurora™ combines RF with pulsed light in order to have a synergistic effect, although it has not yet been confirmed. Both of them can treat wrinkles and vascular lesions. Neither of these devices should be used on the eyelids within the orbital rim in contrast to RF devices, which can be used.

Aluma™ (Lumenis Inc., Santa Clara, CA) combines RF and vacuum suction. Another FDA-approved RF device for treating wrinkles and rhytids is the Accent XL® (Alma Lasers, Caesarea, Israel). It combines two RF modes into a single device. Each proprietary mode – bipolar and unipolar – is delivered by a discrete handpiece to distribute therapeutic heat at different tissue depths within the body. Refirme™ will be further discussed later in this chapter as one example of a bipolar system.

The result of the RF procedure is eyebrow lift, reduction in static wrinkles of the periorbital area and face, softening of nasolabial folds, improvement of jowls and neck skin laxity, and face contour renewal.

MECHANISM OF ACTION

Incision, excision, ablation or coagulation of the targeted tissue is achieved by RF surgery, which traditionally utilizes a wave of electrons to cause heating of tissues. In particular, in aesthetic rejuvenation, RF creates an electrical field, which is alternated rapidly from positive to negative, causing molecules that are charged to move within this field. Resistance to this movement or rotation creates heat. Heat is described by Joule's law:

$$H = j^2/s$$

where j is the density of electrical current and s is the electrical conductivity. The value opposite to conductivity is named resistance or impedance.

Bone has higher impedance and, therefore, electrical current does not penetrate bone. Dry skin and subcutaneous fat tissue have high impedance, and for this reason dry skin must be hydrated to allow passage of electrical current into the underlying tissues.

The thermal effect is determined by the formula:

$$(J) = I^2 \times R \times T$$

where I is the current, R is the impedance of tissue and T is the time of application. Immediate heat-induced changes in collagen structure and long-term dermal collagen remodeling are believed to induce tissue tightening.

Specifically, a certain threshold of heating creates a breakage of intramolecular bonds in the collagen fibrils. In this way, collagen fibrils change shape from a crystalline triple helical structure to a coil structure, becoming shorter,[3] as explained in the infrared section.

The amount of collagen contraction is determined by time and temperature. Low temperatures are desired to avoid pain and burns, but enough heat is required to achieve this controlled collagen denaturation. No single shrinkage temperature exists. According to histopathologic findings, the heating of the dermis at a level of 2–3 mm beneath the surface results in a tissue temperature of 55–70°C. The shrinkage temperature of collagen is believed to be 57–61°C.[4] At these temperatures controlled

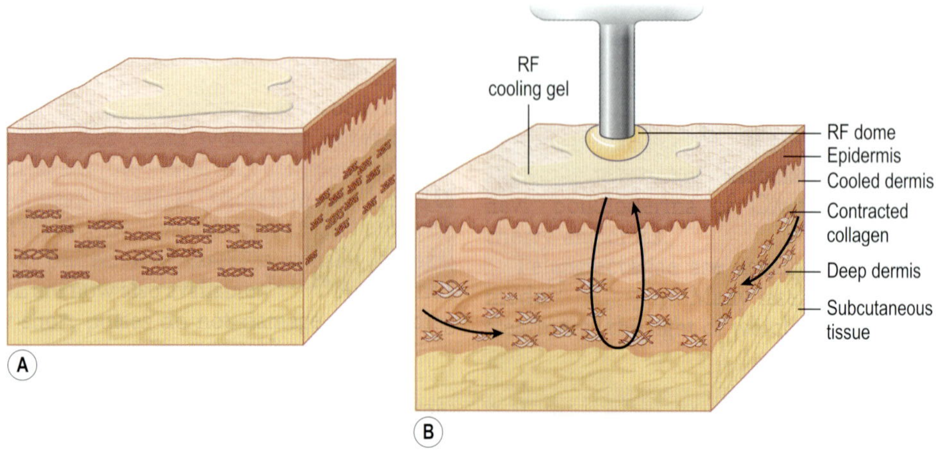

Fig. 7.12 *A*, Schematic diagram demonstrating the heat shrinkage of collagen from a structured triple helix to a random-coil structure. *B*, Schematic diagram demonstrating the heat shrinkage of collagen from a structured triple helix to a random-coil structure during RF application.

denaturation of a small amount of collagen can be achieved, resulting in modification of dermal collagen and shortening of the fibrous septae extending from the dermis into subcutaneous tissue (Fig. 7.12).[5]

This tightening is more efficient if the energy is delivered to special anchoring points, which vary from patient to patient. Their selection is based on the fact that there are vectors pulling the tissues of the face up according to the collagen's contraction. These vectors are based on the insertion points of the superficial musculoaponeurotic system (SMAS).[6] For example, the anchoring point for smoothing nasolabial folds is in the preauricular area.

According to studies, it seems that this heat acts only in collagen in dermis and does not destabilize hyaluronic acid in the matrix and probably does not alter enzymes at the neuromuscular synapses, which are under the subcutaneous tissue; therefore RF can be used in patients who have had hyaluronic acid fillers and botulinum toxin treatment.[7,8]

Initial protocols using single-pass high-energy settings were associated with higher incidences of side effects such as erythema, edema, blistering and subcutaneous fat necrosis. Now the concept is that we use pain as an indicator, marking the highest amount of energy that should be avoided in all cases. Multiple treatments also tend to give better results than a single treatment.[6,9]

Multiple passes with low-energy settings are preferred, which is probably safer, more tolerable and efficacious than a single pass with high-energy settings. Zelickson et al. observed that a greater number of low-energy pulses produced acute morphologic changes similar to those produced by a single higher-energy pulse.[9] The usual energy levels range from 79 to 100 J/cm^2 in ThermaCool® and from power setting 12–40, Cut mode, in Radiage® (now renamed Pellevè™), depending on the area of the face and tolerance of the patient. Finally, another level of action of RF is fat lysis. In particular, by concentrating the heat in deeper level with stacking pulses, unwanted fat in the submental area can be reduced, which can paradoxically work in an opposite direction if you remove fat from wrong places.[10]

INDICATIONS AND CONTRAINDICATIONS

The best candidates for skin tightening treatment are patients aged 35–60 years, having mild-to-moderate skin laxity.

Ideally, non-smokers should have relatively good skin tone, modest photodamage and average amounts of subcutaneous fat present. Previous use of fillers is not a contraindication.

Good candidates are those with fine lines or wrinkles on the face who desire a subtle and natural improvement in their appearance and skin tone, with minimal down time and minimal risk.

On the other hand, patients who have orbital fat prolapse and generalized excessive skin laxity and those having unrealistic expectations or seeking impressive results are not considered good candidates.

Absolute contraindications for this procedure are pacemakers and defibrillating devices in the patient. It is not wise to treat patients with a tendency to hypertrophy scarring or koebnerizing dermatoses, or while on Isotretinoin (Accutane) treatment, or within a year of such treatment.

PREPARATION AND RF SKIN-TIGHTENING TECHNIQUE

Photographs and baseline wrinkle evaluation using the Fitzpatrick Wrinkle Classification System (FWCS) (Table 7.5) should be obtained. Patients should have realistic expectations because the results tend to be subtle and gradual and may not even be noticed by the patients themselves. Dramatic improvement is rare but can be seen even after one treatment session. Immediate results can be seen, depending on technique and perhaps many other, as yet unidentified, factors. If patients have realistic expectations and adequate photographs are secured, the index of patient satisfaction is much better. The degree of clinical improvement on treatment efficacy of treated areas such as glabellar, forehead and lower eyelid wrinkles, crow's feet, nasolabial folds, and midface laxity can be assessed using the FWCS on pre- and postapplication photographs.

Remove any cosmetic agents or other facial emulsions on the skin. Make-up or oily material changes the impedance of the skin surface.

The first step in using the Ellman Surgitron Dual RF S5 device is to place the return electrode/antenna plate on the back of the patient's head. Later the skin should be covered with Ellman RF cool gel.[11] This lowers the skin temperature by 7–8°C. The purpose is to protect and prevent overheating of the epidermis and at the same time deliver the RF energy to the warmer deep dermis to allow thermal changes. For practicing the control of the foot pedal, we should use a 10 mm Wrinkle Treatment Handpiece connected to an Ellman Surgitron Dual RF S5 device with the power level set at 2 (Cut mode). The depth of the heating is dependent on the treatment settings. The settings for energy delivery, the treatment dome tip size and the impedance of the skin tissue all impact the treated area. Neither topical anesthesia nor sedative are given pretreatment.

Before delivering an Ellman RF skin-tightening treatment, a test touching of the RF is done on the back of the patient's hand. This is done to determine the average power setting for commencing the RF treatment and is based on the patient's impedance and resistance. Every patient's threshold is different, and this is a very good method to determine the base power setting. Move the energized dome tip in an oval motion over the top of the hand, applying slight pressure on the tip.

The intensity of the treatment is controlled by the patient; it should be of bearable warmth, and there should be no uncomfortable hot feeling. The sensation should be what the patient can tolerate comfortably. Settings may vary due to the skin location and the skin thickness. Patients should be informed that for maximum benefit the sensation should feel as though the skin were heating to the brink of pain, but be tolerable, and then subside. Areas of thin skin against bone such as the temple, malar, mastoid and mandibular areas are more sensitive and require less energy.

When using the machine on a patient's face the authors recommend starting with the cheek area.

The device is set at a range of power setting of 12–40 (Cut mode) and adjusted to the maximum level of tolerance.

When treating the eyelid and forehead areas, the authors turn the power down to a lower setting and use fast, quick movements, as this area is less fleshy and the skin heats up more quickly.

Table 7.5 The Fitzpatrick wrinkle classification system

Class	Wrinkling	Score	Degrees of elastosis
I	Fine wrinkles	1–3	Mild (fine textural changes with subtly accentuated skin lines)
II	Fine to moderate depth wrinkles	4–6	Moderate (distinct popular elastosis [individual papules with yellow translucency under direct lighting] and dyschromia)
III	Fine to deep wrinkles with or without redundant skin folds	7–9	Severe (multipapular and confluent elastosis [thickened yellow and pallid] approaching or consistent with cutis rhomboidalis)

Cheek and neck flaccidity, when improved, gives the general aspect of rejuvenation (Figs 7.13 and 7.14). Treatment of the cheek starts at the preauricular area, crossing below the malar eminence and stopping at the nasolabial folds. The jawline includes the areas stretching from the posterior angle of the mandible along the jowls to the lateral chin.

The upper neck treatment includes the area from the inferior border of the mandible down to the level of the thyroid cartilage. The midline submental soft-tissue region is also included (Fig. 7.15). The most important thing to remember is not to take the electrode off the skin when your foot is activating the pedal, as it causes a shock to the patient.

After the RF tightening treatment, a cold pack or an ice roller can be used over the treated skin area to lock the unraveled collagen into position.

OPTIMIZING OUTCOMES

- Areas of thin skin against bone such as temples, malar, mastoid and mandibular areas are more sensitive and require us to use less energy.
- After the procedure, the physician must ask if there are areas of lingering burning sensation.
- The patient is asked to apply ice cubes wrapped in gauze directly against the area that burns until the burning sensation has disappeared. This may avoid a real burn.

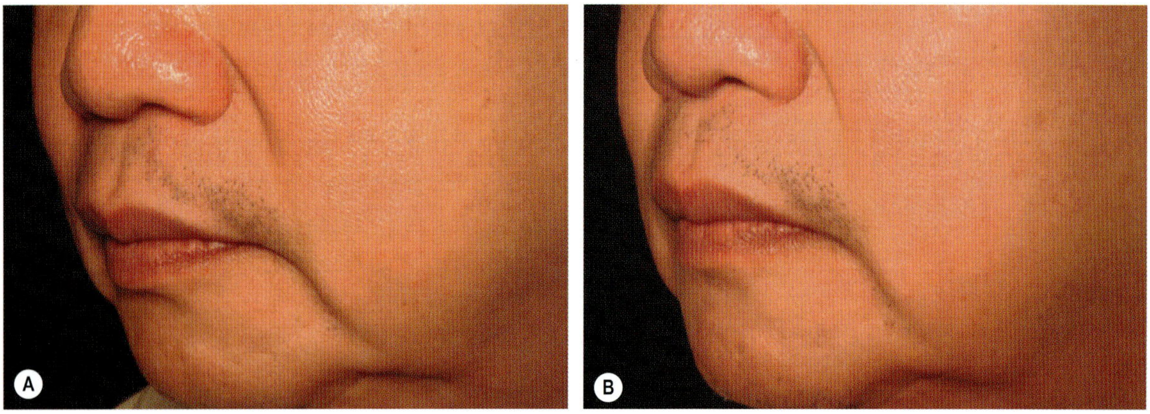

Fig. 7.13 *A*, Pretreatment. Cheek laxity. *B*, After two treatment sessions showing nasolabial fold diminished in depth and improvements in oral commissures and marionette lines.

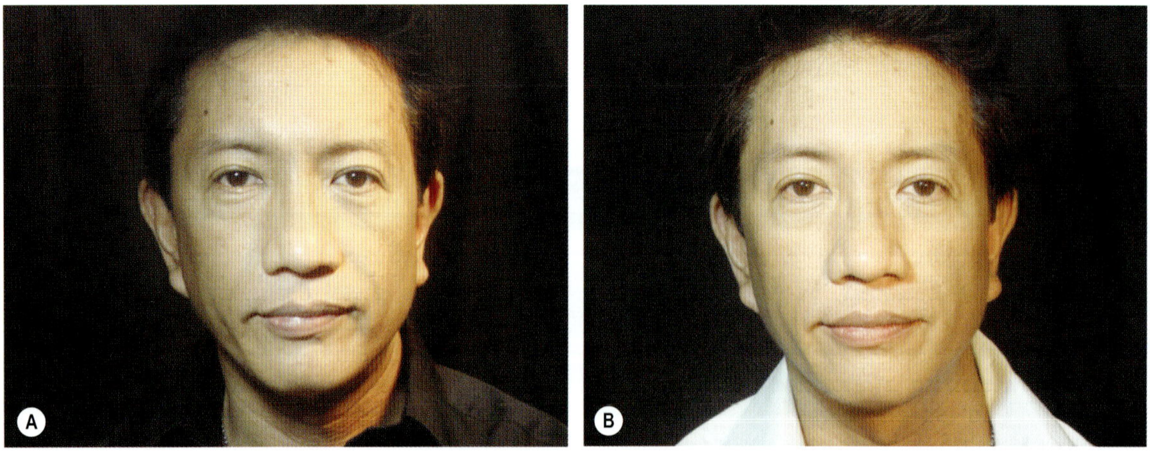

Fig. 7.14 *A*, Pretreatment frontal view of the patient. *B*, 6 months post-treatment of the patient showing tissue tightening of the cheeks, with improvement in the nasolabial fold, cheek contour, marionette lines and the jaw line.

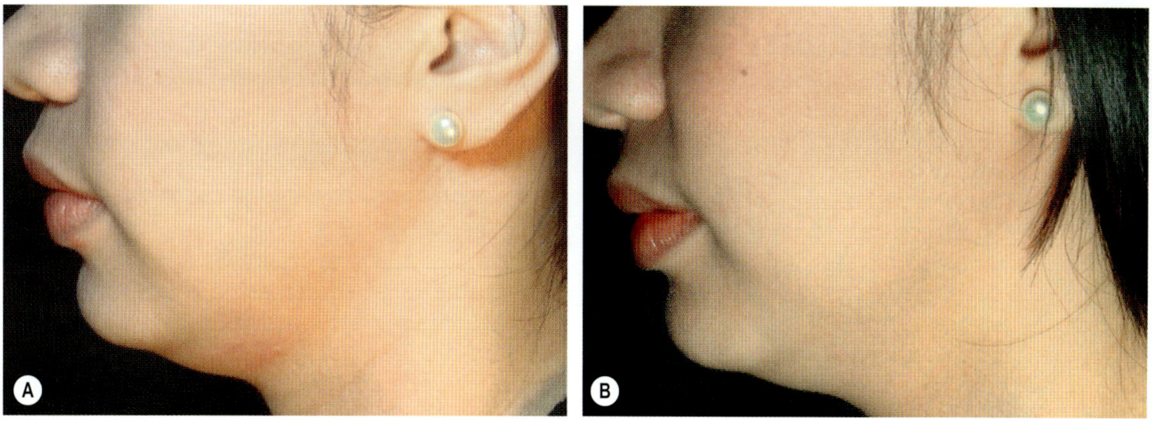

Fig. 7.15 *A*, Pretreatment. *B*, After three treatment sessions of the neck to the submental area showing decrease in submental fullness.

- The skin should be inspected for areas of redness, dusky gray color, pale wheal-like papules or red squares.
- Areas of dusky gray color almost always progress inexorably to a second-degree superficial burn. They are uncommon.
- Contraction of elastin will occur after 7–10 days, and newly produced collagen resumes in a steady way. New application can be made after 1 week.

COMPLICATIONS AND SIDE EFFECTS

The most commonly noted adverse reactions were transient erythema lasting for a few hours to a day, tolerable pain during the procedure described as a warm sensation and mild edema lasting for 1–2 days. Lower settings and multiple passes are advised to reduce the risk of adverse events such as severe pain, blistering, burns, bruising and scarring, and late side effects such as cutaneous depressions, which can occur weeks or months post RF application as a result of overheating of adipose tissue and fibrous septae. Mild depressions resolved spontaneously; however, severe contour irregularities and scarring may be improved with subcision, autologous fat transfer or cosmetic fillers.[12] Fortunately, there were no scarring, burns, bruising or dysesthesia noted in any of our patients.

POSTOPERATIVE CARE

Apply a bland moisturizer, and no other postoperative care is required.

REFERENCES

1 Garito J. *Inventor; Dual RF Radiowave Device*. Assigned to Ellman International Inc; 2008 US Patent 5,954,686, 21 September 1999.
2 Bosniak SL, Javate RM, Aquino MS, et al. Radiosurgery: a new approach to eyelid, orbital, and lacrimal surgery. *Int J Aesthetic Restorative Surg*. 1995;3:9–15.
3 Ross VE, McKinlay JR, Anderson RR. Why does carbon dioxide resurfacing work? A review. *Arch Dermatol*. 1999;135(4):444–454.
4 Zelickson BD, Kist D, Bernstein E, et al. Histological and ultrastructural evaluation of the effects of a radiofrequency-based nonablative dermal remodeling device: a pilot study. *Arch Dermatol*. 2004;140(2):204–209.
5 Biesman BS, Baker SS, Carruthers J, Silva HL, Holloman EL. Monopolar radiofrequency treatment of human eyelids: a prospective, multicenter, efficacy trial. *Lasers Surg Med*. 2006;38(10):890–898.
6 Alam M, Levy R, Pajvani U, et al. Safety of radiofrequency treatment over human skin previously injected with medium-term injectable soft-tissue augmentation materials: a controlled pilot trial. *Lasers Surg Med*. 2006;38(3):205–210.
7 Semchyshyn NL, Kilmer SL. Does laser inactivate botulinum toxin? *Dermatol Surg*. 2005;31(4):399–404.
8 Fritz M, Counters JT, Zelickson BD. Radiofrequency treatment for middle and lower face laxity. *Arch Facial Plastic Surg*. 2004;6:370–373.
9 Finzi E, Spangler A. Multipass vector (mpave) technique with nonablative radiofrequency to treat facial and neck laxity. *Dermatol Surg*. 2005;31:916–922.
10 Dawson E, Willey A, Lee M. Adverse events associated with nonablative cutaneous laser, radiofrequency, and light-based devices. *Semin Cutan Med Surg*. 2007;26:15–21.
11 Garito J. *Inventor; Non-Ablative Skin Tightening RF Electrode And Procedure*. Assigned to Ellman International; 2008 US Patent 11/709,692, 23 February 2007.
12 Narins RS, Tope WD, Pope K, et al. Overtreatment effects associated with a radiofrequency tissue-tightening DEVICE: Rare, preventable, and correctable with subcision and autologous fat transfer. *Dermatol Surg*. 2006;32:115–124.

Bipolar radiofrequency

Neil S Sadick

The ReFirme™ ST Applicator (Syneron Medical Ltd., Yokneam, Israel) is a combination of broadband IR (700–2000 nm) and bipolar RF energies. The author uses the ReFirme to non-ablatively improve both skin laxity and rhytids. The RF energy provides deep tissue heating, whereas IR energy heats the dermal ground substance because it is absorbed by water and possibly by collagen as well. This combination of optical and RF energy is an example of electro-optical synergy (ELOS), which is believed to permit the use of lower levels of both types of energy, thus lowering the risk of adverse effects.[1,2] To optimize outcomes, patients usually require three to five treatment sessions 4–6 weeks apart. Erythema and edema during and after the treatment are transitory and usually do not require treatment. Slight lifting of the lax areas should be evident at the final treatment.

PRETREATMENT CARE

- Avoid skin irritation and intentional tanning.
- Use sunscreen when exposed to the sun.
- Discontinue irritant topical agents for 2–3 days (before treatment visit).
- Arrive at the physician's office with cleaned skin.
- Remove all lotion, make-up, perfume, powder and bath/shower oil from areas to be treated.
- Avoid topical anesthetics unless directed by a physician.
- Inform the treating clinician of dental crowns, caps, braces or other metal implants.

TREATMENT PROCEDURE

The recommended treatment parameters are shown in Table 7.6. Settings are guidelines and should be adjusted according to individual responses to test spots. Topical anesthesia is not required.

1. Obtain a photograph of each side of the face before treatment.
2. Ask the patient to sit up for treatment.
3. Apply conductive gel to the treatment area.
4. Place applicator perpendicular to the skin using full contact and slight pressure.
5. Treat one side of the face (or any area of loose skin) to use as a reference endpoint during subsequent passes.
6. For the first pass, cover the complete area with 30–50% overlap. Do not use the autorepeat mode on bony, thin or delicate areas of skin.
7. Make consecutive passes with 30–50% overlap on vector zones of 20–30 pulses each. One side of the face typically requires approximately 400 pulses. Make passes until you see sustained tightening and edema. Erythema is often present at this endpoint as well.
8. If patient voices discomfort or the skin responds excessively to treatment, reduce the energy level and, if necessary, change the cooling level to the strong setting. Use patient tolerance as a guide.
9. Do not stack pulses, lest a blister develop.
10. Treat the other side of the face with 400 pulses. The total number of pulses for the entire face should be approximately 800.

POSTREATMENT CARE

After treatment with the ReFirme, patients should:

- apply sun block (SPF 30 or higher) to the treated area and avoid intentional suntanning for several days
- apply cold compresses to the treated area to reduce swelling and redness, and apply hydrocortisone or antibiotic ointment if prescribed by the physician
- wash the treated area gently for 3 days without harsh or abrasive products
- avoid hot baths, saunas or exposure of treated area to excess heat for 3 days
- cleanse and pat dry areas with superficial crusts or scabs; do not rub, scratch or remove scabs
- call the physician at the first sign of a blister; apply antibiotic ointment if prescribed.

Table 7.6 Radiofrequency treatment parameters for ReFirme applicator				
Skin type	**Tx area**	**RF energy (J/cm^3)**	**Cooling**	**Number of passes/Tx area**
I–VI	Lower face, under chin	100–120	Normal*	4–7
I–VI	Forehead, bony areas	90–120	Normal*/strong†	2–5

*Equivalent to 10°C.
†Equivalent to 5°C.
RF, radiofrequency; Tx, treatment.

CONCLUSION

The combination of broadband IR (700–2000 nm) and bipolar RF energies has been shown in the author's practice to be a safe and effective modality for the treatment of skin laxity.

REFERENCES

1 Yu CS, Yeung CK, Shek SY, Tse RK, Kono T, Chan HH. Combined infrared light and bipolar radiofrequency for skin tightening in Asians. *Lasers Surg Med*. Jul 2007;39(6):471–475.

2 Gold MH, Goldman MP, Rao J, Carcamo AS, Ehrlich M. Treatment of wrinkles and elastosis using vacuum-assisted bipolar radiofrequency heating of the dermis. *Dermatol Surg*. 2007;33 (3):300–309.

8 Botulinum Toxin for Oculofacial Aesthetic Rejuvenation

Doris M Hexsel, Luitgard Wiest, Mariana Soirefmann

Included on ***DVD***

SUMMARY

Botulinum toxin (BTx) is one of the most revolutionary treatments in facial aesthetics and rejuvenation. The cosmetic use of BTx in the upper third of the face began in the late 1980s and gradually advanced to applications in the mid and lower face, neck and other areas of the body. Its use has permitted a better understanding of the physiopathological process of aging, specifically the role of the muscles. Nowadays, more accurate techniques and the adjunctive use of BTx allow physicians to make more precise applications and achieve better, natural-looking results. Every year, new perspectives on the clinical and cosmetic uses of BTx show the utility and versatility of this therapeutic modality in dermatology and other specialized areas of medicine.

INTRODUCTION

Nowadays, the value of image plays an important role in our society. Since the development of numerous minimally invasive procedures for facial beauty and rejuvenation, it has become easy and safe for patients to improve their appearance. New and less invasive techniques for facial rejuvenation give quick results, with a low incidence of side effects and minimal downtime, as patients can return immediately to their normal daily activities.

Facial wrinkles are caused by several factors, including aging (intrinsic and photoaging), gravity, positional pressure (sleep lines) and facial expressions.[1,2] Repeated muscular contractions involved in facial expression are one of the most important etiologic factors causing facial lines and rhytides, particularly in the upper third of the face. Glabellar, frontal and periorbital are the main areas involved in facial expression. Moreover, these muscular contractions may also contribute to the development of redundancies of the skin over these hyperkinetic muscles and lines. Some dynamic wrinkles that are initially caused by muscular movements become static with the addition of other factors such as chronic solar exposure and the development of cutaneous flaccidity.[3]

Glabellar folds are usually interpreted as suggesting negative feelings, such as sadness, anger[4] and frustration.[5] Although small-to-moderate furrows may be interpreted positively for men, as indicating the ability to concentrate, leadership and even sensitivity, large furrows are more often perceived negatively.[6]

In an attempt to diminish the undesirable expressive rhytides of the face, BTx has been widely used to produce precise and reversible weakness of the hyperfunctional mimetic muscles of facial expression.[7] It is therefore currently considered the best alternative for the treatment of dynamic wrinkles,[8] alone or in combination with other minimally invasive or invasive techniques.[9–11]

BTx injections are of special benefit for patients between 30 and 50 years of age, since the etiology of facial lines in this group is more related to the underlying muscles than to other factors.[1] The treatment of facial expression lines not only represents a matter of aesthetics and vanity, but also leads to improvement of self-esteem.[12]

The medical literature of the cosmetic use of BTx is currently dominated by open-label reports, uncontrolled studies and personal experience reviews. A few double-blind, placebo-controlled studies have been published, some of them in the glabellar area.[5,13–16] In the lateral periorbital area, BTx injections can be safely performed when strict attention is given to the reconstituted BTx pharmacology and to the anatomy of the periorbital muscles, although it is considered an off-label procedure.[17]

HISTORY OF THE COSMETIC USE OF BOTULINUM TOXINS

BTx is known as the substance with the highest specific potency of all natural or synthesized compounds. It is produced by an anaerobic, Gram-positive, rod-shaped organism, *Clostridium botulinum*.

BTx became famous as the cause of botulism and as a biological weapon. Botulism is well known in historical accounts, and has probably been known since the beginning of the human race. In medieval times, it was known in Europe that production of sausages bore a high risk of food poisoning from BTx, so strict guild regulations were imposed on sausage production.

In 1822, Justinus Kerner, a physician in the state of Württemberg in South Germany, provided one of the earliest detailed descriptions of the clinical picture of botulism. He was also the first to speculate on a possible therapeutic use of BTx in conditions like Huntington's chorea.[18] In 1895, Emile Pierre Marie van Emergen identified botulinum neurotoxin as the cause of a botulism outbreak amongst musicians in the Belgian village of Ellezelles. In 1919, the isolation of different BTx types, known as A (BTx-A) and B (BTx-B) was achieved. In 1920, Hermann Sommer of the Hooper Foundation at the University of California concentrated BTx into a relatively pure form. Research and study into the activity of botulinum neurotoxins was stimulated by the events of World War II. Edward Shantz, Carl Lamanna and their colleagues at Fort Detrick successfully isolated BTx-A for the US Army in 1946, and in 1949 Burgen discovered BTx's mechanism of action.

Medical use of BTx began in the 1950s with the work of Vernon Brooks. By the late 1960s, the inhibitory effects of BTx-A on acetylcholine release at the neuromuscular junction were shown in experimental animals. These studies were significantly advanced by ophthalmologist Alan Scott of the Smith-Kettlewell Institute of Visual Sciences in San Francisco in the 1970s. He used BTx-A for treatment of strabismus and blepharospasm. In 1977, the first treatment was attempted in humans.[19]

The batch of BTx-A developed by Schantz under the name of Oculinum in 1979 was approved for human use in 1989, and later acquired by Allergan Inc. Under the name of Botox® it has been used as the primary treatment for focal dystonias since the late 1980s.

In 1987, while treating patients for essential blepharospasm, Jean Carruthers, an ophthalmologist, noted that these patients had significant improvement of dynamic rhytids in the glabella region. Alastair Carruthers, a dermatologist, together with his wife, started systematic studies of BTx for cosmetic use, which were published in 1992, demonstrating the safe and effective use of BTx-A in the treatment of dynamic rhytids in the glabella[20] and bringing in the era of cosmetic use of BTx.

In 1993, Blitzer et al. described the use of BTx for wrinkles of the forehead.[21] Later researchers, such as Arnold Klein, Nicholas Lowe, Patricia Wexler, Richard Glogau and Steven Fagien, contributed publications of their experiences to the widespread use of BTx-A. Subsequently, new indications for cosmetic use such as crow's feet, and new areas as the perioral region and platysma were discovered.[22] Botox® Cosmetic (in other countries Vistabel® or Vistabex®) was approved by the FDA in 2002. Other BTx-A products have been launched into the market in other countries. The most important are Dysport® by Ipsen, Prosigne® by Lanzhou and Xeomin® by Merz.

At first, BTx-A used the principle of identical doses and injection sites for all patients, but in recent years cosmetic treatment with BTx has become much more differentiated and today a more individualized approach prevails, aiming at a global rejuvenation: the BTx 'face lift'. Frequent reports of potential novel uses of BTx-A in facial musculature indicate that we stand at the beginning of its use in aesthetic medicine.

CURRENTLY AVAILABLE BOTULINUM TOXINS

The toxin produced by *Clostridium botulinum* is isolated, purified and stabilized before it can be used as a drug. There are seven different types of BTx, which are known and designated by the letters A, B, C, D, E, F and G. The different BTx types differ slightly in the amino acid sequences of their neurotoxin and in their associated non-toxic proteins. All seven BTx-types share a similar molecular structure and have the same basic mechanism of action: they bind to the same glycoprotein structures and they all block the cholinergic synapse, preventing the release of acetylcholine at the neuromuscular junction of striated muscle fibers, creating a flaccid paralysis of the muscle. Differences in the intracellular protein target or target site cleaved by the light chain of each serotype lead to variations in duration of action and possibly other defects. Only the A and B toxins are available as drugs (Table 8.1).

BTx-B (Myobloc®, Solstice Neuroscience) is less potent than BTx-A in humans and requires approximately 50–150 times the dose of BTx-A to achieve similar results in dynamic rhytides. It appears to have a shorter duration of action than type A, as well as more autonomic side effects. Myobloc® comes in the form of a solution.

Table 8.1 Comparison of different BTx-A

	XEOMIN®	Botox®	Vistabel®	Dysport®/ Reloxin®	Dysport® Cosmetics®	Prosigne®	Neurobloc®/ Myobloc®
Company	Merz Pharmaceuticals	Allergan	Allergan	Ipsen/Medicis	Ipsen/ Medicis	Lanzhou Institute of Biological Products	Solstice Neuroscience
Type	Type A	Type A	Type A	Type A	Type A	Type A	Type B
Approvals	Europe Union, Mexico, Argentina, Brazil	In over 75 countries all over the world	In 16 countries, including the USA, Canada, Italy and France	Dysport: In over 35 countries	Germany, some other European countries and the USA	China, North Korea, Morocco, the Philippines, Indonesian, Brazil, Peru, Ecuador, Chile, Paraguay, Uruguay, Venezuela, Thailand and some others	Europe and the USA
Active substance	Botulinum neurotoxin type A (150 kD)	Botulinum toxin type A complex (900 kD)	Botulinum toxin type A complex (900 kD)	Botulinum toxin type A complex (900 kD)	Botulinum toxin type A complex (900 kD)	Botulinum toxin type A complex (150 kD)	Botulinum toxin type B complex
Comparison of strength of action	1	1:1	1:1	Approx. 1:2.5 to 1:3	Approx. 1:2.5 to 1:3	1:1	1:1000
Indications	Blepharospasm Cervical dystonia	Many indications, including blepharospasm and cervical dystonia	Glabellar lines	Many indications, including blepharospasm and cervical dystonia	Glabellar lines	Blepharospasm, strabismus, hemifacial spasm and other dystonias	Cervical dystonia only
Mode of action	SNAP 25	SNAP 25	SNAP 25	SNAP 25	SNAP 25	SNAP 25	VAMP
Pharmaceutical form	Powder for solution for injection	Powder for solution for injection	Powder for solution for injection	Powder for solution for injection	Powder for solution for injection	Powder for solution for injection	Solution
Units/vial	100	100	50	500	500	100	2500/5000/ 10 000
Volume	max. 8 ml	max. 10 ml	1.25 ml	max. 2.5 ml	max. 5 ml	max. 8 ml	0.5 ml/1 ml/ 2 ml, max. 3.5 ml

Continued

Table 8.1 Comparison of different BTx-A—cont'd

	XEOMIN®	**Botox®**	**Vistabel®**	**Dysport®/ Reloxin®**	**Dysport® Cosmetics®**	**Prosigne®**	**Neurobloc®/ Myobloc®**
Reconstitution	0.9% NaCl solution	0.9% NaCl solution	0.9% NaCl solution	0.9% NaCl solution	0.9% NaCl solution	0.9% NaCl solution	Prepared solution, dilutable
Storage	25°C	2–8°C or freezer −5°C	2–8°C <−5°C	2–8°C	2–8°C	2–8°C	2–8°C, do not freeze
Shelf-life (unopened)	36 months	36 months	36 months	24 months	24 months	36 months	24 months
Shelf-life reconstituted	24 hours	24 hours	24 hours	24 hours	24 hours	4 hours	24 months (closed)
Auxilliary substances	Albumin 1 mg, sucrose 4.7 mg	Albumin 0.5 mg, NaCl 0.9 mg	Albumin 0.5 mg, NaCl 0.9 mg	Albumin 0.125 mg, lactose 2.5 mg	Albumin 0.125 mg, lactose 2.5 mg	Gelatin 5 mg, dextran 25 mg and sacarosis 25 mg	Albumin, NaCl, succinat, octanolat, tryptophan
pH-Wert	5–7	5–7	5–7	5–7	5–7	5–7	5.6
Foreign protein load in dose-equivalence range	0.6 ng/100 U	5 ng/100 U	2.5 ng/ 50 U	5 ng/500 U	5 ng/500 U	4–5 ng/100 U	100 ng/ 10 000 U
Specific activity (MU per ng protein)	166 MU/ng	20 MU/ng	20 MU/ng	100 MU/ng	100 MU/ng	20–25 MU/ng	100 MU/ng

In aesthetic medicine, BTx-A has been used the most so far, although some trials have been undertaken utilizing BTx-B.[23]

MECHANISM OF ACTION

The activity of the different types of BTx is exerted through a multistep process which includes binding to nerve terminals, internalization and inhibition of neurotransmitter release.

The biologically active component is BTx neurotoxin, which consists of two polypeptide chains with molecular masses of 50 kDalton (kD) and 100 kD. These two polypeptide chains are linked together by a single disulfide bond. Thus, BTx neurotoxin is a complex and highly fragile macromolecule. Changes in pH or exposure to light or heat induce changes and finally destruction of the macromolecule, with loss of its biological activity. BTx neurotoxin is associated with various non-toxic proteins, some with hemagglutinating and some with non-hemagglutinating properties.

Clinically, BTx induces a blockade of the cholinergic innervation of the target tissue. When BTx is injected into muscle tissue, muscular paralysis results within 24–72 hours, reaching its maximum effect after 1–2 weeks. The degree of muscular paralysis can be controlled by the amount of BTx administered.

The mode of action of BTx is illustrated in Figure 8.1. BTx neurotoxin with its heavy chain binds to BTx acceptors on the presynaptic nerve membrane. This binding is rapid and irreversible. Subsequently, the light chain is transported into the nerve cytoplasm. The synaptic fusion complex is made up of a group of proteins known as the SNARE proteins (soluble N-ethylmaleimide-sensitive factor attachment protein receptors) that allow the preformed acetylcholine vesicles to dock and fuse to the membrane. This SNARE complex is the location of action for BTx. Inside the nerve ending, the light chains of BTx-A, C and E catalyze the cleavage of SNAP-25 (synaptosomal-associated protein), a 25 kDa protein of the SNARE complex. The different subtypes of BTx have unique areas on the nerve membrane to which they bind and

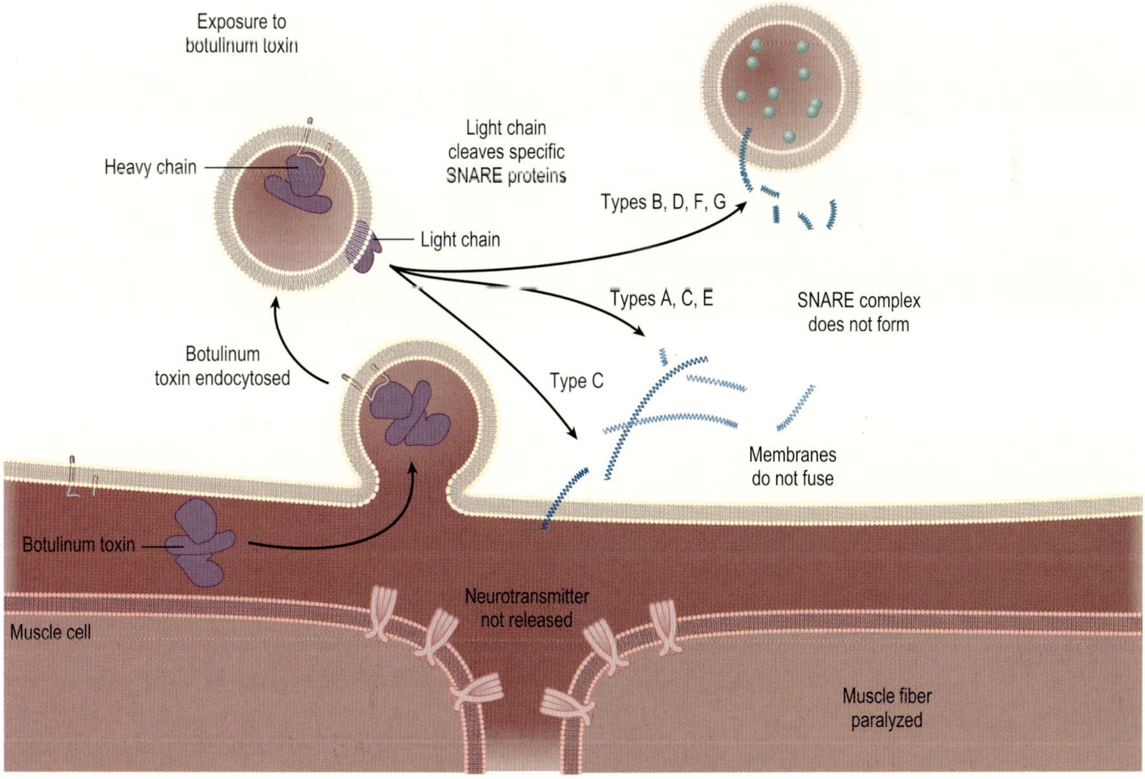

Fig 8.1 Mechanism of action of botulinum neurotoxins. Reproduced with permission from J Am Med Assoc 2001;285(8): 1059–70.

have different proteins within the presynaptic nerve terminal that they cleave. They all have the same mechanism of action: to act as a zinc-dependent endoproteinase and inhibit the release of acetylcholine at the peripheral neuromuscular junction.[24]

The action of BTx within the target tissue decreases over time as the affected axons start to sprout new nerve terminals within 28 days, which continually restore the impaired transmission. During this time the damaged synapse itself will regenerate its function.[25] After 3 months, reinnervation occurs normally and muscles return to their normal function 2–5 months after injection.

The dose of BTx is measured in units of biological activity in a standardized mouse model. One unit (U) of biologic activity is the amount required to kill 50% (lethal dose or LD50) of 18–20 g female Swiss-Webster mice when injected interperitoneally. The dosage units of the different products do not relate to each other. Apart from one clinical trial with methodological shortcomings[26] there are no comparative clinical studies for aesthetic indications. On the other hand, comparison of efficient doses of Botox®[4] and Dysport®[16] for cosmetic applications in the glabella in two controlled studies shows strong evidence of an equivalence of 2.5:1 U between the two products (Dysport® and Botox®). Comparing the studies cited above, the effects obtained with 20 U of Botox® in the treatment of the glabellar area[4] were similar to those obtained with 50 U of Dysport® in the treatment of the same area.[16] These support the clinical evidence that 1 U of Botox® is equivalent to 2.5 U of Dysport® for glabellar lines, giving similar results for efficacy, intensity and duration of paralysis. The manufacturers of Botox®, Dysport® and Xeomin® recommend the reconstitution of their products with 0.9% sterile preservative-free saline.

Since BTx-B is marketed as a solution, it does not have to be reconstituted.

INDICATIONS FOR OCULOFACIAL COSMETIC USE OF BTx-A

The major cosmetic indications for BTx-A use are located in the upper face. This chapter is focused on oculofacial cosmetic uses.

Glabellar Frown Lines

The use of BTx in the glabella can improve brow reposition and delay physiological ptosis of the eyelids and eyebrows, leading to a more jovial appearance and attractive look, retarding the indication of a blepharoplasty.[6,27,28] Glabellar lines, also called 'frown lines', occur as a result of the pull on the skin of the underlying facial musculature, predominantly the procerus and the corrugator supercilli muscles (Fig. 8.2). Glabella is the main indication for BTx treatment.[7,29]

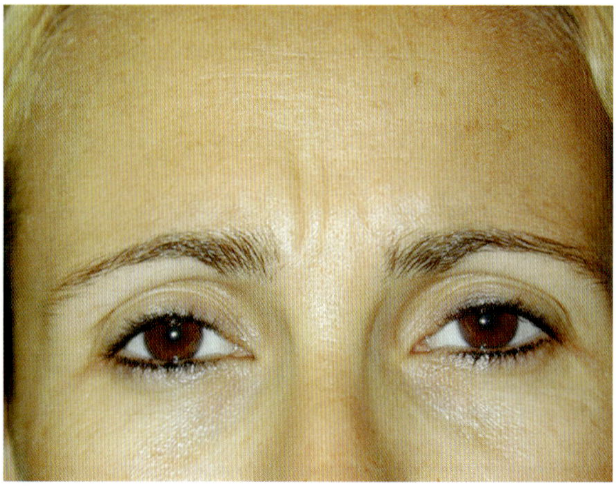

Fig. 8.2 Glabellar lines due to frowning of procerus and corrugator muscles.

Muscles produce the vertical lines of glabella including corrugator supercilli and the medial orbital portion of the orbicularis oculi, both of which move the brow medially, and the depressor supercilli muscle, which pulls the brow inferiorly.[30,31] The procerus muscle pulls the brow inferiorly and produces the horizontal lines of the glabella.[30,31] The sole brow elevator is the frontalis. Injection of BTx into glabellar muscles diminishes the appearance of frown lines, suppresses their mobility and also reduces the expressiveness of eyebrows.[32] Moreover, BTx treatment in the glabellar area is able to produce brow lift[5] (Figs 8.3 and 8.4), change the eyebrow shape[33] and correct eyebrow asymmetries.[34]

Deep glabellar lines can be treated with BTx-A alone or in combination with fillers and/or Subcision® for better results.

Periorbicular Area

Crow's feet result largely from hyperkinetic muscle function of the orbicularis oculi, and experience has shown that chemodenervation of the lateral aspect of this muscle can greatly attenuate the appearance of lateral orbital rhytids, also called 'crows feet wrinkles', without impairing the ability to squint and protect the eyes from foreign bodies or bright

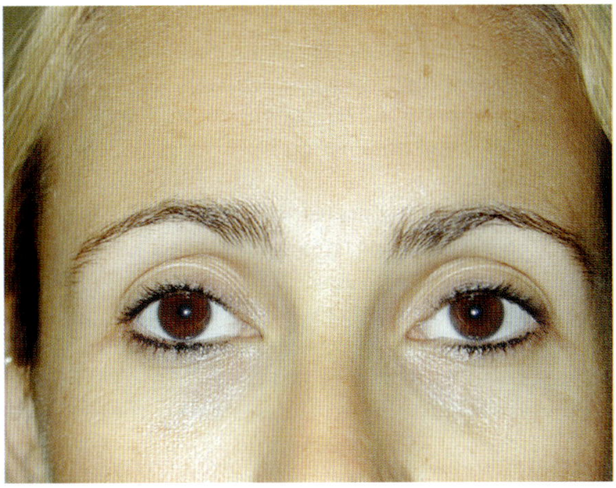

Fig. 8.3 Upper face at rest before injections, showing the original position of eyebrows.

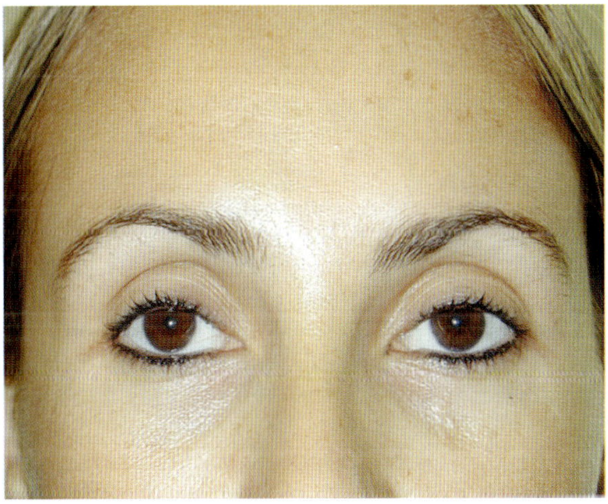

Fig. 8.4 Same patient as Figure 8.3, showing the browlift after BTx injections.

light. The dynamic component of these wrinkles may also be treated with BTx (Figs 8.5 and 8.6).[3]

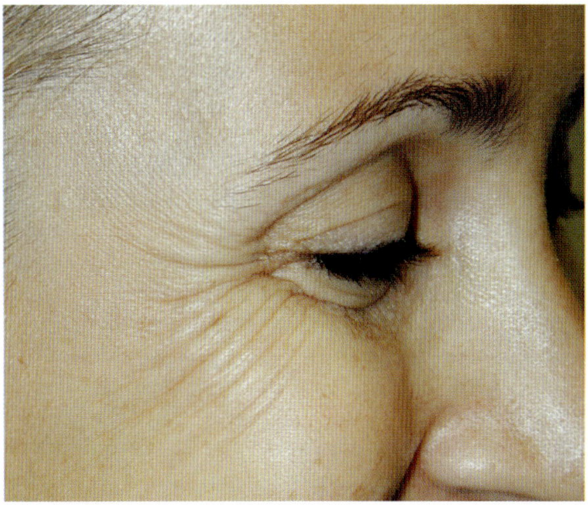

Fig. 8.5 Crow's feet wrinkles, radiating from the lateral canthus, before treatment.

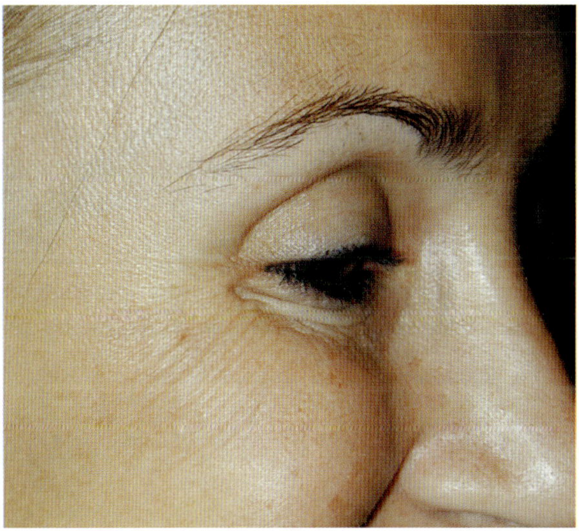

Fig. 8.6 Same patient as Figure 8.4, after treatment with BTx.

PREOPERATIVE CONSIDERATIONS

The following are important preoperative considerations:

- the patient understands the procedure and its limitations
- obtain informed consent and good preoperative photographs (at rest and in movement) have been obtained
- if possible, to discontinue the use of medication/supplementation that might enhance bleeding (anticoagulants, gingko biloba, vitamin E, aspirin) 7–10 days prior to injections
- to discontinue the use of medication that can interfere with BTx-A action (aminoglicosides)
- the individual facial balance, looking at the patient at rest and in movement
- the cosmetic use of BTx-A in patients with pre-existing neuromuscular disorders that alter the neuromuscular junction, such as the Eaton–Lambert syndrome (myasthenic syndrome) and major myasthenia, should be avoided.[7]

TECHNIQUES AND DOSES

Treatment is delivered in an outpatient setting. The patient sits upright on a chair, with the upper part of the body elevated and topical anesthetic is applied. Antisepsis with 70% alcohol or iodinated alcohol is performed before the injections. A marking pen can be used to indicate specific injection points.

Small syringes are preferable for the application of BTx-A. The needle should be oriented in the opposite direction of the ocular globe. Local, light manual compression[6] or the application of cold compresses[6] help to control the size of bruises if they appear during the procedure. Another consideration in this area is to avoid the use of medicines that interfere with blood coagulation.

For glabellar application, BTx-A is slowly injected into the belly of the corrugator muscle, taking care to maintain the needle tip approximately 1 cm superior to the orbital rim. The needle should be positioned perpendicularly and advanced slightly in a vertical direction toward the hairline within the muscle fibers.[6]

One or two injection sites may be used on the belly of the procerus to treat the horizontal lines that appear at the root of the nose. The injection point is in the midline at a point below a line joining the brows and above the crossing point of the 'X' formed by joining the medial eyebrow to the contralateral inner canthus (Fig. 8.7).[6,35,36]

Five-point injections have been described as the standard technique to weaken the entire glabella in women with highly arched brows,[10] as they have less mass in the muscles that produce frowning.[2] If they have more horizontal brows or deep folds they will require a greater quantity of BTx-A, which may be a higher dose or an extra point above each midpupillary line.[10] In men, although the muscles that cause frowning are of greater mass, the accentuated high arching of the eyebrows is unacceptable, as this characterizes a female pattern. To avoid this, an additional dose of BTx-A is injected at the midpoint of each side of the eyebrow, at least 1 cm above the supraorbital prominence.[5]

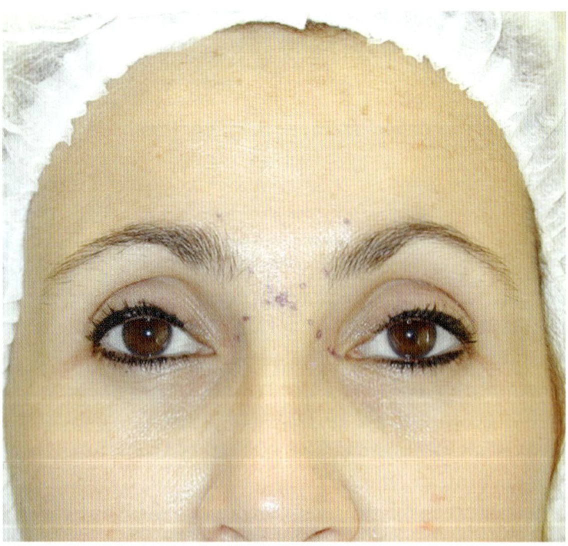

Fig. 8.7 The injection point in the procerus muscle.

Several studies have demonstrated the efficacy and safety of the use of BTx-A in the glabella.[10,16,37–39] The first multicenter, double-blind, randomized, placebo-controlled study proving the efficacy and safety of BTx-A injection for the treatment of glabellar lines was published in 2002.[39] This study described good results with the use of the five-point technique, injecting 4 U of BTx-A (Botox®/Vistabel®) into the midline point of the procerus muscle and two points on either side of the corrugator supercilii, using a total dose of 20 U of Botox®/Vistabel®.[39] A multicenter, double-blind study conducted by Ascher showed that 50 U of Dysport® is an efficacious dose to treat glabellar lines.[16] A study from Monheit and colleagues also concludes that the same dose of 50 U Dysport® gives the most cost-effective results.

Doses and techniques for the application of BTx-A in the glabellar area vary greatly, as treatments must be customized. A randomized study has investigated the efficacy and safety of two injection site patterns of BTx-A (Dysport®) in the treatment of glabellar and central forehead wrinkles. Patients received three injections of BTx-A or placebo in the procerus and corrugator muscles or five injections of BTx-A or placebo in the procerus and corrugator and the two additional sites approximately 1 cm cranial from the corrugator sites.[40] The authors concluded that three central injection sites are essential for the treatment of glabellar wrinkles. The two additional injection sites in the forehead region targeting the frontalis muscle did not improve the efficacy significantly.[40]

For the treatment of periorbital wrinkles, the primary muscle is the orbicularis oculi. This sphincteric muscle sits circumferentially around the eye and has the important function of providing deliberate closure of the eyelids to protect the globe. BTx applications for lateral periorbital wrinkles should be made in the area of the wrinkles, at least 1 cm lateral to the lateral orbital rim in the subcutaneous area (Fig. 8.8).[2,41]

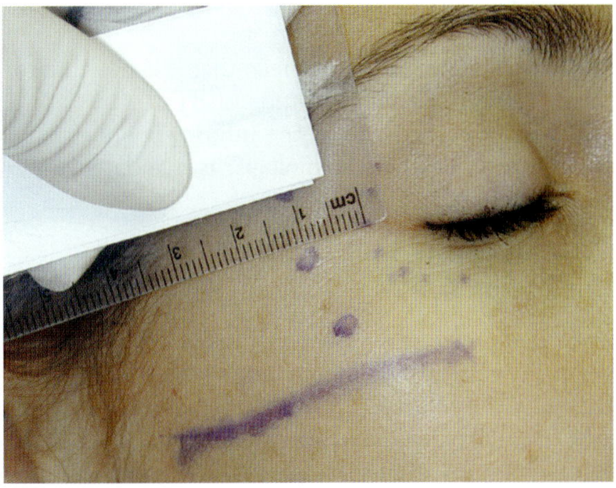

Fig. 8.8 The injection points for lateral periorbital wrinkles. They should be made at least 1 cm lateral to the lateral orbital rim.

Doses for the application of BTx-A in the periorbicular area may also vary. The literature describes doses of Botox® for periorbital wrinkles ranging from 4–5 U/site[42] to 5– 15 U/site,[43,44] distributed over two or three, but sometimes four to five, injection sites. A bilateral, double-blind, randomized study tested placebo against 6, 12 and 18 U of Botox® injected into the periorbital or crow's feet area. All doses were significantly superior to placebo with no clear dose–response relationship.[13] In the periorbital wrinkles, doses of Dysport® may vary from 8[35,45] to 60 U[35,46] and can be distributed over up to five application points.

Intradermic injections of BTx into the pre-septal portion of the lower eyelid reduce some fine wrinkles in this region and augment eyelid opening, especially when combined with BTx treatment of lateral periorbital wrinkles.[47,48] *Patients should be carefully selected for this treatment, as it may aggravate laxity of the lower eyelids.*[49]

In order to slightly weaken and not to cause complete paralysis of the orbicularis oculi, some authors suggest small doses of BTx-A be injected subcutaneously, and not intramuscularly.[50,51] On the other hand, the results from intramuscular or subcutaneous injections of BTx-A of the same doses are similar, due to the diffusion of the product.

POST-PROCEDURE CARE

To minimize the risks of side effects and complications, the treated areas should not be manipulated for 3–4 hours after the injections. It is also recommended that the patient remain in an upright position for this time.[52] The patient should avoid strenuous physical activities for the rest of the day.[53,54] Some authors also recommend that patients contract the treated muscles repeatedly in the first few hours after the injections.[55]

COMPLICATIONS AND SIDE EFFECTS

Complications related to the injection itself include:

- mild stinging, burning or pain
- edema and erythema around injection site
- mild headache.

There are a number of immediate hypersensitivity reactions that are not technique dependent:

- urticaria
- dyspnea
- anaphylaxis.

Particular techniques may cause other reactions, and these are described below.

Ecchymoses and Bruising

Ecchymoses and bruising are caused by deep injections into the crow's feet or into the lower eyelid and may last from 7 to 15 days. For this reason BTx should be injected subdermally and using low dose volumes.

Ptosis of the Upper Eyelid

Ptosis of the upper eyelid is the most significant complication of BTx injections and may be caused by migration of injected BTx through the orbital septum, weakening the elevator palpebrae superioris (Fig. 8.9). If BTx is injected close to the bony supraorbital margin at the midpupillary line where some of the muscle fibres of the elevator palpebrae superioris insert inferiorly to the bony attachment of the

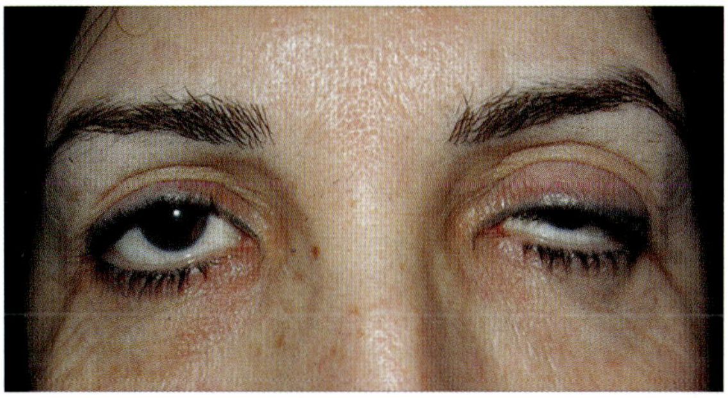

Fig. 8.9 Ptosis of the upper left lid, 8 days after treatment of the glabella with BTx-A.

orbital septum, diffusion into the upper eyelid levator may cause ptosis of the upper eyelid. This may last 2–4 weeks or longer.[22] Instillation of alpha-adrenergic Apraclonidine 0.5% eyedrops, three times a day will stimulate Mueller's muscle to contract, raising the upper eyelid about 1–3 mm.

Brow Ptosis

Older patients frequently compensate for a heavy brow, using the lower fibers of their frontalis to lift the soft tissue of the brow. Brow ptosis is caused by the diffusion of BTx into the low fibers of the frontalis when BTx is injected too rapidly or with too high volumes. A latent eyebrow ptosis can then no longer be compensated by frontalis muscle action.

Lip Ptosis and Possible Oral Incompetence

The zygomaticus major and minor originate at or near the lateral aspect of the superior margin of the zygomatic arch. Injecting the lateral canthus may affect the muscle fibres of some of the levators of the lateral upper lip and the corners of the mouth which may result in lateral upper lip ptosis and possible oral incompetence, causing an asymmetric smile, possible drooling and incontinence. If BTx is injected or diffuses more medially and inferiorly to the superior margin of the zygomatic arch, the central deep levators can be affected, causing possible interference with upper lip competence, including eating and speaking. Injections in this area should be intradermal and of low volume.

Ectropion, Keratitis

In elderly patients with attenuated orbital septa, diffusion of BTx into the superior and inferior palpebral portion of the orbicularis occuli may weaken the lateral tendon, producing lower eyelid ectropion. Prolonged corneal exposure can lead to dry eye and corneal damage. To avoid this, injections should be at least 1.0–1.5 cm lateral to the lateral canthus.

Injecting BTx medial to the midpupillary line of the lower eyelid or involuntary diffusion of BTx in the palpebral portion may weaken the sphincteric function of the palpebral orbicularis occuli, which may impair forced eyelid closure. Weakening the blink reflex may diminish the action of the lacrimal pump and may cause epiphora.[56] A snap test is often recommended prior to injections.

Diplopia

Anatomical considerations mean that it is possible for there to be accidental migration of BTx to the lateral and inferior rectus, and to the inferior oblique. Consultation with an ophthalmologist is mandatory.

Complications that Occur Injecting the Lower Eyelid

In patients who have festooning, pseudoherniation of the infraorbital fat pad can be worsened by injecting BTx into the inferior palpebral orbicularis oculi. This is a particular concern with older patients. This effect may be due to muscular weakness or lymphatic drainage impairment. Flynn et al.[57] found no substantial adverse effects in patients treated with 2 U of Botox® injected pretarsally in the lower eyelid, whereas of those patients who had 4 U injected pretarsally in two divided doses of 2 U each, less than half suffered from 'dry eyes'. With 8 U injected pretarsally into the lower eyelid in two divided doses of 4 U, persistent lower lid edema droopy eyebags and photophobia with difficulty in squinting resulted.

CONCLUSION

Treatment of the facial wrinkles through the use of BTx-A has revolutionized the treatment of facial aging since its first application for cosmetic use by Carruthers and Carruthers in 1992. It represents one of the most important advances in minimally invasive techniques for skin rejuvenation, producing a high degree of patient satisfaction. Moreover, it is a rapid, non-surgical rejuvenation treatment with minimal recovery time.

After 20 years of cosmetic use of BTx and with a large number of published studies suggesting its efficacy and safety, this treatment has become popular and well-established around the world, approved by relevant regulatory agencies, such as the FDA and its counterparts.

Knowledge of muscular anatomy, the physiology of treatment targets, awareness of potential complications and appropriate injection technique are keys to the successful use of BTx.

REFERENCES

1 Said SZ, Meshkinpour A, Carruthers A, et al. Botulinum toxin A. *Am J Clin Dermatol.* 2003;4(9):609–616.
2 Carruthers A, Kiene K, Carruthers J. Botulinum A exotoxin use in clinical dermatology. *J Am Acad Dermatol.* 1996;34:788–797.

3 Kadunc BV. Periorbital wrinkles. In: Hexsel D, Almeida AT, eds. *Cosmetic use of botulinum toxin*. Porto Alegre: AGE; 2002:149–154.

4 Wieder JM, Moy RL. Understanding botulinum toxin. Surgical anatomy of the frown, forehead and periocular region. *Dermatol Surg*. 1998;24:1172–1174.

5 Carruthers JA, Lowe NJ, Menter MA, et al. A multicenter, double-blind, randomized, placebo-controlled study of the efficacy and safety of botulinum toxin type A in the treatment of glabellar lines. *J Am Acad Dermatol*. 2002;46(6):840–849.

6 Hexsel D, Dal'Forno T. Type A botulinum toxin in the upper face. *Clin Dermatol*. 2003;21:488–497.

7 Benedetto A. The cosmetic uses of Botulinum toxin type A. *Int J Dermatol*. 1999;38:641–655.

8 Kede MPV, Sabatovich ODM. Relevance of the cosmetic use of botulinum toxin in facial rejuvenation. In: Hexsel D, Almeida A, eds. *Cosmetic Use of Botulinum Toxin*. 1st ed. Porto Alegre: AGE; 2002:27–31.

9 Klein AW. Treatment of wrinkles with Botox®. *Curr Probl Dermatol*. 2002;30:188–217.

10 Carruthers J, Carruthers A. The adjunctive usage of botulinum toxin. *Dermatol Surg*. 1998;24:1244–1247.

11 Carruthers J, Carruthers A. Botulinum toxin A in the mid and lower face and neck. *Dermatol Clin*. 2004;22(2):151–158.

12 Sposito MMM. Botulinum toxin, muscle relaxation and quality of life. In: Hexsel D, Almeida AT, eds. *Cosmetic use of botulinum toxin*. Porto Alegre: AGE; 2002:28–31.

13 Lowe NJ, Lask G, Yamauchi P, et al. Bilateral, double-blind, randomized comparison of 3 doses of botulinum toxin type A and placebo in patients with crow's feet. *J Am Acad Dermatol*. 2002;47(6):834–840.

14 Keen M, Blitzer A, Aviv J, et al. Botulinum toxin A for hyperkinetic facial lines: results of a double-blind, placebo-controlled study. *Plast Reconstruct Surg*. 1994;94:94–99.

15 Lowe NJ, Maxwell A, Harper H. Botulinum A exotoxin for glabellar folds: a double-blind, placebo-controlled study with an electromyographic injection technique. *J Am Acad Dermatol*. 1996;35:569–572.

16 Ascher B, Zakine B, Kestemont P, et al. A multicenter, randomized, double-blind, placebo-controlled study of efficacy and safety of 3 doses of botulinum toxin A in the treatment of glabellar lines. *J Am Acad Dermatol*. 2004;51(2):223–233.

17 Spiegel JH. Treatment of periorbital rhytids with botulinum toxin type A. *Arch Facial Plast Surg*. 2005;7:198–202.

18 Kerner J. Cotta J, ed. *Das Fettgift oder die Fettsäure und ihre Wirkungen auf den thierischen Organismus, ein Beytrag zur Untersuchung des in verdorbenen Wuersten giftig wirkenden Stoffes*. Tuebingen, Germany: Stuttgart; 1822.

19 Scott AB. Botulinum toxin injection into extraocular muscles as an alternative to strabismus surgery. *Ophthalmology*. 1980;87:(10):1044–1049.

20 Carruthers A, Carruthers JA. Treatment of glabellar frown lines with C. *botulinum* toxin A exotoxin. *J Dermatol Surg Oncol*. 1992;18:17–21.

21 Blitzer A, Brin MF, Keen MS, et al. Botulinum toxin for the treatment of hyper-functional lines of the face. *Arch Otolaryngol head Neck Surg*. 1993;9:1018–1022.

22 Rohrer TE, Beer K. Background to botulinum toxin. In: Carruthers J, Carruthers J, eds. *Botulinum Toxin*. London: Elsevier Saunders; 2005:9–17.

23 Baumann L, Slezinger A, Vujevich J, et al. A double-blinded, randomized, placebo-controlled pilot study of the safety and efficacy of Myobloc (botulinum toxin type B) purified neurotoxin complex for the treatment of crow's feet: a double-blinded placebo-controlled trial. *J Dermatol Surg*. 2003;29(5):508–515.

24 Aoki KR. Pharmacology, immunology, and current developments. In: Benedetto AV, ed. *Botulinum toxin in clinical dermatology*. Abingdon: Taylor & Francis; 2006.

25 de Paiva A, Meunier FA, Molgó J, Aoki KR, Dolly JO. Functional repair of motor endplates after botulinum toxin A poisoning: biphasic switch of synaptic activity between nerve sprouts and their parent terminals. *Proc Natl Acad Sci USA*. 1999;96 (6):3200–3205.

26 Lowe PL, Patnaik R, Lowe NJ. A comparison of two botulinum type A toxin preparations for the treatment of glabellar lines: double-blind, randomized, pilot study. *Dermatol Surg*. 2005;31 (12):1651–1654.

27 Hexsel D, Mattos MISP. Current considerations of aesthetics and facial rejuvenation and their social and psychological implications. In: Hexsel D, Almeida AT, eds. *Cosmetic use of botulinum toxin*. Porto Alegre: AGE; 2002:21–26.

28 Hexsel D, Zechmeister D, Hexsel CL. Perspectives. In: Hexsel AT, Almeida AT, eds. *Cosmetic use of botulinum toxin*. Porto Alegre: AGE; 2002:32–34.

29 Wegerich PB, Rauch L, Ruzicka T. Botulinum toxin A in the therapy of mimic facial lines. *Clin and Experim Dermatol*. 2001;26:619–630.

30 Macedo OR. Patient selection and cosmetic indications. In: Hexsel AT, Almeida AT, eds. *Cosmetic use of botulinum toxin*. Porto Alegre: AGE; 2002:125–130.

31 Sadick N. The cosmetic use of botulinum toxin type B in the upper face. *Clin Dermatol*. 2004;22:29–33.

32 Lackey NJ, Norton SA. Implications of botulinum injection of the brow. [Letter]. *J Am Acad Dermatol*. 2006;54(5):921–922.

33 Levy JL F, Jouves E. Management of the ageing eyebrow and forehead: an objective dose-response study with botulinum toxin. *J Eur Acad Dermatol Venereol*. 2006;20(6):711–716.

34 Finn JC. Botulinum toxin type A: fine-tuning treatment of facial nerve injury. *J Drugs Dermatol*. 2004;3(2):133–137.

35 Carruthers A. Botulinum toxin type A: history and current cosmetic use in the upper face. *Dis Mon*. 2002;48(5):299–322.

36 Carruthers A, Carruthers J. Botulinum toxin type A: history and current cosmetic use in the upper face. *Semin Cutan Med Surg*. 2001;20(2):71–84.

37 Carruthers A, Carruthers J. Prospective, double-blind, randomized, parallel group, dose-ranging study of botulinum toxin type A in men with glabellar rhytids. *Dermatol Surg*. 2005;31(10):1297–1303.

38 Carruthers A, Carruthers J, Said S. Dose-ranging study of botulinum toxin type A in the treatment of glabelar rhytids in females. *Dermatol Surg*. 2005;31(4):414–422.

39 Carruthers JA, Lowe NJ, Menter MA, et al. A multicenter, double-blind, randomized, placebo-controlled study of the efficacy and safety of botulinum toxin type A in the treatment of glabellar lines. *J Am Acad Dermatol*. 2002;46(6):840–849.

40 Rzany B, Ascher B, Fratila A, et al. Efficacy and safety of 3- and 5-injection patterns (30 and 50 U) of botulinum toxin A (Dysport®) for the treatment of wrinkles in the glabella and the central forehead region. *Arch Dermatol*. 2006;142(3):320–326.

41 Edelstein C, Shorr N, Jacobs J, et al. Oculoplastic experience with the cosmetic use of botulinum A exotoxin. *Dermatol Surg*. 1998;24:1208–1212.

42 Garcia A, Fulton JE. Cosmetic denervation of the muscles of facial expression with botulinum toxin. *Dermatol Surg*. 1996;22:39–43.

43 Keen M, Blitzer A, Aviv J, et al. Botulinum toxin A for hyperkinetic facial lines: results of a double-blind, placebo-controlled study. *Plast Reconstruct Surg*. 1994;94:94–99.

44 Blitzer A, Binder WJ, Aviv JE. The management of hyperfunctional facial lines with botulinum toxin. *Arch Otolaryngol Head Neck Surg*. 1997;123:389–392.

45 Tambasco N, Lalli F, Mancini ML, Rossi A. Botulinum toxin in the treatment of facial expression wrinkles (ITA). *Riv Ital Chir Plast*. 1997;29:197–200.

46 Lowe NJ. Botulinum toxin type A for facial rejuvenation. United States and United Kingdom perspectives. *Dermatol Surg*. 1998;24:1216–1218.

47 Louarn CL. Botulinum toxin A and facial lines: the variable concentration. *Aesth Plast Surg*. 2001;25:73–84.

48 Flynn TC, Carruthers JA, Carruthers JA. Botulinum-A toxin treatment of the lower eyelid improves infraorbital rhytides and widens the eye. *Dermatol Surg*. 2001;27(8):703–708.

49 Hexsel D, Mazzuco R, Zechmeister M, Hexsel CL. Complications and adverse affects: diagnosis and treatment. In: Hexsel D, Almeida A, eds. *Cosmetic Use of Botulinum Toxin*. 1st ed. Porto Alegre: AGE; 2002:233–239.

50 Greenway HT, Breisch EA. Superficial cutaneous anatomy. In: Robinson KA, Arndt KA, LeBoit PE, Wintroub BU, eds. *Atlas of Cutaneous Surgery*. Philadelphia: WB Saunders; 1996:5–20.

51 Binder WJ, Blitzer A, Brin MF. Treatment of hyperfunctional lines of the face with botulinum toxin A. *Dermatol Surg*. 1998;24(11):1198–1205.

52 Matarasso SL, Matarasso A. Treatment guidelines for botulinum toxin type A for the periocular region and a report on partial upper lip ptosis following injections to the lateral canthal rhytids. *Plast Reconstr Surg*. 2001;108:208–217.

53 Frankel AS. Botox for rejuvenation of the periorbital region. *Facial Plast Surg*. 1999;15(3):255–262.

54 Maia RB. Post-operative care. In: Hexsel D, Almeida AT, eds. *Cosmetic Use of Botulinum Toxin*. Porto Alegre: AGE; 2002:141–142.

55 Hsu TS, Dover JS, Kaminer MS, et al. Why make patients exercise facial muscles for 4 hours after botulinum toxin treatment. *Arch Dermatol*. 2003;139(7):948.

56 Macdonald MR, Spiegel JH, Raven RB, et al. An anatomical approach to glabellar rhytides. *Arch Otolaryngol Head Neck Surg*. 1998;124:1315–1320.

57 Flynn TC, Carruthers JA, Clark RE. 2003 Botulinum A toxin (BOTOX) in the lower eyelid: dose-finding study. *Dermatol Surg*. 2003;29:943–950.

9 Facial Fillers and Volumizers

Marian Cantisano-Zilkha, Alessandra Haddad

Included on ***DVD***

INTRODUCTION

The aging process is a very complex phenomenon, engendered by genetically determined intrinsic and extrinsic factors. Sun exposure with its cumulative ultraviolet effects, even not related to intrinsic aging, represents the most important leading cause of aging of the skin and its undesirable aesthetic effects. Ultraviolet exposure is aggravated by lifestyle and habits, such as cigarette smoking, poor nutritional practices and chemical exposure to different pollutants and irritants, which lead to biological and immunological changes. As a consequence, we see visible and histological signs of skin aging, such as decreased thickness of the epidermis, dermis and subcutaneous tissue, which are clinically manifested by smile lines, crow's feet and facial creases. Over the last few decades, soft tissue augmentation using injectable fillers, combined with other modalities, has become the standard clinical approach for correcting these age-related defects (Fig. 9.1).[1] Soft tissue fillers can temporarily restore a smoother, younger-looking skin by helping to fill in these lines and creases, to recreate symmetry, volume and a smooth skin surface. The ease of performance, lack of down time and infrequency of complications have increased the popularity and patient acceptance of injectable fillers.[2]

Ideal fillers (SCALES 1953):

- are not modified by liquids or organic tissues
- are chemically inert
- do not cause inflammatory reactions
- are non-carcinogenic or mutagenic
- are capable of resisting to mechanical tensions
- do not produce allergic reactions
- are capable of resisting to mechanical strains
- can be manufactured in different formats
- can be sterilized.

After the decision has been made to perform soft tissue augmentation, selecting the filling substance and proper technique are of utmost importance. However, with so many new products of different nature and longevity, and so many others waiting for approval for use in a particular market, it becomes increasingly important to know the properties, composition and mechanism of action of each particular filler, as well as their interactions and tissue responses. None of the currently available fillers meets all the desired criteria, but, while we still search for the ideal fillers, hyaluronic acid (HA) fillers have become the new gold standard in soft tissue augmentation, fulfilling many of our desired criteria. Although they are very well tolerated, the durability of the HA fillers and, to a lesser degree, collagen fillers varies from several months up to 1–2 years, depending on stabilization methods, molecular size and injection site. In contrast, silicone oil lasts for life and some other synthetic fillers stay for decades.

Whether they are permanent or temporary, all fillers have similar application techniques and are part of the treatment planning for use either alone or in combination with other modalities. In this chapter, we will discuss the current and most recent fillers, FDA and non-FDA approved, their characteristics and skin interactions, different formulations and presentation, best indications (Fig. 9.2), techniques and complications.

EVOLUTION

The implantation of gold plates to correct cranial facial defects was first described by Fallopius in the 16th century.[3] The search for the ideal material for correcting facial skin irregularities has continued for over 500 years. Many injectable or implantable substances that are not compatible with the human skin, or that have been adulterated in their formulation, have been proposed for cosmetically improving soft tissue defects. Over 100 years ago, autologous fat was one of the earliest agents used for soft tissue augmentation.[4] Interest in autologous fat has

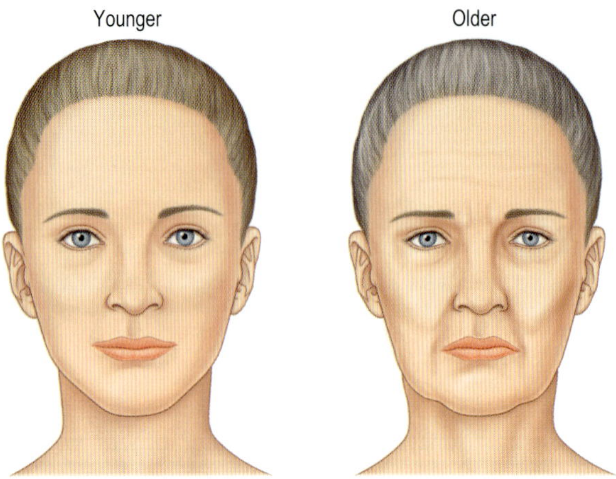

Fig. 9.1 The aging face.

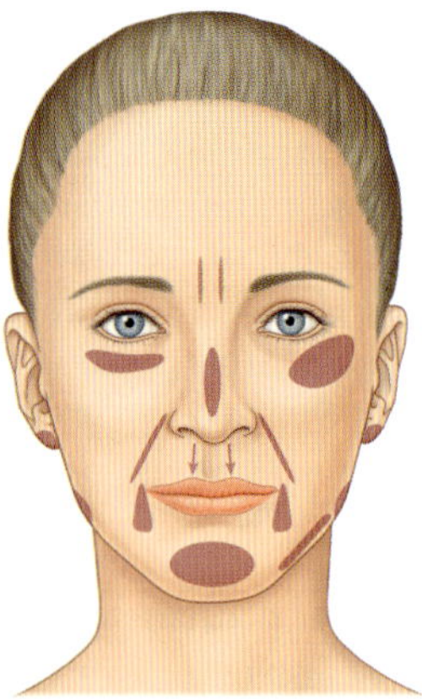

Fig. 9.2 Areas for facial contouring: perioribital augmentation, glabellar, nasolabial and melomental folds, chin and jaw line enhancement, nasal defects, malar enhancement and cheek augmentation.

continued, with the development of new and improved application techniques of structured fat grafting and microinjections (see Chapter 10).

The original concept of tissue augmentation in the modern era involved injecting collagen into the skin. It was believed that the collagen, which has been used for more than 30 years, would incorporate into the skin's own collagen. However, it turned out that collagen only occupies space. That concept continued and was recently altered to include fillers derived from HA, which was also believed to be a passive filler. As it turned out, HA does promote a certain degree of fibroblastic activity.[5] During the last decade, the technology of fillers and volumizers has begun evolving toward using fillers that would induce hyperplasia and make filling more efficient and long lasting.

Silicone is the oldest filling material to be used in the USA. It was first used in 1930. Since1965, both Orenttreich and associates and Barnett have used it for nasolabial augmentation, with good cosmetic results. The FDA has never approved silicone for cosmetic use.

In the 1950s, Gottlieb developed another dermal filler (Fibrel®), a gelatin matrix implant that is now only of historical interest. The principle was to use a fraction of plasma containing fibrinogen and prothrombin to fill up scars and wrinkles. The mechanism of action was based on the normal coagulation and wound healing process, resulting in new collagen formation. Fibrel is no longer available. In 1981, for the first time, a form of xenogenic agent, bovine collagen, received FDA approval.[6] Although those bovine collagen-derived fillers had great potential for hypersensitivity reactions, they had a good safety record and, therefore, have been the most widely used agents for the last 30 years. However, their short duration is a big disadvantage. The HA and hylan fillers represent a big breakthrough for augmentation technology, and they are among the most popularly used dermal fillers. Restylane® (Q-Med, Upsala, Sweden) was the first HA to be approved in the USA in 2003.[7]

CLASSIFICATION

There are many different ways to classify fillers and volumizers, which leads to some degree of confusion. Traditional fillers have been biodegradable, meaning that they are absorbed and eliminated from the body. We will describe the most popular fillers in detail, according to their properties, tissue interaction, source and longevity, application techniques, side effects and complications. Since this is a market that is developing rapidly, there are many fillers waiting for FDA approval and the CE mark in Europe, which is much less rigorous than in the USA. We will discuss the most used fillers with biodegradable and non-biodegradable properties (Table 9.1).

BIODEGRADABLE FILLERS

Collagen Products

For more than 30 years, collagen products have been the most readily available and widely used injectable soft fillers for facial rejuvenation. The main idea was

Table 9.1 Biodegradable and non-biodegradable fillers			
Biodegradable	**Non-biodegradable**	**Slowly biodegradable**	**Biodegradable with fibroplastic properties**
AcHyal	Aquamid	Radiesse	Radiesse
Alloderm	Artefill (Artesense)	New Fill/Sculptra	Hyaluronic Acid/Hylan fillers
Autologen	Bioplastique		New Fill/Sculptra
Cymetra	Evolution		
Bioinblue	Gore-Tex		
Dermal grafting	Meta-Crill		
Dermaplant	Silicone oil (Adatosil, Silikon 1000)		
Elevess	Softform		
Endoplast 50			
Fascian			
Fat			
Human placental collagen			
Hyal system			
Isologen			
Evolence			
Juvederm			
NewFill/Sculptra			
Belotero			
Perlane			
Restylane (family)			
Reviderm			
Surgilift			
Teosyal			
Cosmoderm/ Cosmoplast			
Zyderm/Zyplast			

that once injected into the skin the product would be incorporated into new collagen, producing long-lasting correction. This concept was abandoned when it became apparent that injectable collagen was just a passive space occupier. Collagen products today include human combination collagen, cultured collagen, bovine and porcine, and collagen combined with synthetic and natural substances. Some of them require skin pretesting for hypersensitivity and others do not.

Animal Collagen (Bovine and Porcine) – Xenogenic

Bovine collagen is made from extracted cow skin that is highly purified, sterilized and processed into a liquid form before being used for cosmetic purposes. Because collagen is a protein that is eventually metabolized by the body, bovine collagen injections are not permanent. Three variations of bovine collagen are currently available: Zyderm I,

Zyderm II and Zyplast® (Allergan, Irvine, CA). They are 95–98% type I collagen, and the remainder is type III.

Zyderm I, the least concentrated, is available in a concentration of 35 mg/mL, dispersed in phosphate-buffered physiological saline. It is indicated for superficial rhytids or for layering on top of a deeper filling agent. It should be placed in the superficial papillary dermis. As much of Zyderm I is saline, the treatment area should be overcorrected 150–200%.

Zyderm II is more viscous, with a concentration of 65 mg/mL dispersed in phosphate-buffered physiological saline. It is recommended for the treatment of deeper lines and wrinkles with a deeper placement into the papillary dermis and a recommended overcorrection of 100–150%. It has twice the viscosity of Zyderm I. Both contain 0.3% lidocaine (3 mg/mL) to provide local anesthesia at the time of the injection. They are provided in sterile disposable syringes ready for use and should be kept refrigerated until usage. Each syringe should only be used once. Since they are produced from animal sources, a skin sensitivity test should be performed, at 8 and 4 weeks prior to treatment. Zyderm I and II last for an average of 3 months, but some have been reported to last longer.[8–10]

Zyplast® contains purified bovine dermal glutaraldehyde cross-linked collagen in a concentration of 35 mg/mL because the cross-linkage with glutaraldehyde makes the collagen fibers stronger. Zyplast® is indicated for correction of deeper skin wrinkles and deformities. Since the agent does not decompose at the same rate as non-cross-linked collagen, it lasts longer (more than 3 months). Zyplast® should be injected without overcorrection.

Bovine collagens may be easier to inject in facial areas, such as lip borders, because they are liquid and not thick. They may also be less painful for patients because they are mixed with anesthetics.

Evolence® is a porcine collagen gel implant composed of 35 mg/mL homogenous Type I collagen that received FDA approval in June 2008. It is extracted and purified from porcine tendons, suspended in phosphate-buffered saline (PBS) and cross-linked with a technology that uses sugar (ribose) instead of chemicals – 'Glymatrix' technology. This porcine collagen-derived dermal filler is supposed to be less immunogenic, since the allergenic telopeptides are removed, making it more compatible with human collagen. No pretesting is necessary.

Evolence® is supplied as single-use 1 cm^3 prefilled sterile syringe. It is indicated for dermis correction of moderate-to-deep facial wrinkles and folds, such as nasolabial folds, and meets the criteria for correction lasting from 9 to 12 months.[11] As there has been some postinjection granuloma formation, some doctors do not recommend using it for lips.[12] Patients with a history of dietary porcine allergy should not use Evolence®. Based on preclinical studies, the use of Evolence® in individual patients should be limited to 10 mL over a 1-year period. The safety of injecting greater amounts has not been established.[13]

Other Non-FDA-Approved Xenogenic Collagen

Permacol® (Tissue Science Laboratories, Aldershot, UK), a porcine dermal–collagen matrix graft, is a micronized and cross-linked injectable form of the sheet material used to reconstruct dermal tissue defects. It is produced in a saline vehicle and is available in Europe in 2.5 cm^3 syringes. It is an off-label use because it is approved in Europe for urinary incontinence.

Atelocollagen® (Koken Co. Ltd, Tokyo, Japan) is a collagen-derived filler from breeds of very young Australian calves to decrease the risk of transmission of bovine spongiform encephalitis. It is supplied with 1 cm^3/mg cartridges and is injected with dental syringes. We have not found too much information on Atelocollagen® in the literature.[14]

Allogenic Collagen (Synthetic or Cadaveric)

Human synthetic collagen products are derived from a single human fibroblastic cell culture from a source other than the recipient. They are purified and prepared in the form of a buffered saline suspension, with lidocaine being added to reduce the pain associated with injection. Human synthetic injectable collagen is similar to bovine collagen in its properties and durability, and it is used in much the same way; allergy testing is not required prior to use. There are currently three FDA-approved injectable synthetic human collagen products available in the USA: CosmoDerm1®, CosmoDerm 2® and Cosmoplast™ (Allergan, Irvine, CA), and unlike Dermalogen™ and Cymetra®, which are described below, they are not cadaveric.

CosmoDerm 1® and CosmoDerm 2® have the same indications as the bovine collagens, Zyderm I and Zyderm II, and similar longevity. CosmoDerm 1® has a concentration of 35 mg/mL and CosmoDerm 2® has a concentration of 65 /mL; they are not recommended for individuals who have severe allergies that include a history of anaphylaxis to bovine or other collagen products.

Cosmoplast™ is a concentration of 35 mg/mL of human-derived collagen, which is cross-linked with glutaraldehyde and recommended for correcting deeper wrinkles – the FDA approved both CosmoDerm® and Cosmoplast™ on March 11, 2003. They do not require a pretreatment skin test. Because of the flow characteristics and lidocaine content of the cell culture collagen products, there may be some practical advantages to combining these products with HA injections. For instance, using Cosmoplast™ to first outline upper lip borders may facilitate augmentation of the body of the lip with Restylane®.

Cadaveric collagen products are allograft materials that are derived from tissue banks and subject to FDA screening for transmissible diseases. Cadaveric collagen products are tightly regulated by the FDA, as is other donated tissue. They are intact human collagen fibers or acellular dermal matrix from cadavers for human implants. There are three products: Alloderm®, Cymetra® and Dermalogen™.

Alloderm® and Cymetra® (LifeCell Corporation, Branchburg, NJ) are approved by the FDA for cosmetic corrective use. They are harvested from donated and acellular human donor tissue, freeze dried and processed to eliminate infections, and available from most tissue banks. Alloderm is indicated for transplantation to repair dermal tissue and is widely used to treat full-thickness burns as well as soft tissue augmentation. It requires surgical implantation. Cymetra® is a micronized form of Alloderm® that is more suitable for injection. Both Alloderm® and Cymetra® are rehydrated with saline solution or lidocaine in the physician's office 1 hour prior to injection. Cymetra® is injected deep into the dermis for lip augmentation and to treat rhytids and scars. Since the material is still viscous and generally requires a 23–26-gauge needle for injection, regional blocks are recommended. The manufacturer does not require pretesting for allergies, but 2.1% of patients develop temporary local reactions.[15] Host tissue incorporation, with fibroblast in-growth, and collagen deposition are seen 1 month after implantation.[16] Cymetra® has been contraindicated in patients with history of autoimmune connective disorder.

Dermalogen™ (Collagenesis, Beverly, MA) is another injectable human dermal implant material made from a suspension of pooled human cadaver collagen.[17] It is the allogenic version of Autologen (discussed below). Apparently, development of new collagen and neovascularization is possible, but it is a long process requiring many sessions and is very expensive. Although they are, theoretically, non-immunogenic and incapable of potential allergic reactions, these cadaveric agents have lost their initial appeal, and the two injectable forms (Cymetra® and Dermalogen™) are no longer available.

Autologous Collagen

Although autologous human collagen is derived from the patient's own collagen, this is still technically difficult to produce with consistency and with adequate volume. These products are ideal because there is no immunological response and less chance of infectious complications.

Autologen™ (Collagenesis Inc., Beverly, MA) is collagen harvested and reformulated from the patient's own skin so allergic reactions are considered impossible. Theoretically, it should last longer than other biological fillers. The patient's own skin is harvested during a previous procedure – such as blepharoplasty, facelift or another operation in which skin is removed – and sent to a commercial laboratory where the collagen is extracted, sterilized and prepared for reinjection. The amount of collagen available for injection is limited by the amount of skin removed and the quality of the skin. A total of two to four injections of Autologen may be performed at 1–3-month intervals. If not needed, the remaining processed liquid collagen can be stored for 5 years. Autologen™ injections seem to last longer than bovine collagen injections, but longevity varies. Unfortunately, the company manufacturing Autologen™ is no longer in business.

Isolagen® (Isolagen Inc., Houston, TX) is another autologous collagen that has been temporarily taken off the market pending FDA approval. It is composed of injectable autologous fibroblasts cultured for 4–6 weeks from a 3 mm punch biopsy taken from postauricular skin. Like Autologen™, the patient's own collagen is harvested, purified and packaged in a suspension for injection into the skin. A minimum of three injections, given at 2-week intervals, is recommended. A 70% improvement can be expected following the third injection and, because live cells are used, improvement may continue for several months after the last injection. Because the material is from the patient's body, little risk of allergic response exists. Phase III clinical trials are taking place, for FDA approval. Research has shown it to be effective, and it can last for up to 4 years.[18] Several other autologous and allogenic collagen products have been intermittently available. They initially require multiple injection sessions to attain an acceptable result and the residence time is limited.

Recombinant Collagen

Recombinant collagen is still in initial FDA trial phases, for non-cosmetic applications.

Collagen combined with different materials is discussed under non-biodegradable fillers (Artefill®, FDA approved since 2005, and its precursor Artecoll®) (Table 9.2).

HYALURONIC ACID AND HYALURONANS

HA is a naturally occurring substance found in the skin and connective tissues of all mammals that plays an important role in keeping tissue lubricated. Because it is a uniform, unbranched linear polysaccharide with a simple chemical structure that is identical in all species and tissues, it can be considered an ideal biomaterial.[19] HA supports collagen and elastin fibers and helps retain moisture to give skin its characteristic texture. To produce a gel suitable for use as an injectable filler, HA is chemically modified by cross-linking the molecules. It can be used to fill out facial lines and remove wrinkles, and for soft tissue augmentation, such as lip plumping (Fig. 9.3). Injectable HA fillers remove wrinkles immediately, and the results last longer than other biodegradable fillers. Because HA is a natural substance, hyaluronic fillers are associated with fewer hypersensitivity reactions than other collagen products.[20] Although they can be either animal based or non-animal based, no pretreatment skin testing is required. Most of the HA preparations are synthesized by bacteria, purified and cross-linked to provide a variety of viscosities for injection. The FDA has approved Restylane®, Perlane®, Captique®, Juvéderm™, Hylaform®, Hylaform Plus® and Elevess® HA gels for use in the USA. With the exception of Hylaform® and Hylaform Plus®, which are derived from the rooster combs, they are all non-animal stabilized HA (NASHA™) fillers.

Recent studies have shown that HAs also induce a certain degree of fibroplasias.[5] To minimize the probability of protein impurities bound to the entangled HA, they are biosynthesized from a non-animal source and stabilized with relatively few cross-links in a continuous three-dimensional molecular network to create a gel that can take any form or shape.[21]

The longevity of the HA products depends on the size of the gel particle, the concentration, the area to

Table 9.2 US FDA approved collagens

Type	Collagen concentration	Indication	Volume (cc)	Placement	Overcorrection	Year approval
Zyderm I	35 mg/mL bovine	Fine superficial lines	0.5, 1.0,1.5	Superficial papillary dermis	150–200×	1981
Zyderm II	65 mg/mL bovine	Mild/moderate rhytids, scars	0.5, 1.0	Mid dermis	100×150×	1983
Zyplast	35 mg/mL bovine (cross-linked glutaraldehyde)	Deep lines and folds	1.0, 2.0, 2.5	Deep dermis	None	1985
CosmoDerm1	35 mg/mL human derived	Fine/superficial rhytids	1.0	Superficial papillary dermis	150–200×	2003
CosmoDerm2	65 mg/mL human derived	Mild/moderate rhytids, scars	0.5, 1.0	Mid-dermis	100–150	2005
CosmoPlast	35 mg/mL human derived	Deeper rhytids and folds	1.0	Deep dermis	None	2003
Evolence	30 mg/mL porcine derived	Fine to mild wrinkles	1.0	Mid dermis	None	2008

Cosmoderm, Cosmoplast and Evolence: no pretesting necessary

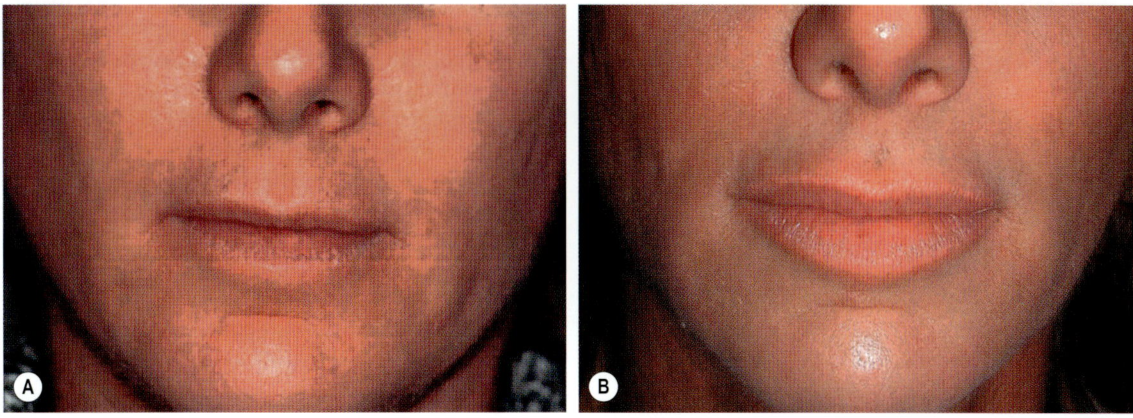

Fig. 9.3 *A*, Before Restylane® injection for lip augmentation on the vermilion border and on the 'body' of the lip. *B*, After Restylane® injection for lip augmentation on the vermilion border and on the 'body' of the lip.

be injected and the presence of inflammation in the area. In healthy tissue, the extracellular capacity to degrade HA (into carbon dioxide and water) is extremely low. Because the molecule is extremely hydrophilic and the amount of HA in the gel bead is about five times larger than needed to maintain its volume, NASHA™ gels will remain approximately the same size and shape despite continuous degradation. The excess material allows the gel bead to last longer, a process called isovolemic degradation. The limited cross-linking allows for significant ability to absorb water and maintain volume.[21] HAs are hyaluronans, whether or not they are derived from bacterial fermentation or an animal.

Restylane® (Q-Med, Upsala, Sweden or, in the USA, Medicis, Scottsdale, AZ) was the first HA to receive USA FDA approval, in December 2002. For many, it is considered the 'ideal filler.' It has 20 mg/mL of HA with a gel bead size of 250 μm and 100 000 units per mL. Restylane® is indicated for fine and moderate lines and wrinkles, and for lip augmentation and tear trough defect repair.[22] The authors have used HA to reshape nasal deformities while a patient was contemplating corrective rhinoplasty (Fig. 9.4). All the Restylane® products have a concentration of 20 mg/cm^3, but the particle size varies. It is dispensed in a 1.0 cm^3 and 0.5 cm^3 prepacked syringe, with a 30-gauge × 1.5-inch-long needle. Restylane Fine Lines® has 20 mg/mL of HA with a gel bead size of 100 μm and 200 000 units per mL. It is good for very fine perioral lines and temporary correction of double Asian eyelid creases (Fig. 9.5), with great patient satisfaction level and instant gratification. Restylane Lipp® was designed for the vermilion border of the lip or to create more volume. Restylane SubQ® is the thickest version of the Restylane® family with cosmetic indication. It is a volumizer, with 1000 gel particles per milliliter.

Perlane® (Q-Med, Upsala, Sweden), which gained USA FDA approval in 2006, has 20 mg/mL of HA

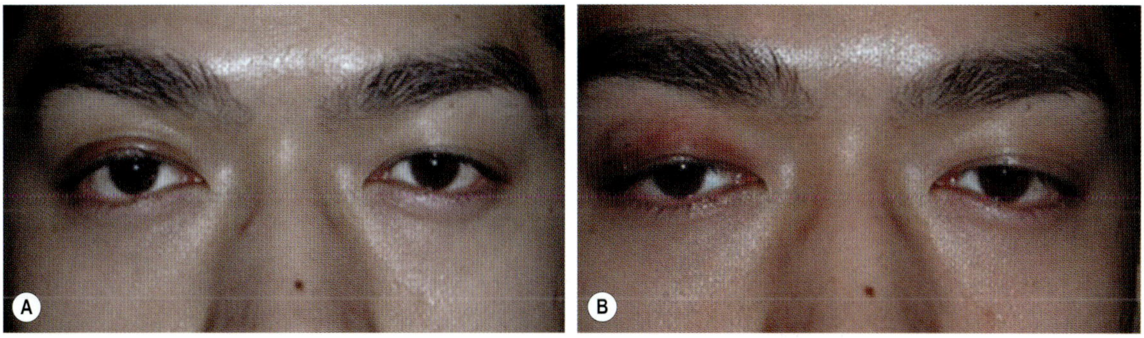

Fig. 9.4 *A*, Double eyelid crease on Asian eyelid. *B*, Immediately after Restylane® injection there is bilateral eyelid symmetry.

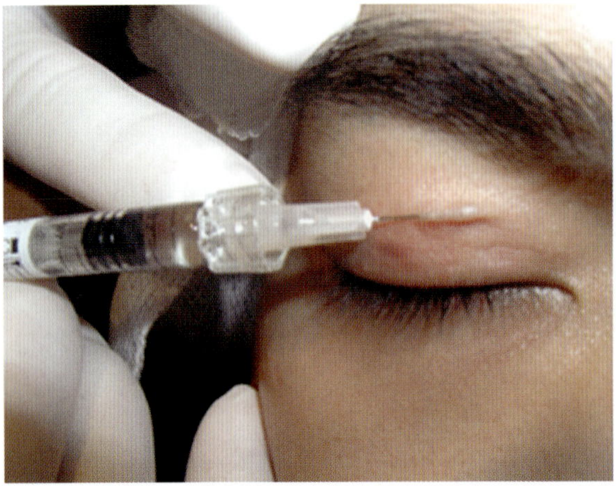

Fig. 9.5 Technique of injection very superficially on the double crease with the purpose of camouflaging the crease and giving instant gratification to a very common Asian eyelid problem.

with a gel bead size of 1000 μm and 10 000 units per milliliter. It is dispensed in a 1.0 cm^3 and 0.5 cm^3 prepacked syringe, with a 27-gauge × 1.5-inch long needle. It is indicated for deeper defects and for broader areas such as nasolabial folds, malar enhancement and other facial irregularities.

Captique® (Genzyme and Allergan, Irvine, CA) received FDA approval for cosmetic use in August 2004. It is a product derived from bacterial fermentation (non-animal) HA. Captique® is plant based. No pretest is needed. Captique® is a clear gel that is indicated for injection into the mid-to-deep dermis for correction of moderate-to-severe wrinkles.

Juvéderm™ (Genzyme, Framingham, MA, and distributed by Allergan, Irvine, CA) was approved by the FDA in June 2006 for treating facial wrinkles and folds.[23] It is developed by bacterial fermentation and differs from the other HA products because it is a homogeneous gel, with the highest concentration of cross-linked HA (above 90%) of any dermal filler currently available. According to the manufacturer, because of its soft consistency, Juvéderm creates a smooth, natural look and a feel that lasts longer, and requires fewer touchups following the initial treatment. In Europe, Juvéderm™ is available in five formulations: Juvéderm™ 18, 24, 24 HV, 30 and 30 HV. HV indicates a higher viscosity and a greater degree of cross-linking for that product. They all have a concentration of 24 mg/mL of HA and are differentiated by the degree of cross-linking. The FDA approved three formulations for Juvéderm™, offering physicians the flexibility to tailor treatments to the particular needs of each patient. They are JuvédermUltra™ 24 HV, recommended for contouring and volumizing facial wrinkles and folds; JuvédermUltra Plus™ 30 HV, recommended for deeper folds and wrinkles; and Juvéderm 30™, for subtle correction of facial wrinkles and for lip augmentation (Fig. 9.6) and folds.

Elvess® (Anika Therapeutics Inc., Woburn, MA) was approved by the FDA in December 2006. It is a sterile, non-pyrogenic gel implant, composed of hyaluronan produced by *Streptococcus equi* (bacterial fermentation), which is cross-linked and suspended in a buffer solution at a concentration of 28 mg/mL, with 0.3% lidocaine HCl, and contains sodium metabisulfite as an antioxidant. It is indicated for injection into the mid-to-deep dermis for the correction of moderate-to-severe facial wrinkles and folds (such as nasolabial folds). It is contraindicated for patients with a history of allergies to sulfites (although rare) or for patients with severe allergies manifested by a history of anaphylaxis. It is the only HA filler to have local anesthetic in its formulation.[24]

Hylaform® and Hylaform Plus® (Allergan, Irvine, CA) are sterile, non-pyrogenic, viscoelastic,

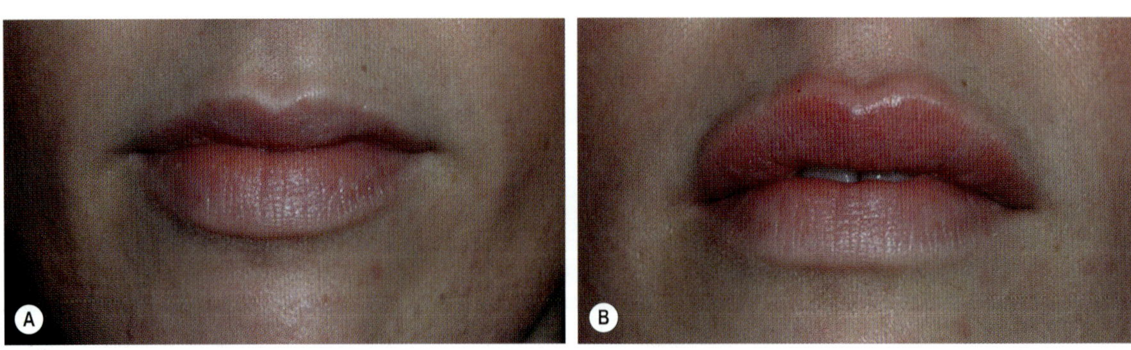

Fig. 9.6 *A*, Before Juvederm™ injection on vermilion border and 'body' of upper lip. Courtesy Dr Yoannis Glavas. *B*, Immediately after Juvederm™ injection.

transparent gel implants composed of cross-linked molecules of hyaluronan. (These products are derived from minced rooster combs, which consist predominantly of HA, and may contain avian protein.) In theory, this extraction technique could subject them to a higher level of impurities or contaminants. Although no allergy tests are needed before treatment with these products, individuals with avian allergies may not be good candidates.

In their composition, they have 5.5 mg/mL of HA and 20% cross-linking. Hylaform Plus®, which is used much like Perlane®, has a larger gel particle and is more viscous than Hylaform®, which is used much like Restylane®. No long-term studies have been conducted to determine the longevity of these products, but it appears to be less than that of Restylane® and Perlane®.[21]

Hylaform® was approved in April 2004 to correct superficial defects and fine wrinkles, and lasts for 6–8 months. Hylaform Plus® was approved in October 2004 to correct moderate-to-severe irregularities and folds and has an average duration of 8–9 months.

HA, derived from rooster combs (Biomatrix, Inc., Ridgefield, NJ), has been used for almost three decades by ophthalmic surgeons during intraocular procedures. One of the authors (MCZ) participated in its early development with Dr Stephen Bosniak (NY, NY) in the reconstruction of sockets of owl monkeys that had become disfigured in fights while in captivity. It was used to enhance and replace volume in the reconstructive and cosmetic areas during unpublished Hylan B gel monkey studies, conducted from 1990 to 1995 (Figs 9.7 and 9.8). It is contraindicated for both monkeys and humans with a history of hypersensitivity to avian protein.

There are many more fillers approved in Europe and South America than there are in the USA.

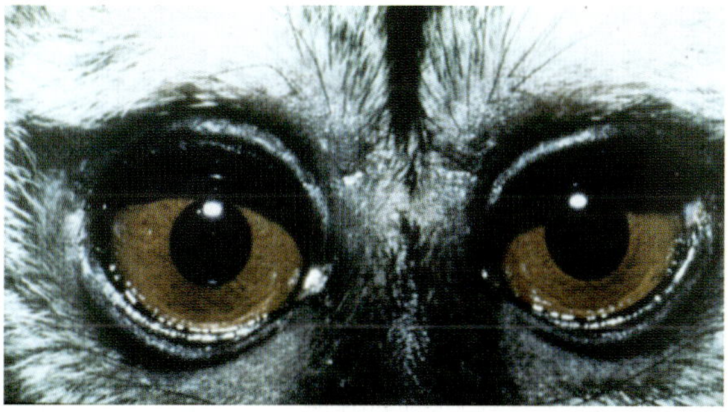

Fig. 9.7 Owl monkey.

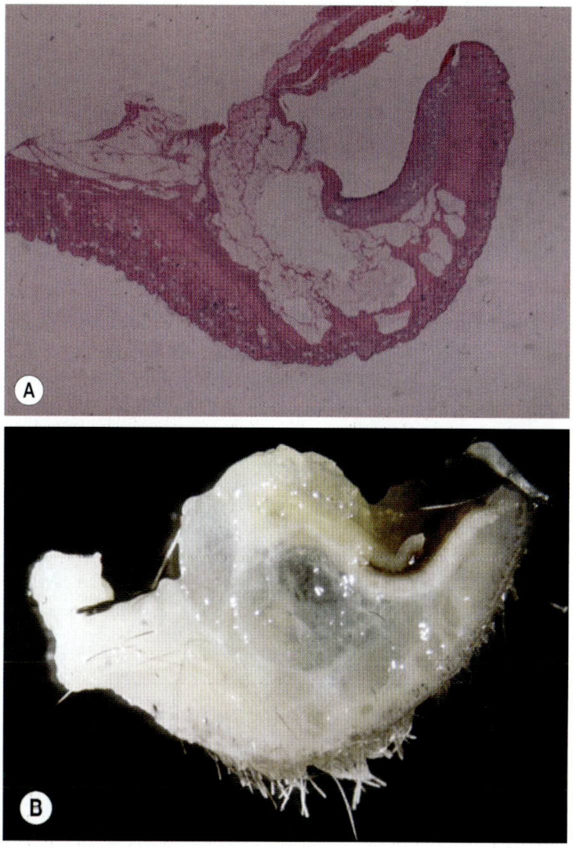

Fig. 9.8 Macroscopic and microscopic specimen of superior sulcus of owl monkeys. The superior orbital sulcus had been injected and reconstructed with cross-linked HA while in captivity in 1990–1995, Biomatrix, Ridgefield, NJ, in preliminary studies of Hyalan B gel as an injectable for socket reconstruction and wrinkle softening. Material still present after 1 year of injection, no inflammatory reaction. It camouflages the crease and gives instant gratification to a very common Asian eyelid problem. Courtesy of Dr Stephen Bosniak and Dr Marian Zilkha.

Following are a few HA products that are not approved for use in the USA.

Belotero® or Esthelis® (Anteis, Switzerland) is a monophasic, non-cross-linked HA that is marketed in some countries in Europe. Designed by HA biofermentation, it is completely biodegradable and biocompatible. It is created using Cohesive Polydensified Matrix®, a technology that gives this product great elasticity and easy flow through the needle. It is available in two forms. Belotero Basic® is meant for treating deeper furrows, lip augmentation, facial outlines, nasolabial folds, glabellar lines and facial depressions. Belotero Soft® is designed to treat perioral lines, lip commissures and forehead wrinkles.

Teosyal®, manufactured by Swiss laboratories Teoxane, consists of several monophasic HA-based products of non-animal origin. It is produced by bacterial fermentation of streptococci bacteria and has a reduced protein and bacterial endotoxin level, resulting in fewer hypersensitivity reactions. It has many different uses depending on the defect and area to be treated. One of the authors (MCZ) has used it in her Brazilian clinic for more than 2 years, with great patient satisfaction and no significant complications, other than from the injection technique (mild swelling and minimum bruising). It has different presentations, according to different sizes of the beads, for superficial, medium or deep placements. It has the same indications as products from the Q-Med family.

Surgiderm®, manufactured by Corneal Development, France, is marketed in five forms, with different degrees of cross-linking.

POLY-L-LACTIC ACID

Poly-L-lactic acid (PLLA), Sculptra®, has been used for many years in resorbable sutures, plates and screws for orthopedic use, and neurological and craniofacial surgery. It is a biodegradable, biocompatible synthetic polymer derived from the alpha-hydroxy-acid family. It has been marketed in Europe since 1999 under the name NewFill®. As a cosmetic injectable, Sculptra® is used to provide volume restoration in those patients with subcutaneous atrophy. It received USA FDA approval in 2004 (Sanofi-Aventis, Paris, France) for the correction of HIV lipoatrophy. It is also used off-label for the correction of lipoatrophy of aging. PLLA is thought to correct lipoatrophy by inducing neocollagenesis via an unknown mechanism. It is believed that this augmentation results from the formation of new, native collagen rather than inhibition of collagen degradation. Increased levels of type I collagen have been identified in histologic sections of treated skin. Breakdown of PLLA into lactic acid occurs slowly over the course of approximately 2 years.

PLLA is different from currently available fillers in that it requires multiple treatments before a true correction is obtained. It should be viewed as a progressive volumizer rather than a wrinkle filler. Immediately following treatment, patients will appear corrected; however, this is due to edema from the injected solution, and it dissipates within a few days after treatment. Most patients will require approximately three to six treatment sessions for adequate correction. Patients with severe lipoatrophy may require more sessions. Current evidence suggests that PLLA is a long-lasting filler that persists for approximately 2 years. However, in our experience, many patients maintain correction for up to 3 years.

Technique

Because PLLA is different from currently available fillers, in that it requires multiple treatments before a true correction is obtained, its technique will be discussed separately.

PLLA is stored as a freeze-dried product that requires reconstitution. The manufacturer recommends that it be reconstituted with 3–5 mL of sterile water. The authors prefer to reconstitute at least 24 hours prior to injection with 5 cm^3 of sterile water. Prior to injection, 2 cm^3 of plain lidocaine is added, for total dilutional amount of 6 cm^3. Each vial is thoroughly mixed using a vortex and the material is drawn up into two 3 cm^3 syringes. A 1-inch, 27-gauge needle is attached to the loaded syringe.

Prior to injecting PLLA, the laboratory vortex is also used to mix the syringes so that a uniform suspension is maintained.[25]

The most common area to be augmented is the cheek. Some advocate augmentation of the temple and hands, but the authors feel that the risk of subcutaneous papules is too high in this region. Once the area to be injected has been outlined, the syringe is advanced into the subcutaneous tissue while the injector's non-dominant hand stretches the skin. The product is then evenly deposited into the subcutaneous tissue using fan-like movements with the linear retrograde technique pivoted around each injection point. This process is repeated at approximately two to four other injection points until an equal amount of PLLA has been placed in the outlined areas. When inserting the needle, one feels a loss of resistance when the subcutaneous space has been entered. Strict attention must be paid to inject PLLA in the subcutaneous layer and not in the dermis. Dermal injections can lead to post-treatment papules and irregularity. It is equally important to cease injection before removing the syringe, in order to avoid inadvertent dermal injection. Care should also be taken to avoid treating above the orbital rim or below the mandible. Needle clogging can occur, so extra needles should be kept on the treatment tray. During a given treatment session, the authors typically inject 0.5 vial per cheek for mild lipoatrophy and 1 vial per cheek for moderate-to-severe lipoatrophy. An assistant massages the treated areas for 5 minutes immediately after treatment. The patient is instructed to self-massage the area for 5 minutes per day for approximately 1 week. In addition, patients are instructed to apply ice to the treated areas post injection.

Complications and Contraindications

There are no absolute contraindications to injection of PLLA. Relative contraindications include active infection or inflammation in the area to be injected. In addition, patients who are using anticoagulants should be warned that they may experience an increased risk of bruising or hematoma formation. This warning should apply to any injectable. Common adverse effects following treatment include inflammation, bruising and edema in approximately 5–10% of patients. Because PLLA is a synthetic, non-animal-based polymer composed of the same material that is commonly used in absorbable sutures, there is minimal risk of an allergic reaction. In some patients, dermal or subcutaneous papules can occur months later (Fig. 9.9). This is thought to be due to uneven subcutaneous placement or inadvertent dermal injection of PLLA. These papules, however, are usually small and non-visible. They can be minimized by ensuring even placement of PLLA in the subcutaneous tissue and massaging the treated areas following treatment.

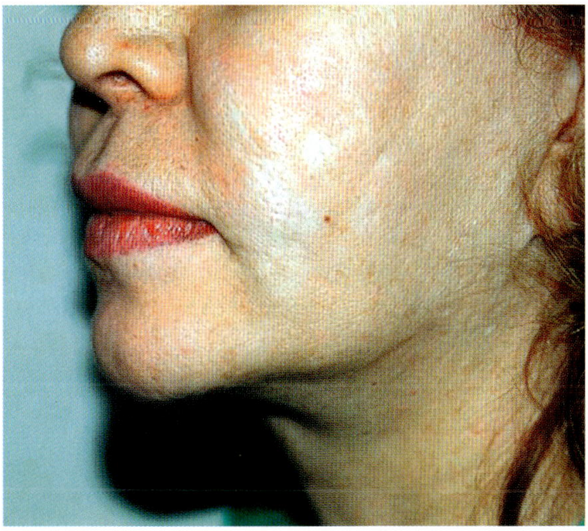

Fig. 9.9 Nodular formation 2 months post Sculptra® injection on cheeks. Courtesy of Dr Alessandra Haddad.

SYNTHETIC CALCIUM HYDROXYLAPATITE

Synthetic calcium hydroxylapatite (CaHA; Radiance® FN, Radiesse®; BioForm Inc., Franksville, WI) is a high-density, low-solubility bioceramic compound of microspheres in a water-based gel carrier. The FDA originally approved it for such uses as treating vocal cord insufficiency, augmenting the neck of the bladder to treat urinary incontinence and treating periodontal defects. It was also used as a radiological tissue marker. In late 2006, the FDA approved Radiesse® for long-lasting correction of moderate-to-severe facial wrinkles and folds, and correction of facial lipodistrophy on HIV-positive patients. It acts as a scaffold for stimulating collagen production. It is used most commonly for nasolabial folds[26] (Figs 9.10 and 9.11) and marionette lines, malar and jaw enhancement, tear trough deformity, areas of bone depression or bone erosion, depressed scars, and in areas requiring soft tissue filling. Sklar and White reported treating 64 patients over a period of 6 months.[27] All patients showed clinical improvement, a high level of satisfaction and minimal side effects (bruising, swelling, lip nodules and tear through overcorrection). The authors do not personally recommend Radiesse® for lip augmentation due to visible nodular formation. When treating tear trough correction Radiesse® has to be placed deeply over the periorbital periosteum. When this is not done correctly, the white color of the product can be visible under the skin. Because Radiesse® is completely biocompatible, no pretreatment allergy testing is required (Table 9.3). Radiesse comes in presentation of prepacked 1.5 cc, 0.8 cc and 0.33 cc, for big, moderate and touch up corrections, respectively. The FDA just approved its dilution on 0.2 cc lidocaine, and the technique uses a female-to-female Luer lock connector (Baxa®, Englewood, Co). It has decreased patients' discomfort during treatment and no topical anesthesia or overcorrection is required.

NON-BIODEGRADABLE AND COMBINATION FILLERS

Non-biodegradable fillers and combination fillers that mix biodegradable and non-biodegradable substances are the 'permanent fillers.' These injectables are made from a variety of materials, ranging from polymethylmethacrylate (PMMA) to silicone. Most of these substances are designed to be encapsulated by one's own body collagen and remain as a permanent to semipermanent solution for tissue deficiencies and simple cosmetic enhancement. Many are not yet available in

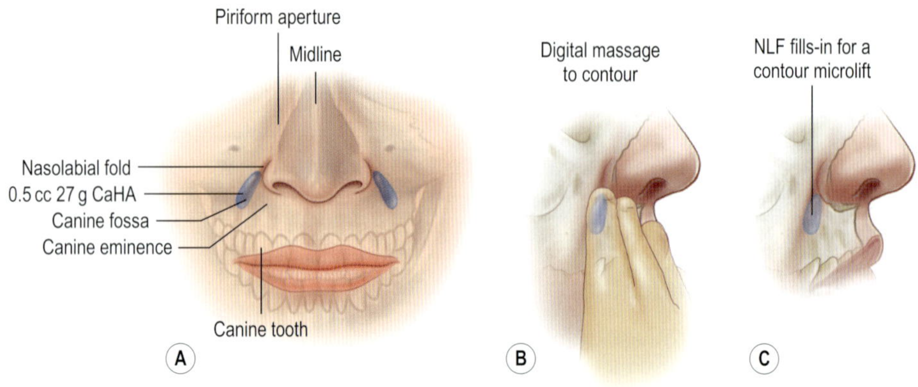

Fig. 9.10 Fosa caninae technique.

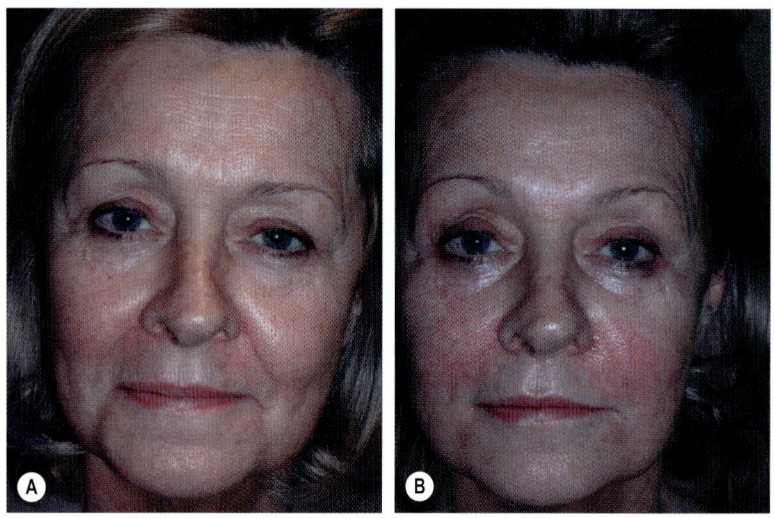

Fig. 9.11 *A*, Before Radiesse® injection on fossa caninae and melomental areas. *B*, Immediately after Radiesse® injection on fossa caninae and melomental areas.

the USA – at least not with FDA approval. The American Society for Aesthetic Plastic Surgery keeps track of what injectables and dermal fillers are approved on the FDA website (www.fda.gov).

Silicone

The clinical use in humans of pure silicone (polymers of dimethylsiloxane) preceded controlled studies in animals. In the 1960s, Dow Corning produced medical-grade silicone for lubricating and coating containers, and for use in skin lotions. It was not intended to be injected into human tissue. Very quickly, liquid silicone for injection purposes became very popular in Asia, Europe and Latin America. The first significant injections of silicone was in Japan, but it was, reportedly, adulterated with olive oil.[28] In the USA, Conway and Goulian reported injecting silicone into the breast and face.[29] In 1965, the FDA declared that injectable silicone was a drug and required Dow Corning to file an investigational new drug application for injectable silicone. In spite of its long history of use for soft tissue augmentation, silicone was never approved by the FDA for that purpose. There are two products available in the USA that are FDA-approved for ophthalmic use. They are Adatosit-5000® and Silikon®. To prescribe silicone injections for soft tissue augmentation constitutes an off-label use.

Despite many problems with product quality, injectable silicone gained popularity throughout the world, and the technique of injecting it into the dermis and subcutaneous tissue in small amounts (microdroplets) – with 1–2 mm of separation[30] at

Table 9.3 Biodegradable fillers FDA approved in the USA (non-collagen derived)

Product	Source	Approved indication in U.S.	FDA approval	Duration	Injection needle
Restylane®	Bacterial fermentation NASHA technology	For the correction of moderate to severe facial wrinkles and folds and lips	December 2003	6–8 months	30 gauge
Perlane®	Bacterial fermentation NASHA technology	FDA approved; designed for shaping facial contours (such as in the cheeks and chin), correcting deep folds	May 2007	9–12 months	27gauge
Captique™	Hyaluronan-synthesized via bacterial fermentation	For the correction of moderate to severe facial wrinkles and folds	December 2004	4–6 months	
Juvéderm 30 HV®	Produced by bacterial fermentation	For the correction of moderate to severe facial wrinkles and folds	June 2006	9–12 months	27 gauge
Juvéderm 24 HV®	Produced by bacterial fermentation	For the correction of moderate to severe facial wrinkles and folds	June 2006	6–8 months	30 gauge
Juvéderm 30®	Produced by bacterial fermentation	For the correction of moderate to severe facial wrinkles and folds	June 2006	9–18 months	27 gauge
Hylaform®	Animal derived from rooster combs	For the correction of moderate to severe facial wrinkles and folds	April 2004	4–6 months	30 gauge
Hylaform Plus®	Animal derived from rooster combs	Shaping facial contours (such as in the cheeks and chin), correcting deep folds and for lip augmentation	October 2004	6–8 months	27 gauge
Elevess®	Produced by bacterial fermentation	Correction of moderate to severe facial wrinkles and folds	October 2004	6–8 months	30 gauge
Slowly biodegradable filters					
Sculptra™	Poly-L-lactic acid	For the restoration and/or the correction of lipoatrophy in patients with HIV	August 2004	1–2 years	26 gauge
Radiesse™	Calcium hydroxylapatite microspheres suspended in an aqueous gel	Long-lasting correction of moderate to severe facial wrinkles and folds, such as nasolabial folds. Radiesse also received a second FDA approval for the long-lasting correction of facial fat loss (lipoatrophy) in people with human immunodeficiency virus (HIV)	December 2006	1–2 years	27 gauge

each treatment site – has become crucial for successful treatment. A fibroplastic reaction to the foreign material is responsible for the permanent progressive result, and that is why we should make an attempt to undercorrect the patients. The technique should be repeated every 6 months until the desired effect is obtained. The adverse effects of silicone injected in humans are inflammation, hardness, ulceration, migration, change in coloration and granulomas. In the case of silicone injection for breast augmentation, the migration of silicone particles in axillary lymph nodes has been reported.[31,32]

Artefill® (Artes Medical, USA) is the latest generation of Artecoll®, which is available in Europe. It is a suspension of PMMA beads, 32–40 μm particles in size, in 3.5 bovine collagen suspension. Artefill® has been FDA-approved since 2005. Since it is the only permanent filler with FDA approval for facial use, proper patient selection is of utmost importance.

Like other bovine collagen preparations, Artefill® has to be tested prior to injection to rule out an intolerance to bovine protein. To diminish their electrostatic force, the beads are polished. This has decreased the frequency of granulomas, which was relatively high with the old preparation (Artecoll®). Pollack recommends a conservative approach with small volume (undercorrection) and long interval between injections.[33] Artefill® is injected into the immediate subdermis or at the deepest dermal level, for deep rhytids and folds. Patients with thin skin, defects that are not well defined or large pores are not good candidates, since it can lead to lumpiness, beading and rigging. In general, two or three treatments are necessary, depending on the area corrected. There is an immediate filling effect, due to the collagen in the preparation, which is slowly resorbed in 2–3 months and then substituted by a neosynthesis of collagen, stimulated by the microspheres of PMMA that are encapsulated by the body's own collagen. This process takes from 2 to 4 months.

The results are reported to be good and permanent. However, when granulomas develop, they should be carefully, and immediately, treated with intralesional triamcinolone. According to Acalay et al. they resolve well.[34] Care should be taken to prevent skin atrophy due to the steroid treatment. Surgical removal of granulomas is difficult and can be mutilating. Recently, granuloma formations associated with Artecoll® and Artefill®, which occurred many years after their injection, have been observed following a laser skin resurfacing and during an interferon treatment for viral hepatitis. It is therefore suggested that patients undergoing any immunomodulating therapy should be asked if they have had previous injection of long-lasting or permanent fillers. For lip augmentation, where there seems to be a higher incidence of beading, Carruthers and Carruthers recommend pretreating the orbicularis oris with botulinum toxin.[5] In the opinion of the authors, since we do not like to compromise safety for longevity, better alternatives than Artefill® are available today for lip enhancement.

OTHER NON-FDA-APPROVED PERMANENT FILLERS

Artecoll® (RMI, The Netherlands) is approved in Europe and Canada, and comprises 30–60 μm PMMA beads, 3.5% bovine collagen and 0.3% lidocaine. As mentioned previously, it is the precursor of Artefill®, FDA-approved in 2005. Acalay and colleagues have reported late-onset granuloma formation[34] (Fig. 9.12).

Bioalkamide® (Polymekon, Italy) is another homogenous permanent gel preparation of polyalkylimide. As with the other permanent gel preparations, it gives good results when it is tolerated. However, allergic reactions appear to be common and may come with huge edematous swelling and/or granuloma formation. Allergic reactions may be treated with steroid injections. In addition, incision and expression works remarkably well with this gel.[2] Bioalkamide® has CE Marking as a humanitarian-use device (HUD) for treating severe lipodistrophy.

Aquamid® (Contura International A/S, Soeborg, Denmark) is made of hydrophilic polyacrylamide, which can absorb between 300 and 400 times its original weight in water. It has also been used for over a decade as a filler in cosmetic applications, nasolabial folds, lip augmentation and facial irregularities. Although the results are permanent, they are, reportedly, reversible with dilution and aspiration. Nodular formation and abnormal swelling have been reported from 1 week to a year following its injection.[35]

Bioplastique® is injectable solid silicone microspheres suspended in a polyvinylpyrrolidone carrier that is used as a contouring injectable.[36] It has CE Marking.

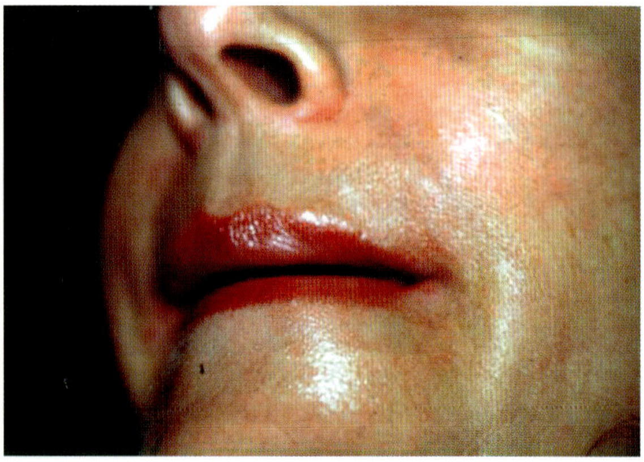

Fig. 9.12 Granuloma formation on upper lip post Artecoll® injection. Courtesy of Dr Alessandra Haddad.

Biopolimero®, also known as silicone oil, comes in 350, 1000 and 5000 centistokes. The higher the number, the more viscous the oil. This product is permanent and difficult to remove.

Dermagen® is a mineral-based dermal filler that comprises silica and oxygen.

DermaLive® or DermaDeep® is a French injectable implant manufactured by Derma Tech and, reportedly, distributed in over 40 countries. It is a HA-based dermal filler with added acrylic hydrogel (a non-resorbable component). This product comprises positively charged, porous, polyvinyl microspheres suspended in a polyacrylamide gel. The microspheres are manufactured of the same suture material already used very successfully in microsurgery. After injection, the hydrophilic acrylic hydrogel attracts a great amount of water and forms minute particles that stimulate collagen synthesis, thus sustaining a very long-lasting effect. It is not degradable by the human body. If side effects occur, they will remain as long as the material is in the skin.

There is a very high risk of granuloma formation, which starts as small palpable nodules that most patients can feel as hard nodules even before they become obvious for other people (Figs 9.13 and 9.14). Surgical removal is the treatment, but once the patient reacts with granulomas, they will continue to develop new nodules that have to be removed. Histopathologically (Figs 9.15 and 9.16) well-demarcated foreign-body granulomas are seen with a fibrous pseudocapsule and polygonal foreign bodies in a dense granulomatous and partly fibrous tissue. Areas of necrosis develop, and fistula formation is not rare.[2] Apparently, a bacterial biofilm may

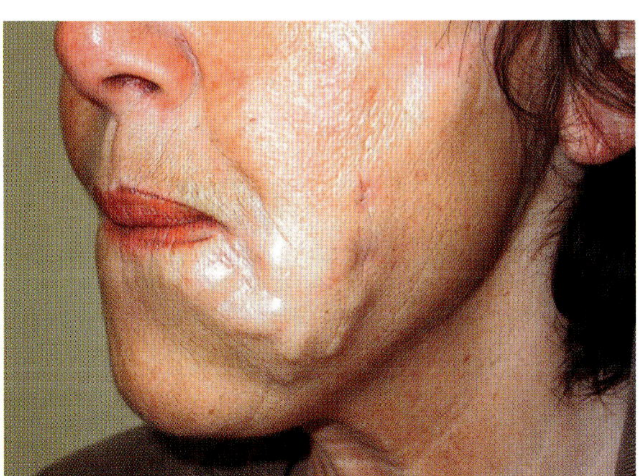

Fig. 9.13 Well-demarcated foreign-body granulomas post Dermalive® injection. Courtesy of Professor Eckart Haneke.

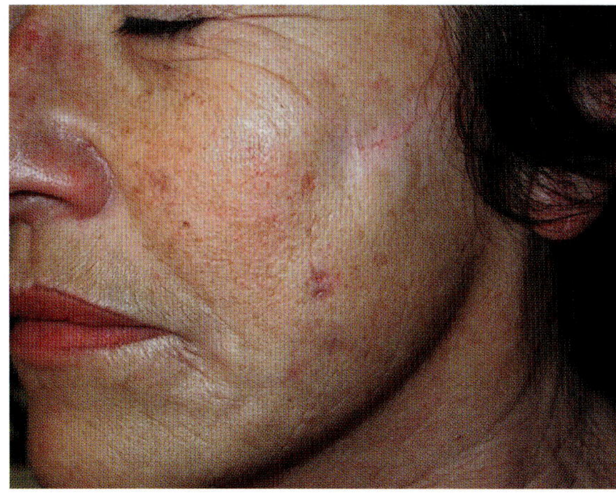

Fig. 9.14 Postsurgical extirpation of granulomas. Courtesy of Professor Eckart Haneke.

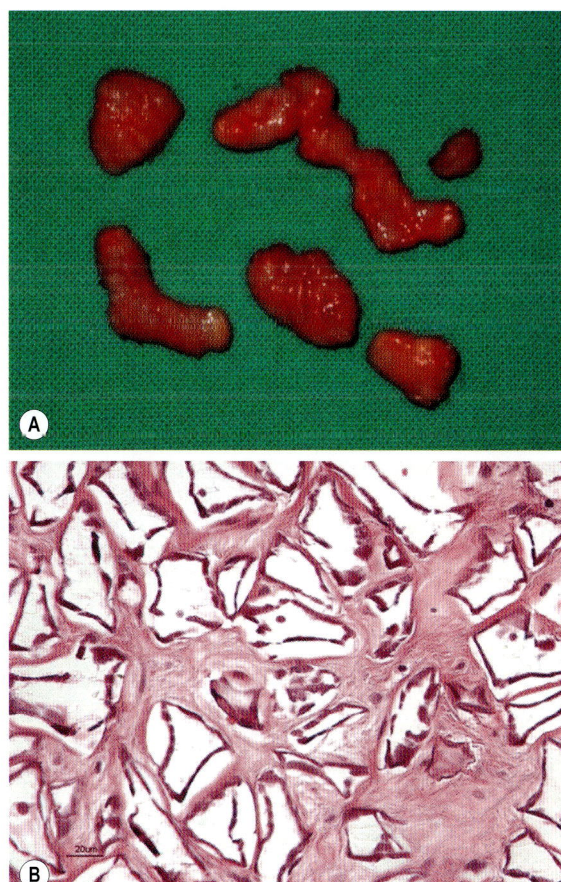

Fig. 9.15 Macroscopy of granulomas.

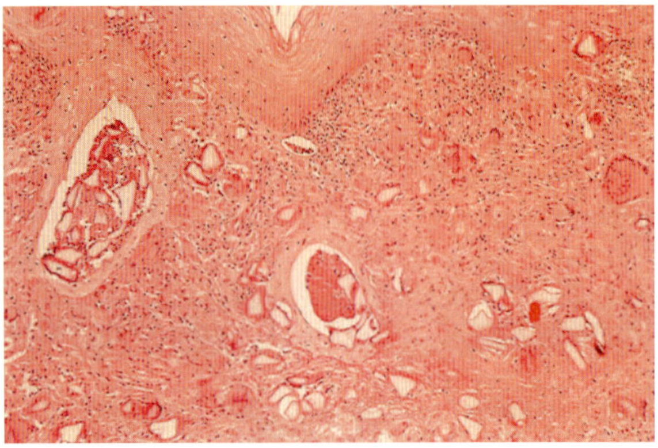

Fig. 9.16 Microscopic aspect of fibrous pseudocapsule and polygonal foreign bodies in a dense granulomatous and partially fibrous tissue. Areas of necrosis develop and fistula formation is not rare. Apparently, a bacterial biofilm may form on the surface of the acrylic particles. Courtesy of Professor Eckart Haneke.

form on the surface of the acrylic particles. It is thought that this phenomenon may be the reason for late abscess formation following injection of these fillers.

They should not be injected over other products; if a temporary injectable has been given before, it has to be fully dissipated before injecting the acrylic hydrogel. Since complications such as infection and local inflammation are rather common, the treatment area should not be touched, and, if the area has to be cleaned, it should be done with a sterile gauze pad and rubbing alcohol. Cosmetic creams or moisturizers should not be applied, and the injection site should be kept free of cosmetics, oils, etc. for at least 12 hours. Failure to do so can result in infections and abscesses (Fig. 9.17). These products can be found in Australia, the UK and Africa, and throughout Europe and Asia. It has CE Marking. DermaDeep® is intended for the deepest layers of the skin to correct tissue deficiencies or for tissue contouring; DermaLive® is intended for more superficial layers. Both products are not suitable for superficial wrinkles.[2]

Evolution® consists of polyvinylhydroxide microspheres suspended in acrylamide. The product is generally well tolerated, but it can also induce a foreign body reaction. Results reportedly last 2–3 years or more.

Metacrill®, made in Brazil by Metacril, comprises PMMA microspheres suspended in a clear carrier made from carboxymethylcellulose.

Outline®, manufactured in France, is made up of positively charged hydrophilic polyacrylamide gel with an unknown percentage of residual unpolymerized acrylamide monomer. Its pH is 7.4. It comprises only positively charged hydrophilic polyacrylamide gel. The positive charge attracts the negatively charged HA and other glucosaminoglycans. Outline is presented in three forms and can be injected into the mid-dermis, deep dermis and just below the dermis.[2]

General Treatment Techniques

Regardless of which dermal filler is used, the choice of the product and the correct depth of application are critical for the optimum result.

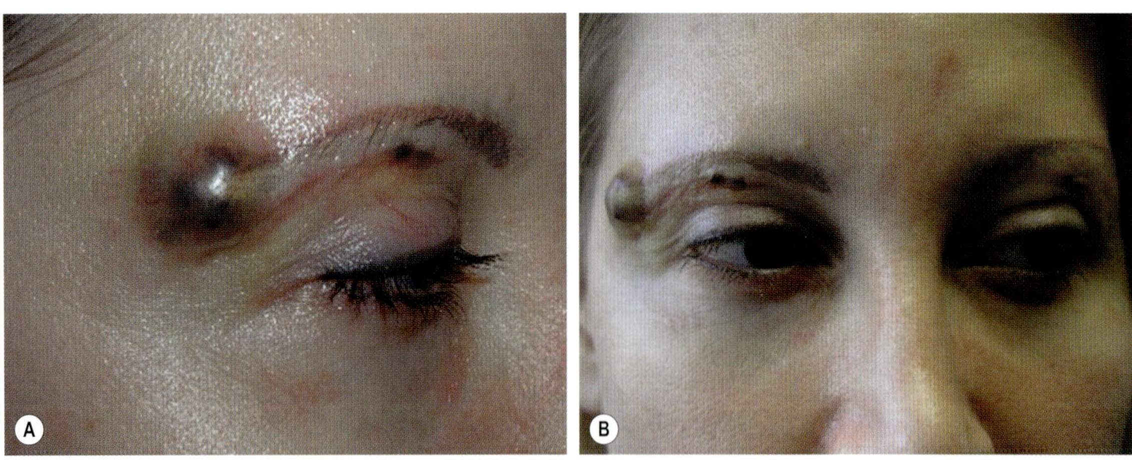

Fig. 9.17 *A*, Patient at 6 months post injection with Dermalive® in Paris, as an attempt to elevate her eyebrows. Necrotic and painful inflammatory granuloma formation secondary to the injection. Removing the necrotic material by surgery is the only treatment indicated. Courtesy of Dr Marian Cantisano-Zilkha. *B*, Frontal view of same patient. Courtesy of Dr Marian Cantisano-Zilkha.

Patients are treated while sitting in an upright position. They are given three sublingual arnica montana C5 pellets immediately before the injections and advised to continue taking them four times daily for 3 days. The areas to be injected are first cleansed to remove make-up, and a headband is applied to keep the hair away. Photographs taken before and after the injection are paramount for future publications or for comparative purposes. As mentioned previously, most collagen products (except Evolence® and Sculptra® when reconstituted) contain lidocaine in their formulations, which reduces the discomfort associated with injection. In contrast, most HA products (except Elevess®) do not contain anesthetic agent; therefore we should apply either topical anesthetic or regional blocks, or inject the area around the treatment site with local anesthetic in a 'field block' fashion (such as mini-dental blocks or 'depression blocks'), taking care not to create too much tumescence and distort the defect. The peripheral nerve blocks (supra- and infraorbital, and mental) will provide deeper anesthesia, but some degree of distortion.

If a topical anesthetic is used, Natragel™ (Gel Concepts LLC., Whippany, NJ) is applied, for a deeper penetration of the material and some vasoconstrictive effect. Ice may be applied before and after injection.

Four different implantation techniques are generally used: linear threading, serial puncture, fanning and cross-hatching. Regardless of the technique being used, the injection should be administered slowly to minimize discomfort, bruising and adverse outcomes secondary to technique injection.

Serial puncture is technically the easiest method because the needle tip does not move during injection. The needle enters the skin to the desired depth, a small amount of filler is deposited, and the needle is withdrawn. It is a favorite technique for beginners. It can be a good technique for glabella, distensible acne scars and lip augmentation, right on the bulk of the mucosa, or to create definition, to the philtrum (Fig. 9.18). The injection sites should be close together, to prevent gaps, and the skin should be tightly pulled from the injection site. After the injection, the area should be gently massaged to create a smooth layer.

The linear threading is the most popular technique. It involves holding the needle parallel to the length of the wrinkle on the dermal level or fold that is being treated, piercing the skin, creating a tunnel, advancing the needle and injecting the material in either a retrograde or an anterograde fashion, making sure to stop injecting before withdrawing the needle. This technique is ideal for vermilion border, nasolabial folds and tear trough deformities.[22] We should also use the 'Restylane push technique,'[26] where we apply a certain amount of the filler over the periosteum, in a retrograde fashion, and then gently massage it over the defect (Fig. 9.19).

The fanning and cross-hatching techniques are variations of linear threading. They can be used in areas where a larger volume of filler is needed or when a multicontoured area is being filled with a product such as Sculptra®, which was previously described (Fig. 9.20).

The puncture and linear threading techniques are the most used techniques for soft tissue augmentation (collagen, HA, L-polylactic acid, calcium hydroxylapatite and the non-biodegradable products). The fanning and cross-hatching techniques are also suitable for HA products and L-polylactic acid therapies, and, often, when a broad area of defect is covered. (This technique is described separately because of its uniqueness of reconstitution, which is the key for success.)

COMPLICATIONS

Complications can be technique dependent, filler dependent or both. Once you carefully and consciously choose the best and safest filler for the particular area to be injected, the most frequent reasons for patient dissatisfaction are inappropriate placement or superficial placement. To further reduce the chance of problems, there are general

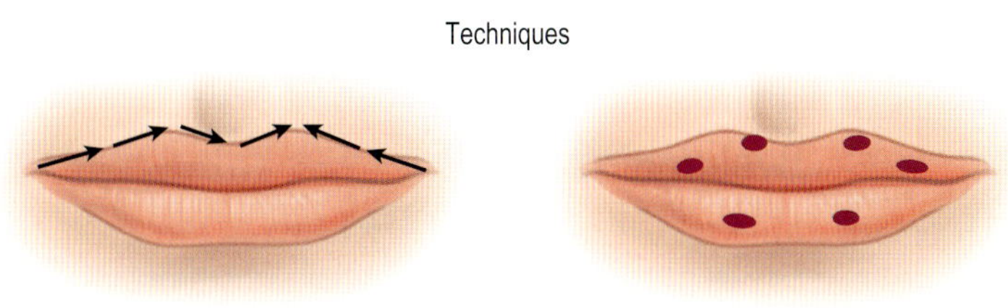

Fig. 9.18 Serial and puncture techniques for lip augmentation.

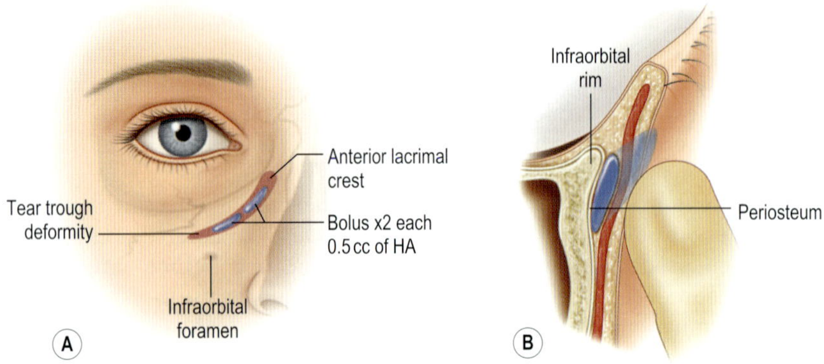

Fig. 9.19 Treatment of tear trough deformities.

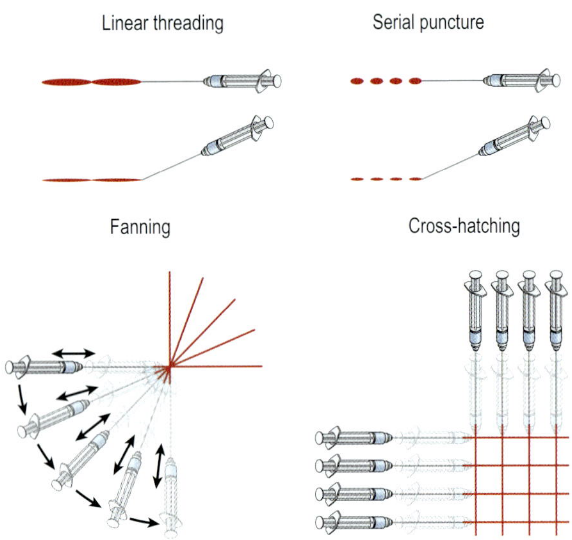

Fig. 9.20 Injection techniques.

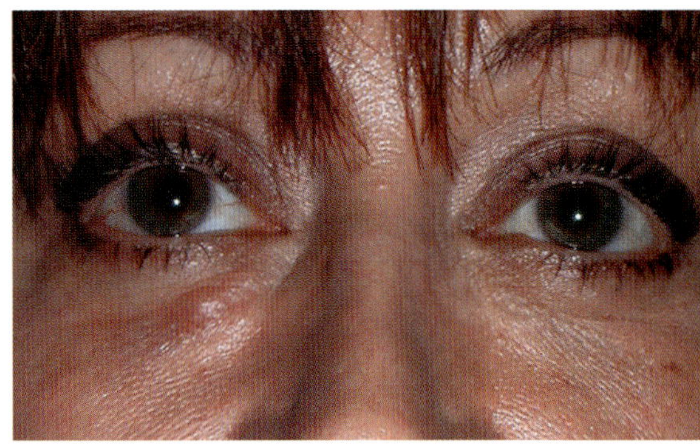

Fig. 9.21 Superficial placement of HA on right lower lid. This can be easily corrected with diluted injection of the enzyme hyaluronidase. Courtesy of Dr Marian Zilkha.

guidelines related to the injection technique, the site of correction and volume techniques. You may even combine chemically different fillers and still be very safe. Due to the reversibility of HA, complications from these fillers can be easily corrected (Fig. 9.21), with diluted intradermal or subcutaneous injections of hyaluronidase (Hydase®, Vitrase®), on the site to be corrected. Sensitivity to any of the currently approved FDA products is quite rare and can usually be managed with antiinflammatory agents. Infection is also quite uncommon and can usually be managed with either antibiotics or antivirals, depending on the clinical features. The most concerning complication of fillers is cutaneous necrosis.[37,38]

Patients reluctantly accept localized bruising and puncture marks at the injection sites. They can be minimized with the use of topical vasoconstricting anesthetic agents, cutaneous pre- and postinjection cooling with Natragel® masks and ice, and applying postinjection pressure.

In areas such as the glabella, there is a danger of creating local vascular occlusion with local development of necrosis and retinal vascular obstruction, therefore some practitioners completely avoid injecting that area. The authors recommend soft biodegradable fillers, low volumes, slow injection technique and keeping injections on a very superficial dermal plane.

Hyaluronic Acid

Mild transient localized erythema is the exception rather than the rule following HA implantation. Local areas of hardening and gel aggregation at the injection sites can often be palpated for several days. Although they are rarely visible, the patient should be told that this is not unusual and will become less apparent with time. Following lip augmentation, superficial injections can leave more visible lumps. Because the product is very hydrophilic, any localized irritation and increased secondary edema will amplify their prominence. To avoid this, patients should be instructed not to rub the areas with their tongue. In areas of superficial implantation or translucent skin, the gel may be visualized as a gray shadow through the skin. Most female patients prefer the correction of the cutaneous depression and do not object to the grayish shadow, the Tyndall effect. However, they must be advised of it before the treatment.

Localized edema following implantation is usually not problematic and may even accentuate the correction (Fig. 9.22). The authors instruct patients that if the correction is less evident in 5–7 days, this is not because the gel has dissipated but because they need more volume implanted. Patients are asked to return in 7–10 days for a possible touch-up. During 1996 and 1997, the authors saw two cases of sterile, suppurating granulomas with onsets 10–14 days following the initial injections. One required incision and drainage, the other was self-limited, with complete resolution after 16 days. No other similar reactions have been seen with Restylane® or Perlane® since 1997.[38–40] Delayed reaction to Hylaform® or Hylaform Plus® may be somewhat different because they are cross-linked products of avian origin. In areas where there has been an over-filling, or where the implantation of HA has been too superficial, patients may not want to wait for the naturally occurring breakdown. These areas can be injected with diluted dose of hyaluronidase (Hydase® or Vitrase®) and the defect dissipates within 24 hours.

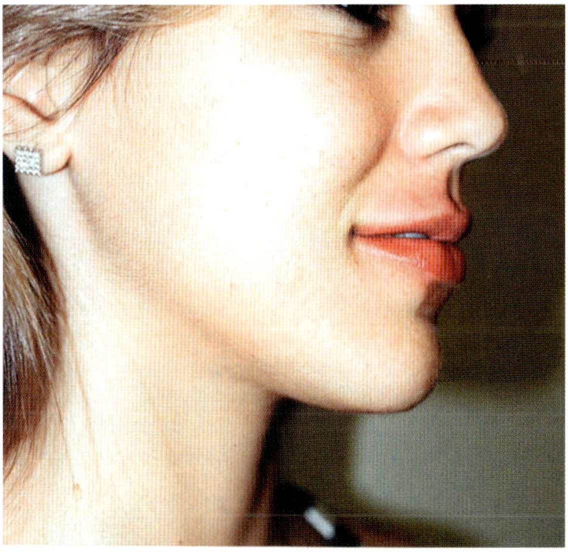

Fig. 9.22 Angioneurotic edema post hyaluronic lip injection. Courtesy of Dr Alessandra Haddad.

Collagen

Even the patients with two negative skin tests may eventually exhibit an inflammatory response following implantation and require corticosteroid injections; these patients may develop localized atrophy at the injection sites or develop subcutaneous scarring in the long term. This becomes evident when other products are used for volume augmentation at a later date. There has also been some controversy regarding sequential collagen implantation and the development or exacerbation of autoimmune and collagen-vascular diseases.[40–42] Although patients with known inflammatory responses to collagen are discouraged from undergoing further treatments with human fibroblast-derived collagen, it is hoped that these products will produce less inflammatory responses in fewer patients (Table 9.4).

Non-biodegradable Fillers

An Internet search for fillers reveals a great number of preparations, most of which have no FDA or EU approval. Their production standards and quality are sometimes questionable. However, because they are usually sold at a much lower price, they are tempting for some users and potential patients.

Table 9.4 Adverse sequelae and complications associated with collagen injections
Bovine and human:
Redness, edema, bruises
Infection, herpetic or acneiform eruption
Contour irregularity (wrong placement)
Intravascular injection, tissue necrosis, blindness
Bovine:
Hypersensitivity reaction: cyst, granuloma

The authors expressively warn against the use of unapproved fillers even though they may come with a 'certificate of good production' and claims of perfect purity and good tolerability. The physician always remains legally responsible for what he or she does. Patients seeking, and paying for, aesthetic procedures to improve their appearance will not hesitate to litigate, and it will be the physician's problem to prove that approved, top-quality products were used.

Bacterial infections are late adverse events associated with gels and particulate preparations that may become clinically evident as soon as 1–2 weeks, or as late as years after injection. The bacterial cultures often remain negative or may grow so-called non-pathogenic bacteria that are part of the normal resident flora of the skin and/or oral mucosa. Histologically, the lesions are similar to whatever preparation was used: foreign body granuloma containing gel particles, macrophages, lymphocytes, often granulocytes, rarely bacteria, sometimes central necrosis and fistula formation. An early clinical symptom may be a deep-seated tingling followed by swelling. Such an infection will disappear when a degradable substance has been injected, but any infection that develops after non-degradable filler injection requires high-dose antibiotic treatment for at least 2 weeks without prior steroid injections. If non-steroidal antiinflammatory drugs, steroids or low-dose antibiotics were given before the antibiotic treatment, these have to be extended over a month or even longer. Although the material is highly biocompatible and does not move in the tissue, it is an excellent growth medium for many kinds of bacteria. Microscopic examinations suggest that they may form a biofilm on the surface of the polyacrylamide particles. Sometimes, one or more surgical interventions may be necessary and sometimes they can be mutilating (Figs 9.23 and 9.24).

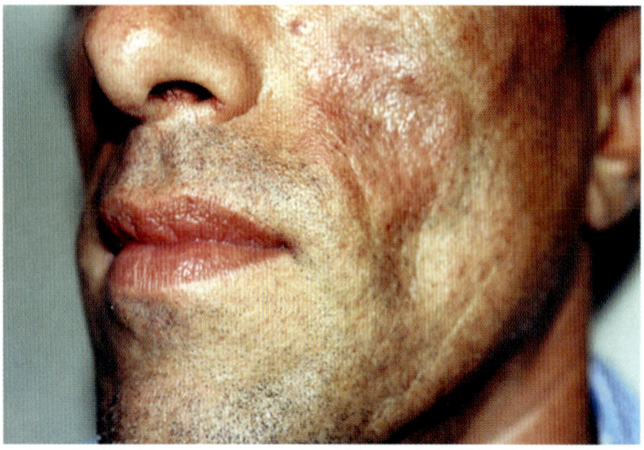

Fig. 9.23 Metacril on cheeks, on facial lipodystrophy; palpable nodular formation. Courtesy of Dr Alessandra Haddad.

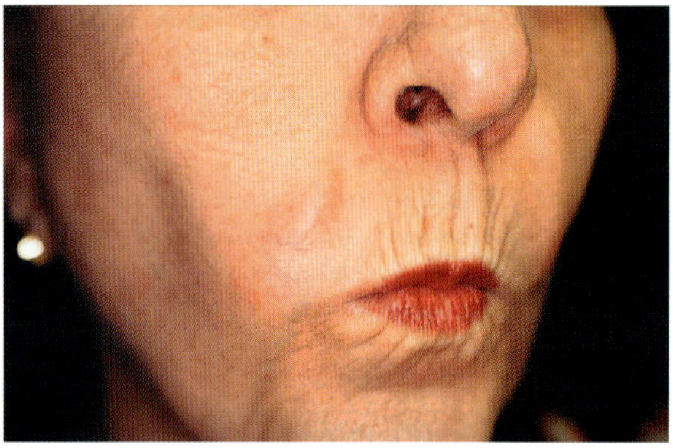

Fig. 9.24 Metacril on nasolabial folds – palpable and painful nodular formation. Courtesy of Dr Alessandra Haddad.

Products containing PMMA microspheres should not be used in the periorbital area because there are the possibilities of a retrograde venous injection and a central retinal vein occlusion with secondary blindness. Although the exact percentage has not been published, many of these patients develop granulomas. Considerable granuloma formation has also been observed many years after PMMA injection after the patient received interferon injections for the treatment of chronic hepatitis C.[42,43] The authors have seen several patients, referred from Europe, who have developed skin ulcerations. The products using bovine collagen to suspend the microspheres may also have complications secondary to bovine collagen use. Products containing HA in suspension may also have complications secondary to the source of HA.

Poly-Lactic Acid

Poly-lactic acid has to be reconstituted and mixed very well before use. If it is not mixed thoroughly enough at least 24 hours prior to injection and not sufficiently diluted, there may be an increased incidence of granuloma formation. It is very important to know how to differentiate granuloma formation from the accumulation of too much material that has not been totally reconstituted, creating clogs of polylactic acid. In my (MCZ) 6 years of highly successful clinical experience with the use of such a material, I have learned that a practical way to know if the suspension is well mixed is to carefully follow the steps of reconstitution, and to make sure that the suspension does not clog a 27-gauge needle, which is the recommended size for the injection. Clogging will require frequent changing of the needle and increase the likelihood of irregular injection. After the injection is finished, the authors often massage the area with an antibiotic ointment for 10 minutes to make sure that the product is well distributed. If an inflammatory granuloma formation occurs (Fig. 9.9), injection of diluted steroids is recommended. If too much accumulation of material is observed, the authors recommend injecting distilled water in the lesion to dilute and dissolve it.

Silicone

Using microdroplets of ultrapurified silicone in properly selected patients may avoid the extreme, and often unrepairable, complications associated with its abuse. Large volumes of silicone that have been injected will migrate. With time the spreading of the product makes surgical excision difficult or impossible. Because of the adjacent inflammatory reaction, these masses of silicone will be difficult or impossible to remove without leaving significant soft tissue deformities. In case of siliconomas, a TNF-α inhibitor may be tried.

THE FUTURE

New injectable tissue augmentation materials are already in the pipeline. There is a growing interest in products that are longer lasting, but that do not sacrifice safety for longevity, as previously discussed. The availability of products that have fibroplastic properties, and offer great safety and patient satisfaction, is a reality. There is also a great potential for stem cell implantation in the near future. Products containing a combination of HA and dextranomers have already been tested for longer-lasting corrections of facial surface and contour irregularities.

THE KEYS TO SUCCESS/OPTIMIZING OUTCOMES

- Understanding the differences between fillers.
- Understanding differences between static wrinkles and laxity.
- Correct evaluation of the defect.
- Proper choice of the filler.
- Patients with realistic expectations.
- Good technique for application.

CONCLUSIONS

In conclusion, dermal fillers are a true, real, good option for minimally invasive rejuvenation. The complications with dermal fillers can be well prevented, as long as you select safer fillers, follow low-volume and gentle techniques of injection, and use easily-deployed strategies to minimize their incidence and impact.[43,44]

REFERENCES

1 Terino OE. *Three-Dimensional Facial Sculpting*. New York: Informa Healthcare; 2007.
2 Haneke E. Polymethyl methacrylate microspheres in collagen. *Semin Cutan Med Surg*. 2004;23:227–232.
3 Goldberg DJ. Fillers in Cosmetic Dermatology. Informa Healthcare UK, Series in *Cosmetic and Laser Therapy*. 2006;1:4.
4 Panicacci RS, Grossman K. Facial rejuvenation with autologous fat injections. In: Bosniak S, Antisano VCV, Zilkha M, eds. *Minimally Invasive Techniques in Oculoplastic, Orbital and Reconstructive Surgery*. New York: Theime; 1999.
5 Carruthers J, Carruthers A. *Soft Tissue Augmentation*. 2nd ed., vol. 7. Elsevier; 2008:83 (fillers working by Fibroplasia).
6 Goldberg DJ. Fillers in Cosmetic Dermatology. Informa Healthcare UK, Series in *Cosmetic and Laser Therapy*. 2006;1:6–10.
7 Goldberg DJ. Fillers in Cosmetic Dermatology. Informa Healthcare UK, Series in *Cosmetic and Laser Therapy*. 2006;6:137.
8 Matti BA, Nicolle FV. Clinical use of Zyplast in correction of age- and disease-related contour deficiencies of the face. *Aesthetic Plast Surg*. 1990;24:227–234.
9 Stegman SJ, Chu S, Bensch K, Armstrong R. A light and electron microscopic evaluation of Zyderm collagen and Zyplast implants in aging human facial skin: a pilot study. *Arch Dermatol*. 1987;123:1644–1649.
10 Lemperl G, Morhenn V, Charrier U. Human histology and persistence of various injectable filler substances for soft tissue augmentation. *Aesthetic Plast Surg*. 2003;27:354–367.
11 Narins RS, Brandt FS, Lorene ZP, Maas CS, Monheit GD, Smith S. Twelve-month persistency of a novel ribose-cross-linked collagen dermal filler. *Dermatol Surg*. 2009;34(suppl 1):S31–S39.
12 Braun M, Braun S. Nodule formation following lip augmentation using porcine collagen-derived filler. *J Drugs Dermatol*. 2008; 7(6):579–581.
13 *Instructions for use*. Available at www.evolence.com. Accessed June 27, 2008.
14 Yoshiko M, Fumitaka T, Nobuyoshi Hideo S, et al. Atelocollagen-mediated synthetic small interfering RNA delivery for effective gene silencing in vitro and in vivo. *Nucleic Acids Res*. 2004;32:109.
15 Klein AW. Skin filling. Collagen and other injectables of the skin. *Dermatol Clin*. 2001;19(3):491–508, ix.
16 Sclafani AP, Romo 3rd T, Jacono AA, et al. Evaluation of acellular dermal graft sheet (alloderm) and injectable (micronized Alloderm) forms for soft tissue augmentation. Clinical observations and histological analysis. *Arch Facial Plast Surg*. 2000;2 (2):130–136.
17 Fagien S. Facial soft tissue augmentation with injectable autologous and allogenic human tissue collagen matrix (atuologen and dermalogen). *Plast Reconstr Surg*. 2000;105:362–373.
18 Isolagen and FDA Reach Agreement on Phase III Protocol Design. *Dermatology News*. Oct. 14, 2006.
19 Agerup B, Wik O. *NASHA: the Monograph*. Uppsala, Sweden: Q-Med; 2001.

20 Narins RS, Brandy F, Leyden J, et al. A randomized, double-blind, multicenter comparison of the efficacy and tolerability of Restylane versus Zyplast for the correction of nasolabial folds. *Dermatol Surg*. 2003;29:588–595.
21 Bosniak S, Cantisano-Zilkha M, Glavas JP. Injectable fillers. In: Bosniak S, Cantisano-Zilkha M, eds. *Minimally Invasive Techniques of Oculofacial Rejuvenation*. New York: Theime; 2005.
22 Bosniak S, Sadick N, Cantisano-Zilkha M, Glavas Y, Roy D. Definition of the tear trough and the tear trough rating scale. *J Cosmetic Dermatol*. 2007;6(4):218–225.
23 Approvals FDA. Juvéderm. Available at www.drugs.com. Accessed on February 6, 2007.
24 *Official Site*, www.elevess.com. (accessed October 2008).
25 Leonard AL, Hanke CW. *J Am Acad Dermatol*. 2006;55:511-512. Surgical Pearl: the use of a laboratory vortex for poli-L-lactic acid injection.
26 Ahn MS. Calcium hydroxylapatite: radiesse. *Facial Plast Surg Clin North Am*. 2007;15(1):85–90, vii.
27 Sklar JA, White SM, Radiance FN. A new soft tissue filler. *Dermatol Surg*. 2004;30:764.
28 Rees TD, Platt J, Ballantyne DL. An investigation of cutaneous response to dimethylpolysiloxane (silicone liquid) in animals and humans – a preliminary report. *Plast Reconstr Surg*. 1965; 35:131–139.
29 Conway H, Goulian Jr D. Experience with injectable Silastic RTV as a subcutaneous prosthetic material. *Plast Reconstr Surg*. 1963; 32:294–302.
30 Spira M, Rosen T. Injectable soft tissue substitutes. *Clin Plast Surg*. 1993;20:181–188.
31 Nosanchuck JS. Silicone granuloma in breast. *Arch Surg*. 1968;97:583–585.
32 Symmers WstC. Silicone mastitis in 'topless' waitress and some other varieties of foreign-body mastitis. *BMJ*. 1968;iii:19–22.
33 Pollack S. Some new injectable dermal filler materials. Hylaform, Restylane and Artecoll. *J Cutaneous Med Surg*. 1999;3(suppl 4): S27–S37.
34 Acalay J, Alkalay R, Gat A, Yorav S. Late onset granulomatous reaction to Artecoll. *Dermatol Surgery*. 2003;29(8):859–862.
35 Christensen L, Breiting V, Vuust J, Hogdall E. Adverse reactions following injection with permanent facial filler polyacrylamide hydrogel (Aquamid): causes and treatment. *Eur J Plast Surg*. 2006;28(7):464–471.
36 Ellis DA, Segall L. Review of non-FDA-approved fillers. *Facial Plast Surg Clin North Am*. 2007;15(2):239–246.
37 Hanke CW, Higley HR, Lolivette DM, et al. Abscess formation and local necrosis after treatment with Zyderm or Zyplast collagen implant. *J Am Acad Dermatol*. 1991;25(2 Pr 1):319–326.
38 Bosniak S, Cantisano-Zilkha M. Restylane hyaluronic acid gel for facial rejuvenation: A 4-year experience. *J Cosmet Laser Ther*. 2001;3:192–193.
39 Bosniak S. Cantisano-Zilkha M. Glavas IP. Non-animal stabilized hyaluronic acid gel for facial rhytids ablation: a six-year clinical experience. In press.
40 Cukier J, Beauchamp RA, Spindler JS, et al. Association between bovine collagen dermal implants and a dermatomyositis or polymyositis-like syndrome. *Ann Intern Med*. 1993;118(12): 920–928.
41 Trautinger F, Kokoschka EM, Menzel EJ. Antibody formation against human collagen and C1q in response to a bovine collagen implant. *Arch Dermatol Res*. 1991;283(6):395–399.
42 Fischer J, Metzler G, Schaller M. Cosmetic permanent fillers for soft tissue augmentation: a new contraindication for interferon therapies. *Arch Dermatol*. 2007;143:507–510.
43 Glogau R, Kane M. Effect of injecting techniques on the rate of adverse events in patients implanted with non-animal hyaluronic acid dermal fillers. *Dermatol Surg*. 2008;34(1):S105–109.
44 Cantisano-Zilka M. Understanding the uses of injectable fillers and volumizers. In: Zilka M, ed. *Contemporary Guide to Aesthetic Enhancement*. Newtown, PA: Handbooks in Health Care; 2008.

10 Fat Transfer

Luiz Alexandre Lorico Tissiani

INTRODUCTION

Fat transplants have been used in the aesthetic and reconstructive plastic surgery field for more than a century. In 1893, when Neuber[1] first reported on using fat grafts to treat depressed scars, he concluded that fat specimens could not be bigger than an almond. Since that time, numerous surgeons from different medical specialties have utilized fat tissue in a great variety of pathologies.

Lexer[2] used a block of fat tissue to correct a post-traumatic facial deformity and obtained an initial good result. In the long-term follow-up, he observed high rates of contraction and this fact inspired him to use bigger and bigger blocks of fat tissue. He never analyzed his grafts under the microscope. To improve the integration of fat grafts, May[3] incorporated fascia to fat tissue grafts, and Peer[4] chose to add the dermis to fat tissue. In 1957, Schorcher[5] treated patients with hypomastia using multiple small fragments of fat tissue and observed a 75% loss rate in a 9-month follow-up. Ellenbogen[6] developed the so-called 'fat pearls' with an average size of 8 × 5 mm. He used them in the eyelids and tear troughs, and experienced a 50% loss.

Because so many plastic surgeons have published unsatisfactory results with the use of fat grafts, this technique fell into disgrace for many years until Coleman's first papers were published in the early 1990s.[7,8] His results have given the plastic surgery community a new look at fat grafts. He discovered how to work with fat in a very systematic and reproducible way, which is called 'lipostructure', and has obtained much more favorable results.

In 1998, Lambros[9] published some thoughts about retaining ligaments of the midface as latticework, and its relationship with skin and soft tissues, mainly the fat tissue. There is often a deflation component when the face ages, and this makes volume replacement necessary when rejuvenating a patient's face. The zygomatic area and tear trough are anatomical sites where grafted fat tissue presents very good to excellent survival rates. Conversely, lips and nasolabial folds are the areas with the least graft integration rates.[10]

Considering that fat tissue has been used as a filler, it might be assumed that it has many characteristics of an ideal filler (Table 10.1), and only recently it has been adopted as the main source of adult mesenchymal stem cells.[11,12]

INDICATIONS AND CONTRAINDICATIONS

Fat tissue transplantation can be used whenever the main problem is soft tissue insufficiency caused by surgery, trauma, aging or pathology. In cosmetic surgeries, fat grafts can be used in post-liposuction deformities (Fig. 10.1), in saucer deformity after gynecomastia surgery, and to reestablish, or simply add volume to, all facial areas such as zygomatic (Fig. 10.2), mandibular, mental, temples, lips, nasolabial folds, eyebrows, eyelids, neck, tear troughs, face lifting deformities and acne scars. Cosmetic breast augmentation with fat is possible, but it is a very controversial issue. It deserves a closer evaluation and requires a great knowledge of adipose-derived stem cells (ADSCs) and their handling.

Fat transplants also have many applications in reconstructive surgeries, the most common of which are the Romberg's syndrome (Fig. 10.3) and other pathologies that present with lipodystrophy. Post-traumatic tissue loss in different areas of the body, defects following benign and malignant tumor resections, refinements in breast reconstruction, sequelae of facial paralysis, and sequelae of radiation therapy are all very common reasons for undergoing plastic surgery.[13]

There are very few situations where fat tissue cannot be used. Extreme thinness is the most common contraindication because thin people do not have enough fat tissue to be harvested and grafted. Patients with poor general health are also not candidates for fat grafting.

Table 10.1 Advantages of fat tissue
Low-cost harvesting
Readily and easily obtainable
Possible repeated harvesting
No immune reactions (short or long term)
A source of adipose derived stem cells
Indirect stimulation of angiogenesis

PREOPERATIVE HISTORY AND CONSIDERATIONS

When a patient asks for some facial improvement, it is important to identify exactly what he/she is looking for, what his/her lifestyle is and how long the downtime period can be. Patients with high expectations are tricky, and the surgeon must thoroughly discuss the goals and limitations of the technique. It is also very important to take as many photographs

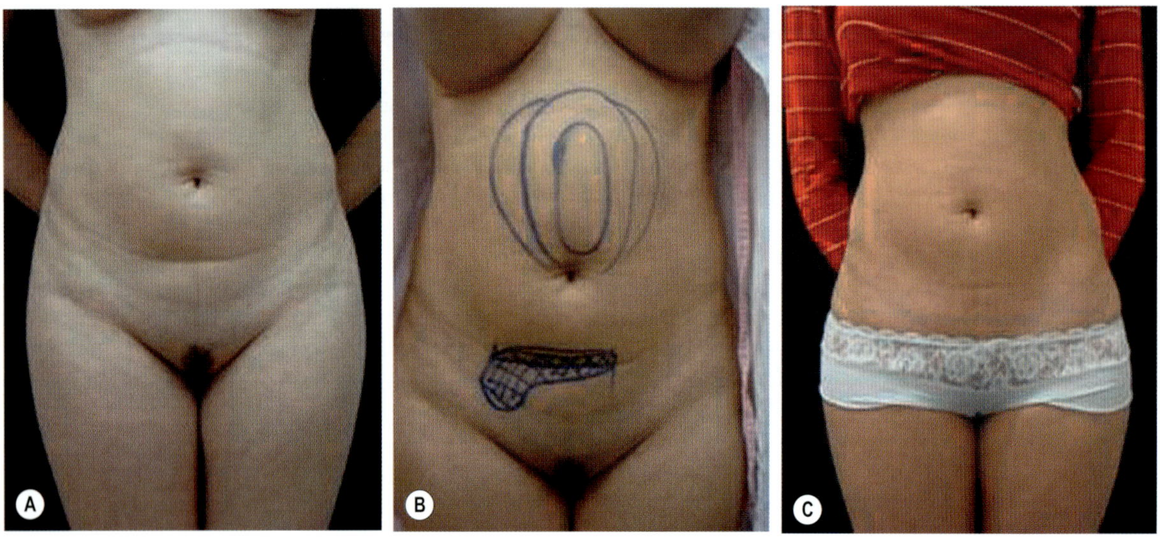

Fig. 10.1 Post-liposuction deformity on the abdomen: preoperative, demarcation and postoperative result after 9 months of structured fat grafting.

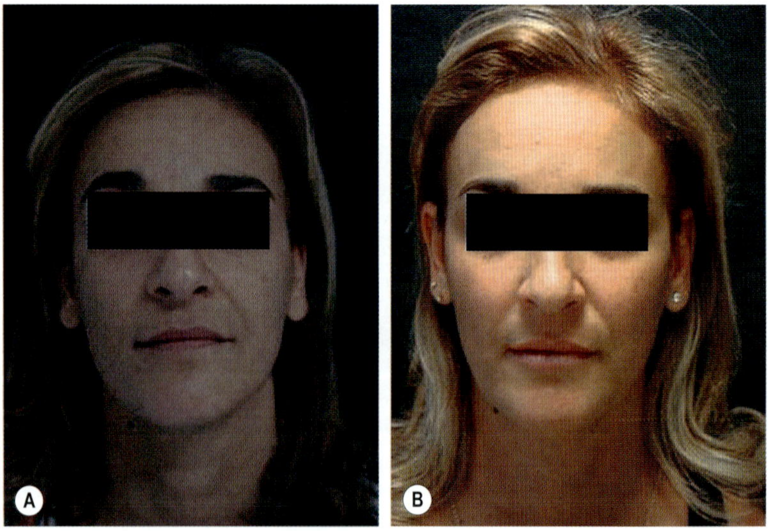

Fig. 10.2 One-year postoperative period of fat grafting to the malar areas and lips.

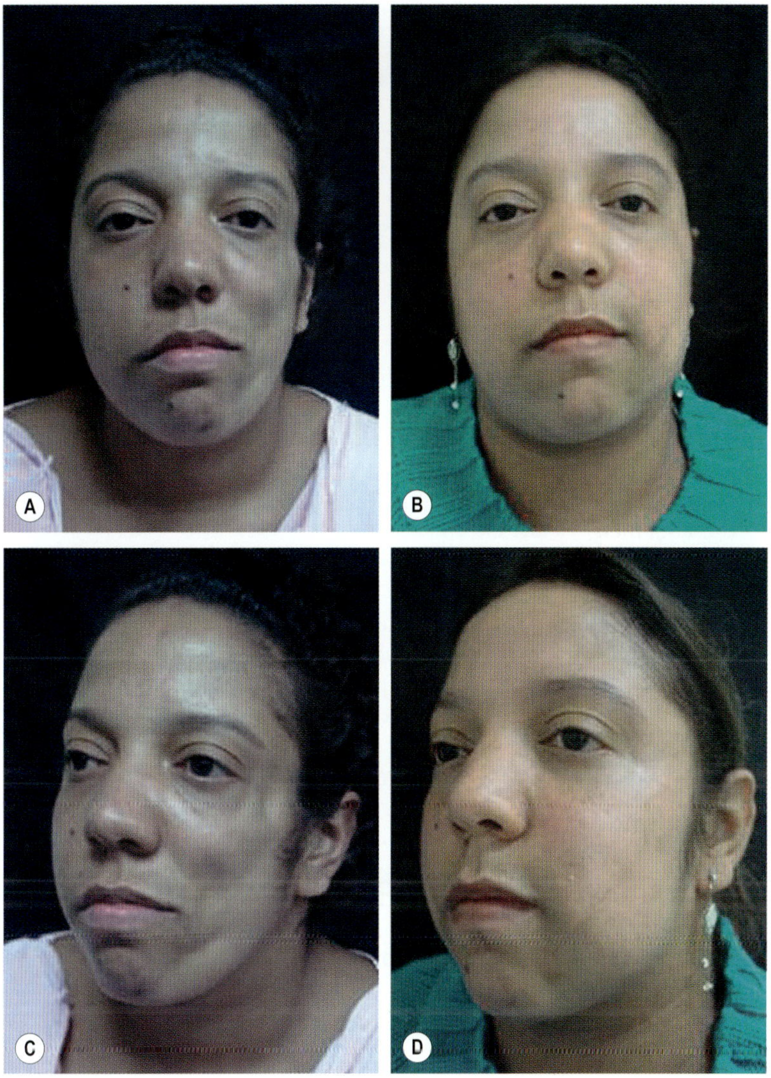

Fig. 10.3 Two years 1-month postoperative two fat grafting sessions for Romberg's syndrome. Patient has put on weight (20 kg) between the first and second procedures. Note the improvement on the periorbital region (lid–cheek junction and temporal fossa).

as possible, from different angles and views, discuss with the patient where the problems are and demonstrate how they will be addressed by making drawings on the photographs. It is a good idea to ask patients to bring you old photographs. This can help you understand how they are aging and can give you clues about what a patient is looking for.

A patient's medical history is a fundamental source of information about pathologies, blood clotting problems, allergies, current medications, previous surgeries and response to anesthesia. It is important to ask about previous cosmetic treatments: when, where, what product was injected, and how often? These questions can give you some information about the patient's self-esteem and may suggest potential problems during fat graft delivery to the host tissue.

On physical examination, check skin quality and sensitivity, mimic musculature work and palpate the whole face in search for small nodules or blurred subcutaneous areas. This can help to identify areas treated with fillers that were missed during the clinical questionnaire.

Do not forget to prepare a good informed consent document with as much information as possible, including a note that a second procedure of fat transfer could be necessary because some absorption might occur. Fat grafts present some volumetric reduction until the sixth month and stabilize by the 12th month. Horl et al.[10] demonstrated this phenomenon very well using magnetic resonance imaging.

OPERATIVE APPROACH

Structured fat grafting involves three important steps: harvesting, preparation and transfer. Fat tissue is obtained through small cannulas (2.5 mm in diameter × 15 cm in length) with two sequenced holes on the tip and under low negative pressure. The plunger of a 10 cm^3 Luer Lok syringe should be pulled back in 2 cm^3 increments. If general anesthesia is employed, a solution of ringer lactate and epinephrine in a final concentration of 1:500 000 is utilized and, if sedation is the option, a solution is made with lidocaine, bupivacaine, sodium bicarbonate, saline and epinephrine.

The abdomen is the preferred donor site. When different areas of the body are compared, some studies show no difference in adipocyte viability and survival rate after harvesting. Usually, the abdomen presents some localized fat and incisions can be placed inside the navel, leaving behind no stigma of surgery.

To optimize centrifugation, syringes full of fat are briefly decanted in a tube rack (Kartell, Labware Division, Noviglio, Italy) before they go into the centrifuge. Plungers are removed and a plastic plug seals the tip of the syringe while a silicone cork closes the upper part. The whole process of centrifugation is completely sterile.

After centrifugation (3000 rpm for 3 min), three well-separated layers are present. The top layer (least dense) is full of oil and cell debris, and the bottom layer is a mixture of blood and anesthetic solution. Both these layers must be discarded by aspirating the oil and draining the blood. The intermediate layer primarily consists of viable fat cells. To check the number of living cells, Boschert et al.[11] specifically subdivided this layer into three parts and concluded that the part close to the bottom layer contained more adipocytes (in number) than the other two parts.

The middle layer is entirely transferred to 1 cm^3 Luer Lok syringes, through a Luer-to-Luer transfer, and grafting maneuvers are started. To do so, microcannulas (which means 'a blunt tip') of 1.0, 1.2 and 1.4 mm in diameter × 7 cm in length, with one hole on the tip, are employed. Multiple layers are done starting deep to the bone, passing through the muscles and ending close to the skin. If necessary, crossing tunnels can be made. The most important thing is to deliver small amounts of fat cells during withdrawal and, usually, to introduce a volume less than 0.1 cm^3, in a radiating pattern during each pass. Needles are never used to graft fat tissue, and 3 cm^3 syringes are not used on the face.

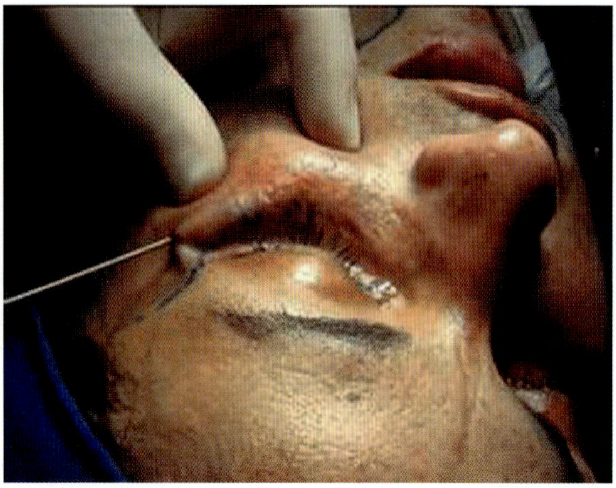

Fig. 10.4 The portal to the orbit is being made with a needle where the microcannula is inserted and positioned under the orbicularis.

To improve tear trough and lid–cheek junction, two portals are done. The first is located lateral to the orbit and approximately 1 cm below a horizontal line that passes at the level of the lateral canthus (Fig. 10.4). The second one is placed at the meeting point of two lines – a vertical one that passes tangential to the lateral limbus and a horizontal one that passes at the level of the nostril sill. The latter portal is also utilized to graft the malar area. Because the portals are made with a 21G needle, there is no need for sutures and there is no scarring (Figs 10.5 and 10.6).

OPTIMIZING RESULTS

Table 10.2 summarizes areas we consider can optimize the results of fat transplantation.

COMPLICATIONS AND SIDE EFFECTS

As in every surgical procedure, structured fat grafting has complications; however, most of them are considered mild to moderate. As the consequence of multiple passes, edema and ecchymosis are present after all surgeries but are considered undesirable side effects rather than complications (Fig. 10.7). Edema and ecchymosis are really troublesome when so much work is done to the eyelids and tear trough because these structures are composed of easily distensible tissues. Corticoids are routinely used during the induction of anesthesia to prevent formation of severe edema.

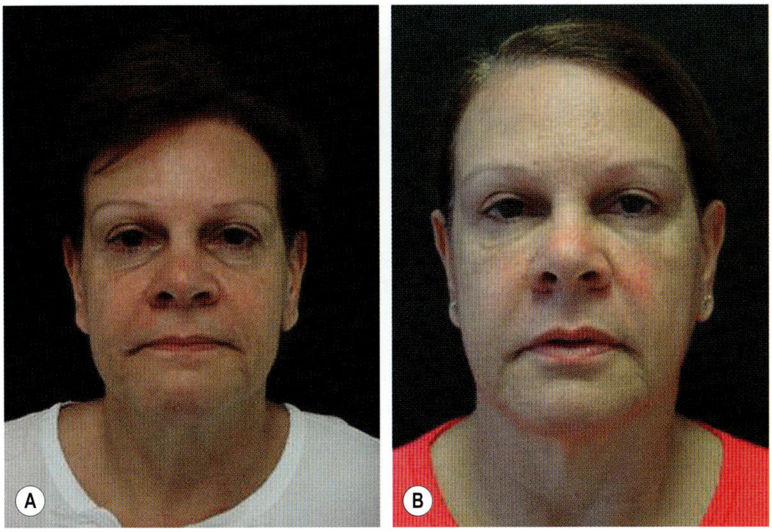

Fig. 10.5 Preoperative and 10-month postoperative of superior and inferior blepharoplasty, with fat grafting into the lid–cheek junction and tear trough.

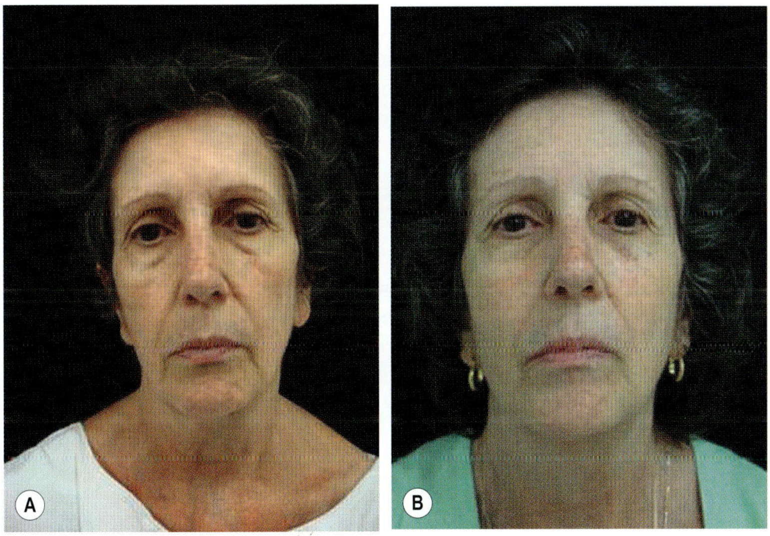

Fig. 10.6 Pre- and postoperative of 10 months of fat grafting into the midface, tear trough, and lid–cheek junction.

When working on the eyelids, irregularities are more likely to happen due to the thin skin.

There are two ways to treat minor irregularities and lumps. First, it is possible to aspirate fat by employing the twist technique (Lambros) or by simply moving the cannula back and forth. Second, it is possible to combine some removal (by suctioning) with grafting to fade the lumps away.

Major asymmetries are rare but possible. Mild ones are more frequent, and care should be taken to avoid them. A meticulous physical examination must be made at the office to detect constitutional or acquired asymmetries and, once detected, they should be rigorously discussed with the patient. Photographs will help the surgeon to show these anatomical differences to patients, and will allow the preparation of an appropriate operative plan. The photographs must be present in the operating room.

Muscle imbalance and nerve paresthesia are occasional and transient symptoms. They indicate that some work was done inside the muscle and that cannula passes caused some trauma to the nerve. Using blunt tip microcannulas eliminates the possibility of causing trauma to a partial or complete section of a nerve, vessel or latticework of the face.

Amaurosis is a very rare and disastrous complication in facial fat grafting. The great majority of cases are related to fat injections in the glabellar area and usually happen due to arterial occlusion. This author discourages fat grafting into the glabella.

Table 10.2 Tips for structured fat grafting

Harvest	Use fine cannulas
	Use low negative pressure
	Use Luer Lok syringe system
Preparation	Provides an excellent cell separation
(centrifugation)	Is a very systematic way to handle fat tissue
	Optimizes volume placement
Grafting	Use microcannulas (blunt tip).
	Use 1.0 cc Luer Lok syringes.
	Take small parcels of fat in each pass
	Make sure there are no lumps
	Avoid external molding
	Structure work with multiple passes
	Use criss-cross only if necessary
	Use needle ports instead of incisions
	Employ knowledge of topographic facial anatomy
	Become familiar with the resistance of different tissues
	Do not use an injector gun

POSTOPERATIVE CARE

As previously mentioned, edema and ecchymosis will always be present in the immediate postoperative period. Usually, ecchymosis subsides in 2–3 weeks, and gross edema subsides in 4 weeks. When treating lips and eyelids, more intense edema and ecchymosis are expected. In the first 2 weeks, cooled devices (gel masks, ice packs and gauzes with chilled saline), applied topically, should be used to reduce edema in the treated area. As soon as the edema subsides, the volume of the tissues reduces dramatically. Antibiotic prophylaxis is employed and painkillers are prescribed to be taken only if necessary. Small dressings on the ports are changed daily in the first week and discontinued after that. Patients must be informed that the final result will be reached within 1 year, but only minor changes will occur after the sixth month. Direct sun exposure must be avoided during the first 6 months. It is very important that you do not omit any information when assuring patients about the postoperative course. The more you inform, the more uneventful the recovery period will be.

CONCLUSIONS

There are hundreds of published papers in the literature in favor of and against fat tissue transfer, and with both favorable and unfavorable results.[14–19] As in all surgical procedures, some techniques are better than others and the best one may not exist. However, when fat grafting is considered, it might be assumed that the

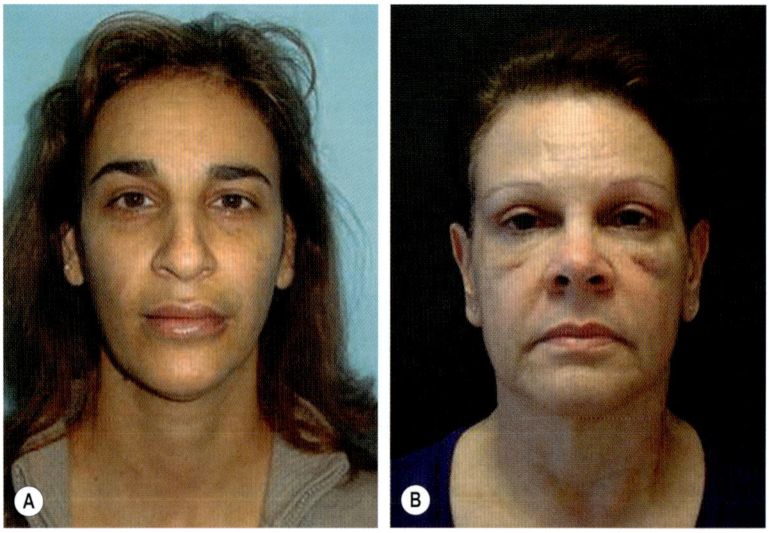

Fig. 10.7 Observe edema and ecchymosis after treating lips and inferior eyelids in recent postoperative periods.

'structured way,' with all its steps, is the gold-standard method of grafting fat tissue. Structured fat grafting is a reliable and reproducible technique.

In this systematized method, surgeons can constantly work in the same manner, and the daily practice can teach them where mistakes were made and where progress needs to be made. Moreover, surgeons of different schools and countries can exchange experiences as the methodology is standardized, and improvements to the technique can be added.

Recently, Coleman[12] published a paper where he emphasized that fat tissue is more than a permanent filler carrying some biological properties.

Fat tissue is currently the main source of adult mesenchymal stem cells, the so-called ADSCs. The presence of these cells in the grafted tissue can answer some questions and issues that, in the past, were obscure. Improvement of skin quality (texture and color), acne scars and radiotherapy damage are now attributed to the presence of these multipotent cells in the fat transplants.

The main reason for making multiple passes while grafting fat tissue is not to possibly enhance the volume to be injected but to improve the contact of fat cells with the host tissue to promote better nutrition, respiration and adhesion of the transplanted cells. Although meticulous and technical work is done, inevitably some cells will die. According to the 'surviving theory' (the most accepted theory to explain how transplanted fat cells survive), transplanted adipocytes, in this stress-induced situation, have the capacity to differentiate into preadipocytes, which are more resilient to hypoxia and nutritional deficiencies. Structured fat grafting provides a favorable microenvironment for mature adipocytes, preadipocytes and ADSCs. That is the reason this technique presents amazing results.[20,21]

To isolate ADSCs, let them multiply on sequenced symmetric mitosis and enrich a regular fat graft with them. Doing this can really improve graft adherence rates. There are four possible ways ADSCs can improve graft adherence:

- ADSCs can differentiate into adipocytes.
- ADSCs can differentiate into endothelial cells promoting angiogenesis and graft survival.
- ADSCs secrete vascular endothelial growth factor (VEGF), which stimulates angiogenesis.
- ADSCs survive as original multipotent cells.

The incorporation of this recent biotechnology to fat grafts has brought a new understanding of fat tissue usage and represents both the present and the future of cosmetic and reconstructive plastic surgery. Surgeons who have been working with fat tissue, and those who intend to, must be open minded to this new era of regenerative medicine.

REFERENCES

1 Neuber F. Fat transplantation. *CHir Kongr Verhandl Dsch Gesellc Chir.* 1893;22:66.

2 Lexer E. Euber freie fettransplantation. *Klin Ther Wehnschr.* 1909;18:53.

3 May A, Knaysi G. On the use of basic dyes for the demonstration of the hydrolysis of fat. *J Bacteriol.* 1941;42(5):587–589.

4 Peer LA. The neglected 'free fat graft': its behaviour and clinical use. *Am J Surg.* 1956;92:40.

5 Schorcher F. Fettgewebsverpflanzung bei zu kleiner Brust. *Munch Med Wochenschr.* 1957;99:489.

6 Ellenbogen R. Free autogenous pearl fat grafts in the face. A preliminary report of a rediscovered technique. *Ann Plast Surg.* 1986;16:179–194.

7 Coleman SR. Long-term survival of fat transplants: controlled demonstrations. *Aesthet Plast Surg.* 1995;19(5):421–425.

8 Coleman SR. Facial recontouring with lipostructure. *Clin Plast Surg.* 1997;24(2):347–367.

9 Lambros V. Fat injection for the aging midface. *Oper Techn Plast Reconstr Surg.* 1998;5(2):129–137.

10 Horl HW, Feller AM, Biemer E. Technique for liposuction fat reimplantation and long-term volume evaluation by magnetic resonance imaging. *Ann Plast Surg.* 1991;26:248–258.

11 Boschert MT, Beckert BW, Puckett CL, Concannon MJ. Analysis of lipocyte viability after liposuction. *Plast Reconst Surg.* 2002;109(2):761–765.

12 Coleman SR. Structural fat grafting: more than a permanent filler. *Plast Reconst Surg.* 2006;118(3S):108S–120S.

13 Billings E, May Jr J. Historical review and present status of free fat graft autotransplantation in plastic and reconstructive surgery. *Plast Reconstr Surg.* 1989;83(2):368–381.

14 Chajchir A. Fat injection: long-term follow up. *Aesthet Plast Surg.* 1996;20:291–296.

15 Ciuci PM, Obagi S. Rejuvenation of the periorbital complex with autologous fat transfer: current therapy. *J Oral Maxillofac Surg.* 2008;66(8):1686–1693.

16 Guerrrerosantos J. Long term outcome of autologous fat transplantation in aesthetic facial recontouring . 16 years of experience with 1936 cases. *Clin Plast Surg.* 2000;27(4):515–543.

17 Jackson I. A successful long-term method of fat grafting: recontouring of a large subcutaneous postradiation thigh defect with autologous fat transplantation. *Aesthet Plast Surg.* 2001; 25:165–169.

18 Niechajev I, Sevcuk O. Long-term results of fat transplantation: clinical and histologic studies. *Plast Reconstr Surg.* 1994;94 (3):496–506.

19 Pu LL, Cui X, Fink BF, Gao D, Vasconez HC. Adipose aspirates as a source for human processed lipoaspirate cells after optimal cryopreservation. *Plast Reconstr Surg.* 2006;117(6):1845–1850.

20 Rigotti G, Marchi A, Galiè M, et al. Clinical treatment of radiotherapy tissue damage by lipoaspirate transplant: a healing process mediated by adipose-derived adult stem cells. *Plast Reconstr Surg.* 2007;119(5):1409–1422.

21 Rohrich RJ, Sorokin ES, Brown SA. In search of improved fat transfer viability: a quantitative analysis of the role of centrifugation and harvest site. *Plast Reconst Surg.* 2004;113(1): 391–395.

22 Sommer B, Sattler G. Current concepts of fat graft survival: histology of aspirated adipose tissue and review of the literature. *Dermatol Surg.* 2000;26(12):1159–1166.

11 Dark Circles: A Combination Approach

Doris M Hexsel, Taciana Dal'Forno, Alessandra Haddad, Marian Cantisano-Zilkha

Included on **DVD**

INTRODUCTION

Dark circles are one of the most common dermatological complaints. The condition is also called periorbital melanosis, periorbital skin hyperpigmentation and infraorbital darkening. Dark circles are defined as unaesthetic blemishes around the eyes, especially at the lower eyelid. This condition is frequently seen in both men and women of all ages.[1] Despite occurring in children and being more prevalent in certain ethnic groups (Middle Eastern and Mediterranean backgrounds), dark circles can be interpreted as an age-related change, since smooth skin around the eyes – the thinnest skin in the body – and skin color uniformity are the main attributes related to perceived age.[2] The physiopathology of dark circles is not yet completely understood.

Three different factors may contribute to the clinical picture of this condition, alone or in combination:

1. Shadows: shadowing is secondary to convexity of the lower eyelid, which in turn is caused by the bulge of the eye, lower lid fat prolapse or excess depth of the nasojugal groove (known more recently as tear trough deformity)(Fig. 11.1).[3]
2. Vessels: a bluish color is secondary to the subcutaneous venous network (Fig. 11.2) while a reddish color is secondary to the visible dermal capillary network (Fig. 11.3).
3. Pigment: the brown color commonly seen in this condition is secondary to superficial melanin (Fig. 11.4) while a brown-blue color is secondary to dermal melanin.[4] These can be more easily seen under a Wood's lamp (Fig. 11.5).

Other etiologic factors are also reported for dark circles, including postinflammatory hyperpigmentation secondary to atopic or allergic contact dermatitis and periorbital edema.[5]

The lower eyelid skin is very thin, and alterations in the blood flow supplying this area can worsen dark circles. Aging, expressed by changes in the pigmentation of the skin, loss of elasticity, worsening of the nasojugal groove and more visible vessels under the skin, can also aggravate the appearance of dark circles.

Very few studies have been published on dark circles, one possible reason being the difficulty in measuring the condition. Ohshima and Takiwaki analyzed dark circles quantitatively using various bioengineering techniques.[6] Two kinds of reflectance meters and image analysis were used to measure erythema index (EI), melanin index (MI) and oxygenation index (OX) in subjects with and without dark circles. Also, the thickness and echo density of the dermis were evaluated using ultrasound echo images. Evaluation of EI and MI by image processing methods also seems suitable for quantitative evaluation of dark circles of the lower eyelid. Dermal thickness of the eyelid skin may also be involved in the appearance of dark circles.

There are also few published studies on the treatment of dark circles in the indexed literature. Proposed treatments usually involve a combination of different techniques: topical therapy, dietary supplements, peelings, fillers, autologous platelet-rich plasma rejuvenation, lasers, carbon dioxide therapy and surgery, and these should be directed to the local skin alterations (blood vessels, pigments, nasojugal groove and surface irregularities). They can be used alone or in combination, according to the patient's needs (Figs 11.1–11.5).

TOPICAL THERAPY

Many active ingredients of commercial products for the treatment of dark circles have not yet been studied to prove their real efficacy. These products generally contain antioxidants, bleaching agents, moisturizers and stimulants of new collagen formation.

A multicenter study investigated an eye cream containing a proprietary mixture of human growth factors

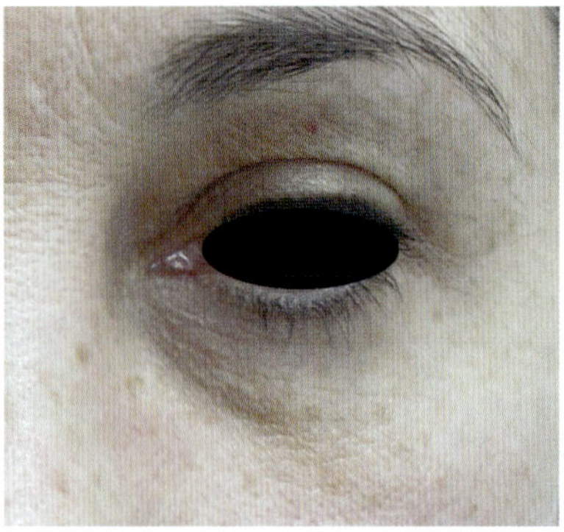

Fig. 11.1 Shadowing secondary to the bulging contour of the lower lid (nasojugal groove).

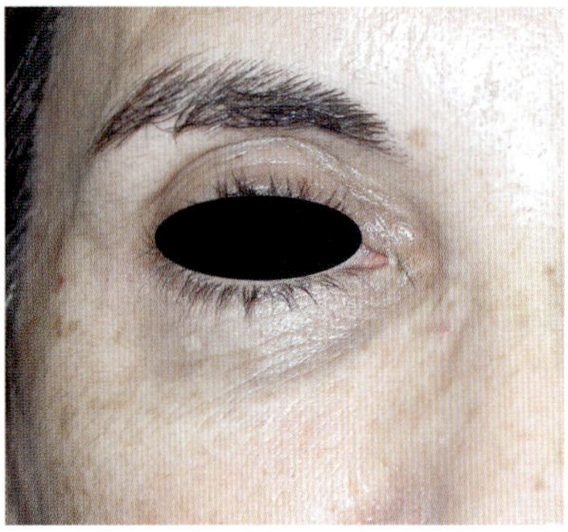

Fig. 11.2 Bluish color secondary to the subcutaneous venous network.

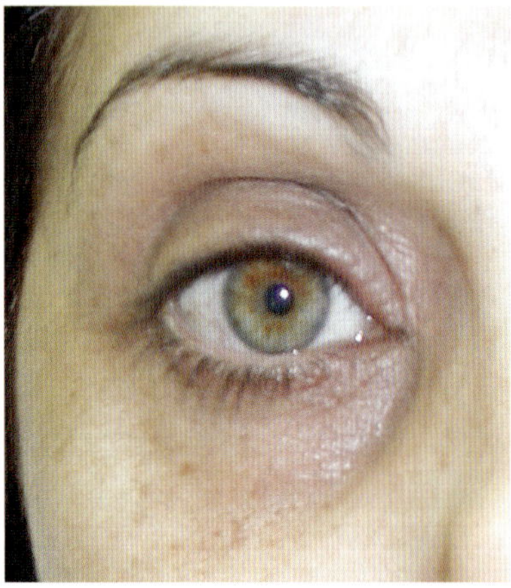

Fig. 11.3 Reddish color secondary to the visible dermal capillary network.

and cytokines in combination with caffeine, bisabolol, glycyrrhinic acid and sodium hyaluronate for periorbital rejuvenation. The study revealed that some clinical signs of aging, including dark circles, showed

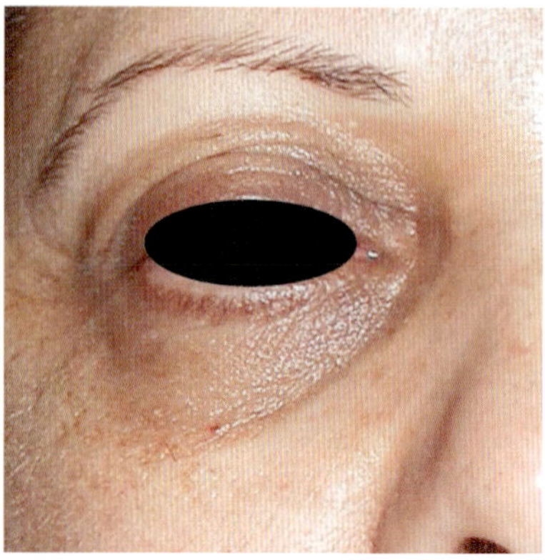

Fig. 11.4 Brown color secondary to hyperpigmentation of the periorbital area.

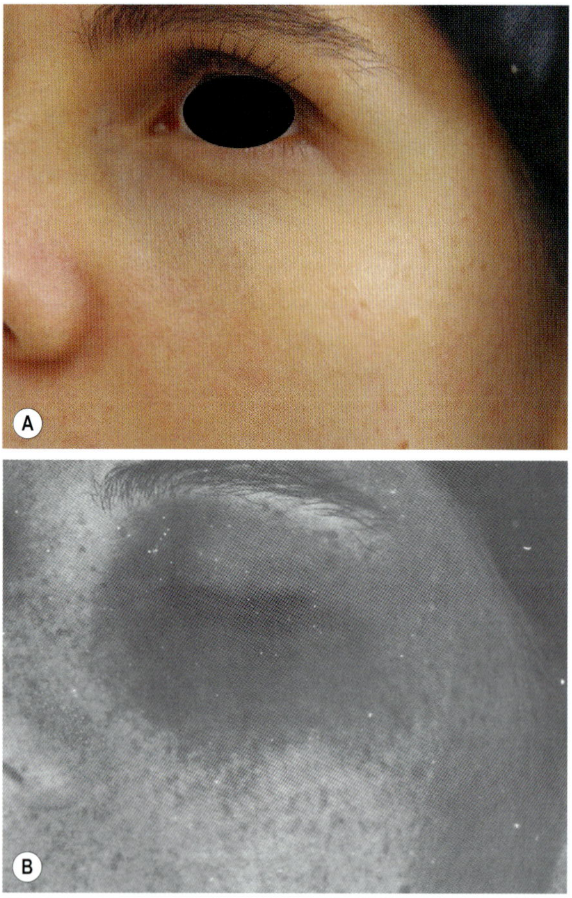

Fig. 11.5 Patient with slight dark circles. *A*, Clinical aspect of patient with slight dark circles. *B*, UV picture of the same patient showing hyperpigmentation in the periorbital area.

significant improvement after 6 weeks of twice-daily application, with excellent tolerability.[7]

A study showed that the use of vitamin K combined with retinol 0.15% for the treatment of periorbital hyperpigmentation was effective in 93% of patients.[8] Another study evaluated a gel containing 2% phytonadione, 0.1% retinol and 0.1% vitamins C and E, which was moderately effective in reducing dark circles when applied twice daily to the lower eyelid site for 8 weeks in healthy Japanese adults.[9]

Cosmetic camouflage, an opaque make-up, is very helpful for patients, especially women, who are familiar with these types of products. Camouflage make-up is usually creamy and comes in a variety of shades to match the natural skin color. Sometimes it is blended with color correctors to achieve a good color match and conceal dark circles.

DIETARY SUPPLEMENT

One study has evaluated the effects of a dietary supplement containing soy extract, fish protein polysaccharides, extracts from white tea, grape seed and tomato, vitamins C and E as well as zinc and chamomile extract on the skin of post-menopausal women.[10] The evaluation after 3 and 6 months of treatment showed significantly greater improvement of skin conditions in the active group in a variety of parameters, including dark circles. This was the first study evaluating the effect of dietary supplements on dark circles, but it may be the beginning of a new research treatment field.

CHEMICAL PEELING

Despite little support in the literature, chemical peeling can be helpful for dark circles. It acts through exfoliation, abrasion and the shedding of superficial skin cells and layers, reducing pigmentation and wrinkles of the skin (Fig. 11.6) around the eyes, significantly improving some cases of dark circles. The choice of the agent, concentration, number of applications and other factors will depend on each patient's needs. The most frequently used peels for dark circles are trichloroacetic acid (TCA) and phenol peels.[11] For further information see Chapter 4.

FILLERS

Injectable fillers can be used alone or in combination with other facial procedures to improve the appearance of dark circles. Addressing the hollowness of the periorbital region by using a filler requires a thorough understanding of the delicate and vascular nature of these tissues. Injectable hyaluronic acid is used to augment the nasojugal groove to eliminate the shadowing that worsens dark circles (Fig. 11.7).[12–15]

Airan and Born first described a technique using injectable non-animal-stabilized hyaluronic acid (NASHA) placed in the subperiosteal plane of the inferior orbital rim using a multiple puncture technique administered under local anesthetic.[16] One year later, Steinsapir and Steinsapir reported a 2-year experience of treating nasojugal grooves with injectable hyaluronic acid. They demonstrated the usefulness of these fillers for the treatment of these grooves, with a low incidence of complications. In the postoperative period, localized swelling, bruising and asymmetry were relatively common. Cellulitis occurred in two cases and migraine in one patient.[12]

Goldberg and Fiaschetti published their experience in periorbital augmentation with 244 hyaluronic acid (HA) injections in 155 patients. One hundred and eight out of 121 patients (89%) who received follow-up visits were satisfied with the cosmetic improvement. For maintenance, the interval to a second injection averaged 6.5 months.

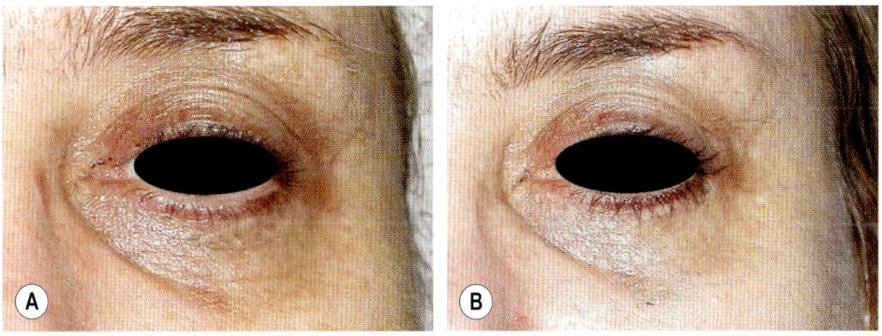

Fig. 11.6 TCA peeling for treatment of photoaging and dark circles. *A*, Before treatment with 30% TCA. *B*, After treatment.

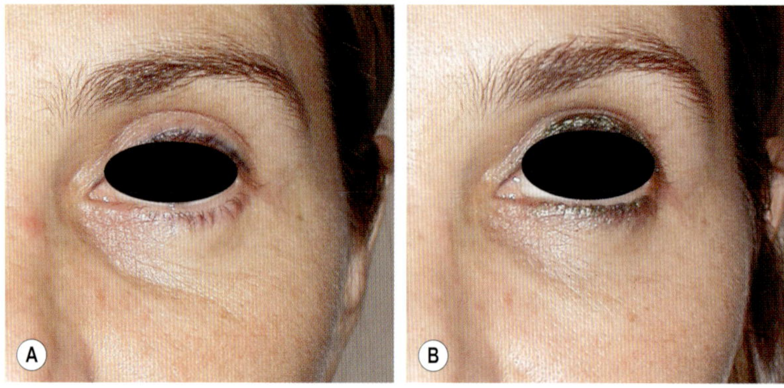

Fig. 11.7 Hyaluronic acid augmentation of the nasojugal groove. *A*, Before treatment. *B*, After treatment.

The authors highlighted that patients with very thin skin, preexisting color problems or preexisting eyelid fluid may not be good candidates for periorbital filling with injectable hyaluronic acid gels,[14] since the high hydrophilic properties of HA may worsen the condition.

Bosniak, Zilkha et al introduced a modified technique using injectable HA gel for augmentation of the lower eyelids in 12 female patients.[17] The technique is applied in the supraperiosteal plane, puncturing the skin twice only with a 0.25 mL bolus of HA, while under topical anesthesia. After the procedure, digital pressure was used when hemostasis was needed and to minimize possible ecchymosis. Ice compresses were applied for 5 minutes post procedure to minimize localized swelling and erythema. The authors called this technique 'hyaluronic acid push' due to the use of digital pressure to push the filler into the desired position to modify the contour. The most common complications were temporary postinjection erythema and edema. These were treated with application of ice compresses and resolved completely over 72 hours. One patient with slight overcorrection and anterior placement of the filler over the anterior lacrimal crest improved with administration of hyaluronidase and massage.

According to Bucky and Kanchwala, autologous fat and alternative fillers, including calcium hydroxylapatite, can be considered as an additional option for the treatment of dark circles, besides contributing significantly to overall facial rejuvenation.[18]

In the infraorbital region, intravascular injection may occur, causing side effects of different degrees of severity, from hematomas to vascular occlusion. These can be avoided by the use of small and delicate cannulas.

AUTOLOGOUS PLATELET-RICH PLASMA REJUVENATION

Autologous platelet-rich plasma rejuvenation is a novel treatment strategy that relies on the natural healing capacity of the synergistic cascade of autologous growth factors.[19] It has been used in clinical practice since the 1990s and has an extremely broad range of healing applications in oral and maxillofacial surgery, cosmetic surgery, cardiovascular surgery, otolaryngology, burns and wound healing, and lately in aesthetics, where it is used to address damaged and aged skin. Platelets, when present in body tissues outside the bloodstream, are activated by various chemicals to release growth factors, which attract stem cells to the site of injury. The growth factors stimulate neo-vascularization and the production of collagen, elastin and new extra-cellular matrix. Platelet-rich plasma is a natural and powerful means of delaying as well as reversing cutaneous aging and due to its importance it is thoroughly discussed in Chapter 13. The significant increase in skin thickness and elasticity as well as the moderate volumetric effect achieved by both intradermal and subdermal injection of platelets provides a safe, natural and long-term solution for skin regeneration and in particular peri-orbital rejuvenation.

LASERS

The ruby or Nd-Yag, the Q-switched alexandrite laser, the carbon dioxide (CO_2) laser and the intense pulsed light (IPL) are the most commonly used lasers in the treatment of dark circles.[4,20] They improve dark circles by acting on specific chromophores, such as water, hemoglobin and melanin.

By targeting these chromophores, they induce vascular and pigment alterations. Furthermore, they stimulate collagen production, thus improving the flaccidity that worsens dark circles. The number of sessions and the results may vary for each patient, according to the type of laser or light source used. The use of sunscreens during treatment is highly recommended to prevent hyperpigmentation after the procedures.

Significant lightening of infraorbital hyperpigmentation was observed in one study, 9 weeks after CO_2 laser resurfacing.[21] This was the first report of the successful use of a non-pigment-specific laser system for the treatment of infraorbital dark circles. Manuskiatti et al. also showed in their study that 75–100% of the patients demonstrated improvement in periorbital hyperpigmentation with a Q-switched alexandrite laser immediately following the use of a pulsed CO_2 laser.[4]

On the other hand, Lowe et al. evaluated the clinical and histological appearance of infraorbital skin pigment in 17 patients with dermal melanin deposition treated with a Q-switched ruby laser.[22] Of those patients treated with a single Q-switched ruby session, 23.5% achieved greater than 50% response. Of those treated twice, 88.9% achieved greater than 50% response.

A total of 18 Japanese patients underwent combined therapy using a Q-switched ruby laser to eliminate dermal pigmentation and topical bleaching treatment with tretinoin aqueous gel and hydroquinone ointment performed 6 weeks beforehand to reduce epidermal melanin. Seven of 18 patients (38.9%) showed excellent clearing after treatment and eight patients (44.4%) were rated as good. Only one patient (5.6%) was rated as fair and none was rated as poor. Postinflammatory hyperpigmentation was observed in only two patients (11.1%). This new treatment was considered effective for improvement of periorbital skin hyperpigmentation, with a low incidence of postinflammatory hyperpigmentation.[23]

Alster and Hirsch evaluated the clinical efficacy and side effect profile of single-pass CO_2 laser skin resurfacing in 52 consecutive patients with skin phototypes I–VI presenting with infraorbital hyperpigmentation.[24] The treatment improved, among other parameters, the appearance of infraorbital hyperpigmentation in all skin types. The severity and duration of side effects and complications are reduced with this technique (compared with multiple-pass procedures with the same device) and may offer a possible solution to the problem of treating patients with darker complexions.

The new fractional devices (CO_2, Erbium:Yag) seem to offer similar results to CO_2 ablative treatments, with less downtime but more sessions required. However, further studies are required to determine the best treatment parameters.

CARBON DIOXIDE INSUFFLATION THERAPY

Carbon dioxide insufflation therapy is an ancient technology that is gaining popularity in Europe and South America for skin tightening and rejuvenation (see Ch. 14). Carbon dioxide insufflation therapy is the cutaneous and subcutaneous administration of CO_2 gas for therapeutic purposes. It originated in the royal spas of France in 1932, where it was used to treat patients affected by peripheral arterial occlusive disease. Studies have demonstrated that subcutaneous CO_2 therapy positively affects local parameters of cutaneous microcirculation, improves cutaneous elasticity and induces localized adiposity cytolysis. In South America, especially in Brazil, and in Europe, CO_2 therapy has been applied to the treatment of stretch marks, hypertrophic scars and cellulite with impressive results. Some other additional medical applications for CO_2 insufflation therapy are:

- peripheral arteriopathies
- microangiopathies
- erectile dysfunction associated with microangiopathy
- psoriasis
- varicose ulcers
- alopecia
- skin laxity
- dark undereye circles
- acute arthritis neuropathies
- sports medicine applications.

The possible positive effect of CO_2 therapy on microcirculation, skin elasticity and localized adiposities leads us to believe that it may be a valuable adjunct in the treatment of physiologic aging changes of the periorbital area and dark circles, and that it will enhance the effects of current non-invasive and minimally invasive treatments. Several studies are currently ongoing around the world to scientifically document the safety and effectiveness of this adjunct therapy, which seems to be a very promising addition to our current range of rejuvenation procedures.

SURGERY (BLEPHAROPLASTY)

Successful outcomes have been obtained in the improvement of the appearance of dark circles with transconjunctival blepharoplasty associated with phenol chemical peels in patients with Fitzpatrick phototypes I–IV, with a low incidence of complications.[25]

CONCLUSION

Dark circles represent a common unaesthetic condition caused by multiple etiologic factors, which may vary from patient to patient. The treatment of dark circles should be directed to the factors responsible for the clinical manifestations of each patient, such as blood vessels, pigmentation and skin irregularities. Thus, the treatment response can also vary from patient to patient. Some treatments are very effective for some patients, but not for all. Further studies are needed to improve understanding of the causes of this condition and to develop more effective therapeutic options.

REFERENCES

1 Baumann L. Disorders of pigmentation. In: Baumann L, ed. *Cosmetic Dermatology*. New York: McGraw-Hill; 2004:63–71.

2 Nkengne A, Bertin C, Stamatas G, et al. Influence of facial skin attributes on the perceived age of Caucasian women. *J Eur Acad Dermatol Venereol*. 2008. (Epub ahead of print).

3 Sadick NS, Bosniak SL, Cantisano-Zilkha M, Glavas IP, Roy D. Definition of the tear trough and the tear trough rating scale. *J Cosmet Dermatol*. 2007;6(4):218–222.

4 Manuskiatti W, Fitzpatrick RE, Goldman MP. Treatment of facial skin using combinations of CO_2, Q-switched alexandrite, flash-lamp-pumped pulsed dye, and Er:YAG lasers in the same treatment session. *Dermatol Surg*. 2000;26(2):114–120.

5 Freitag FM, Cestari TF. What causes dark circles under the eyes? *J Cosmet Dermatol*. 2007;6(3):211–215.

6 Ohshima H, Takiwaki H. Evaluation of dark circles of the lower eyelid: comparison between reflectance meters and image processing and involvement of dermal thickness in appearance. *Skin Res Technol*. 2008;14(2):135 141.

7 Lupo ML, Cohen JL, Rendon MI. Novel eye cream containing a mixture of human growth factors and cytokines for periorbital skin rejuvenation. *J Drugs Dermatol*. 2007;6(7):725–729.

8 Elson M, Nacht S. Treatment of periorbital hyperpigmentation with topical vitamin K/vitamin A. *Cosmetic Dermatol*. 1999;12 (12):32.

9 Mitsuishi T, Shimoda T, Mitsui Y, Kuriyama Y, Kawana S. The effects of topical application of phytonadione, retinol and vitamins C and E on infraorbital dark circles and wrinkles of the lower eyelids. *J Cosmet Dermatol*. 2004;3(2):73–75.

10 Skovgaard GR, Jensen AS, Sigler ML. Effect of a novel dietary supplement on skin aging in post-menopausal women. *Eur J Clin Nutr*. 2006;60(10):1201–1206.

11 Gatti JE. Eyelid phenol peel: an important adjunct to blepharoplasty. *Ann Plast Surg*. 2008;60(1):14–18 discussion 1920.

12 Steinsapir KD, Steinsapir SM. Deep-fill hyaluronic acid for the temporary treatment of the naso-jugal groove: a report of 303 consecutive treatments. *Ophthal Plast Reconstr Surg*. 2006;22 (5):344–348.

13 Kane MAC. Treatment of tear trough deformity and lower lid bowing with injectable hyaluronic acid. *Aesth Plast Surg*. 2005;29(5):368–372.

14 Golberg R, Fiaschetti D. Filling the periorbital hollows with acid hialuronic gel: initial experience with 244 injections. *Ophthal Plast Recontr Surg*. 2006;22(5):335–341.

15 Stephen B, Neil S, Marian C, Ioannis PG, Deborshi R. The hyaluronic acid push technique for the nasojugal groove. *Dermatol Surg*. 2008;34(1):127–131.

16 Airan LE, Born TM. Nonsurgical lower eyelid lift. *Plast Reconstr Surg*. 2005;116:1785–1792.

17 Bosniak S, Sadick NS, Cantisano-Zilkha M, Glavas IP, Roy D. The hyaluronic acid push technique for the nasojugal groove. *Dermatol Surg*. 2008;34(1):127–131.

18 Bucky LP, Kanchwala SK. The role of autologous fat and alternative fillers in the aging face. *Plast Reconstr Surg*. 2007;120 (6 suppl):89S–97S.

19 Kakudo N, Mitsui T, Kushida S, Notodihardjo FZ, Kusumoto K. Proliferation-promoting effect of platelet-rich plasma on human adipose-derived stem cells and human dermal fibroblasts. *Plast Reconstr Surg*. 2008;122(5):1352–1360.

20 Fodor L, Ramon Y, Fodor A, Carmi N, Peled IJ, Ullmann Y. A side-by-side prospective study of intense pulsed light and Nd:YAG laser treatment for vascular lesions. *Ann Plast Surg*. 2006;56(2):164–170.

21 West TB, Alster TS. Improvement of infraorbital hyperpigmentation following carbon dioxide laser resurfacing. *Dermatol Surg*. 1998;24(6):615–616.

22 Lowe NJ, Wieder JM, Shorr N, Boxrud C, Saucer D, Chalet M. Infraorbital pigmented skin. Preliminary observations of laser therapy. *Dermatol Surg*. 1995;21(9):767–770.

23 Momosawa A, Kurita M, Ozaki M, et al. Combined therapy using Q-switched ruby laser and bleaching treatment with tretinoin and hydroquinone for periorbital skin hyperpigmentation in Asians. *Plast Reconstr Surg*. 2008;121(1):282–288.

24 Alster T, Hirsch R. Single-pass CO_2 laser skin resurfacing of light and dark skin: extended experience with 52 patients. *J Cosmet Laser Ther*. 2003;5(1):39–42.

25 Epstein JS. Management of infraorbital dark circles. A significant cosmetic concern. *Arch Facial Plast Surg*. 1999;1(4):303–307.

12 Minimally Invasive Laser Lipolysis for Facial and Neck Rejuvenation

Bruce E Katz, Jason C McBean

Included on **DVD**

INTRODUCTION

Laser lipolysis is a new minimally invasive method for liquefying fat and tightening the skin. The Food and Drug Administration approved the first laser lipolysis device in October 2006 for the surgical incision, excision, vaporization, ablation and coagulation of all soft tissues.[1] Liposuction is an extremely common cosmetic surgical procedure with over 450 000 operations performed in 2007, according to the American Society of Aesthetic Plastic Surgery.[2] It is also fast becoming a preferred method for facial and neck rejuvenation, given the low operative risk, absence of scarring and fast recovery times. The drawbacks associated with traditional liposuction include increased blood loss, ecchymosis, long recovery time with increased postoperative discomfort, skin laxity as well as pulmonary emboli, seromas and visceral perforations.

Since the inception of a 1064 nm pulsed Nd:YAG laser system (SmartLipo, manufactured by Deka, distributed by Cynosure, Westford, MA) in 2006, several additional devices have been introduced to the market. At the time of this publication, these include additional 1064 nm laser devices (Prolipo® by Sciton, Palo Alto, CA, and Lipolite® by Syneron, Irvine, CA), a 1320 nm laser (CoolLipo® by Cooltouch, Roseville, CA), a 980 nm diode device (Lipotherme® by Osyris, Helemmes, France), and a new combination 1064 nm/1320 nm sequential firing laser (Smartlipo Multiplex® by Cynosure, Westford, MA).

These newer technologies are indicated for laser lipolysis as well as improvement of flaccidity. Laser lipolysis addresses the drawbacks mentioned above: increased blood loss, ecchymosis, long recovery time and skin laxity. It achieves these improvements by creating lipolysis, coagulating small blood vessels and inducing new collagen formation, the end result being reduced adiposity, skin retraction and decreased flaccidity.

EQUIPMENT AND LASER SPECIFICATIONS

The standard laser lipolysis device is a pulsed 1064 nm Nd:YAG system. The pulse width is 150 μs and the repetition rate 40 Hz. The power output goes as high as 18 W. The key features of this technology include the short pulse duration that creates a high peak power and the high repetition rate (Fig. 12.1).

Laser lipolysis utilizes a gradient pulse delivering high peak power. Other laser systems use a gated or standard pulse delivery system that delivers energy over a longer period of time, leading to potential collateral tissue damage. The peak power of laser lipolysis leads to adipocyte rupture without charring of adjacent tissue.

In this procedure, energy is transmitted to the subcutaneous tissue through a 300 or 600 μm fiber. The 300 μm fiber is used for machines with power wattage up to 10 W, whereas the 600 μm fiber is used for 18 W and higher. The fiber is seated in a 1 mm diameter stainless-steel microcannula of variable lengths, depending on the treatment location. The fiber optic is extended 2 mm beyond the end of the cannula and cleaved cleanly prior to operating. A guiding red light, referred to as the 'He:Ne beam' (helium and neon), aids the surgeon in precisely visualizing the subcutaneous laser fiber location while operating. A 1.5 mm incision, #11 blade stab or 18-guage needle is enough to introduce the cannula, which is then guided through the fat at various depths, including the subdermal layer.

The exact mechanism of action of lipolysis and collagen stimulation is still under investigation. A proposed theory involves photothermal heating and photomechanical effects that disrupt adipocyte membranes, thereby breaking them into smaller particles that are then removed by suctioning or reabsorbed through the lymphatic system. The localized heating induced by the laser also denatures existing collagen, allowing for the stimulation of new collagen and collagen retraction. In addition to lipolysis and collagen stimulation, the laser also coagulates blood

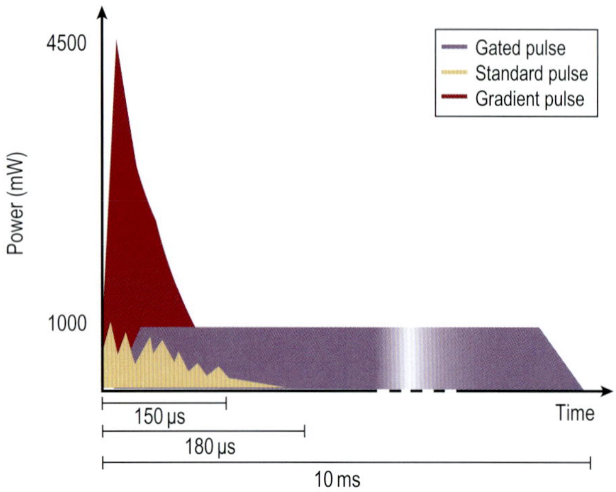

Fig. 12.1 High peak power of laser-assisted lipolysis.

vessels, which, when combined with the hemostatic effects of tumescent anesthesia, leads to marked improvement of ecchymoses, seromas and edema.

INDICATIONS AND CONTRAINDICATIONS

Indications and contraindications are shown in Box 12.1.

Laser lipolysis is a body-contouring technique for relatively healthy individuals. Laser lipolysis should be limited to patients who fall into the American Surgical Association class I, II or, rarely, III (Box 12.2).

Physicians should obtain a complete history and physical evaluation, particularly regarding recent pregnancy and weight patterns. The surgeon should also verify baseline laboratory data to evaluate liver function and to test for presence of hepatitis pregnancy, occult infection or blood discrasias.

BOX 12.1 INDICATIONS

- Small localized areas of unwanted adiposity
- Mild to moderate skin laxity

CONTRAINDICATIONS

- Impaired liver function, hepatitis C, chronic hepatitis B, alcoholic liver disease
- Acute infections
- Current pregnancy or pregnancy within the 3 months prior to surgery
- Allergy to lidocaine or epinephrine
- Thin areas with severe dermatoheliosis with little subcutaneous adipose tissue

BOX 12.2

- Class I = normal healthy patients
- Class II = mild systemic disease that results in some functional limitation
- Class III = moderate to severe disease, which results in some functional limitation
- Class IV = systemic diseases that pose constant threats to life and are functionally incapacitating
- Class V = moribund and not expected to survive 24 hours with or without surgery.

Lawrence N, Leonhardt J, Liposuction. In: Robinson JK, Hanke W, Sengelmann R, Siegel. Surgery of the Skin: Procedural Dermatology Spain: Elsevier Mosby; 2005. p. 517

Prior to surgery, it is important to determine whether the patient is an appropriate candidate for laser lipolysis. The ideal candidate is one who has small, localized areas of adipose tissue and mild-to-moderate skin laxity. Patients who have severe skin laxity with minimal adipose tissue, thin 'crepy' skin, prominent submental salivary glands or retrognathia are less ideal candidates with features that may hinder optimal results. Those who demonstrate thin 'crepy' skin or severe laxity in the absence of subcutaneous adipose tissue are at an increased risk of thermal burns. These patients are candidates for skin-tightening devices (see Chapter 7).

The indications for laser lipolysis as it pertains to facial and neck rejuvenation continue to evolve. Historically, liposculpture of the cervical and submental regions were reserved for younger patients with good skin tone. Now, laser lipolysis alone or combined with suction-assisted lipoplasty provides excellent results for patients in their 50s, 60s and even 70s. Generally, laser lipolysis is indicated for patients who have small unwanted localized areas of adipose tissue and mild-to-moderate skin laxity.

Cervical and submental regions are ideal locations for laser lipolysis for several reasons. As highlighted by Zins et al., numerous authors have noted that neck skin, as opposed to facial skin or skin elsewhere, has a unique ability to contract.[3] This clinical observation, while not entirely understood, has prompted many surgeons to opt for more conservative neck rejuvenation, favoring liposculpture over platysmaplasties and neck lifts.[3] Due to the additional contractile effect produced by the laser, surgeons are now noting dramatic improvement in the postoperative cervicomental angles of their patients.

Additionally, the cervical and submental areas are small and therefore can be easily accessed via few, inconspicuous incisions. Also, the risk of lidocaine toxicity is reduced due to the smaller volumes necessary to achieve adequate anesthesia.

There are no contraindications specific to laser lipolysis when compared to traditional tumescent liposuction. The same considerations with regard to tumescent anesthesia and lidocaine toxicity apply.

PREOPERATIVE HISTORY AND CONSIDERATIONS

The preoperative evaluation also involves obtaining adequate history, physical examination, and laboratory data in order to ensure the suitability of the liposuction candidate. Patients with a preexisting cardiovascular or respiratory condition may require medical clearance by their primary-care physicians, cardiologist or pneumonologist. Naturally, patients may downplay the severity of their health conditions for an elective cosmetic procedure.

The physician should be particularly aware of those patients with impaired liver function, hepatitis C, chronic active hepatitis B and alcoholic liver disease because lidocaine is metabolized by the cytochrome P450 enzymes of the liver. While patients with liver disease are at an increased risk of developing lidocaine toxicity, treatment of small areas such as the neck, submental areas and face inherently limit toxicity risk due to the small volumes necessary to achieve adequate anesthesia. Laboratory evaluation should include complete blood count with platelets, serum chemistries, partial thromboplastin time (PTT), prothrombin time (PT), human immunodeficiency virus (HIV), hepatitis B and C panel, and pregnancy test.

A surgical history is also important. Patients with prior surgeries or liposuction may have increased scarring, making passage of the cannula difficult. In these scenarios, one may discuss the prior case with the previous surgeon. The age of scars is also important information to obtain from the patient. Older scars tend to be softer and may be suctioned through, while newer scars should be suctioned around.[4]

Once informed consent is obtained, a baseline patient weight and vital signs are obtained. The weight is used to determine the optimum, safe maximum volume and concentration of tumescent anesthesia. The recommended maximum dose of lidocaine for tumescent anesthesia is 55 mg/kg as per the American Academy of Dermatology. Cardiac monitoring with pulse oximetry and supplemental oxygen should be available and a plan for medical emergencies should be established.[5]

The patient may be photographed using standard lighting and positioning. The patient may be seated or standing, and images should be taken from the front, at 3/4 view and from the side (profile) (Fig. 12.2). It is important to standardize images as much as possible to ensure a correct comparison of before and after images. Excellent clinical photographs are critical because many patients forget their presurgery appearance and are impressed by the change after seeing the before images. Patients are informed that the images are confidential and sign a release if used for research or publication purposes. The images are also vital for medical–legal purposes.

Perioperative medications vary by clinician preference and patient requirements. Some clinicians provide an anxiolytic such as lorazepam or midazolam prior to the procedure. Clonidine, an alpha-2 adrenergic receptor, used as antihypertensive, may be employed for its additional sedative effect and to temper tachycardia resulting from epinephrine used in the tumescent anesthesia. Intramuscular narcotics such as meperidine may be employed to dampen the discomfort of the infused tumescent anesthesia. Finally, an antihistamine such as hydroxyzine is often employed for additional sedation and to offset potential nausea or dermatitis produced by the above medications.

OPERATIVE APPROACH

After the patients are photographed, they are marked with a surgical marker. Meticulous marking is paramount because once the anesthesia is administered anatomical landmarks may be lost. Closely follow the contours of the adipose areas when marking to facilitate smooth transitions between anatomic units. Mark the borders of the mandible, being careful to include the fuller areas of the jowls and submental fat pads. Stay medial to the anterior border of the sternocleidomastoid muscles to avoid vital vessels and nerves (Fig. 12.3).

Once the patient is marked and receives the perioperative medications, the nursing personnel prepares the entire area with a surgical antimicrobial cleanser. Small incisions are made with a 1.5 mm punch, an 18-gauge needle or a #11 blade. The incisions are made in three locations: just inferior to the angle of the mandible bilaterally and in the submental crease. The authors' preferred method is to use a 1.5 mm punch (Fig. 12.4) due to ease of creating a uniform hole, which relaxes in the direction of normal skin tension lines. We do not suture these small incisions to allow natural drainage of the infiltrated solution,

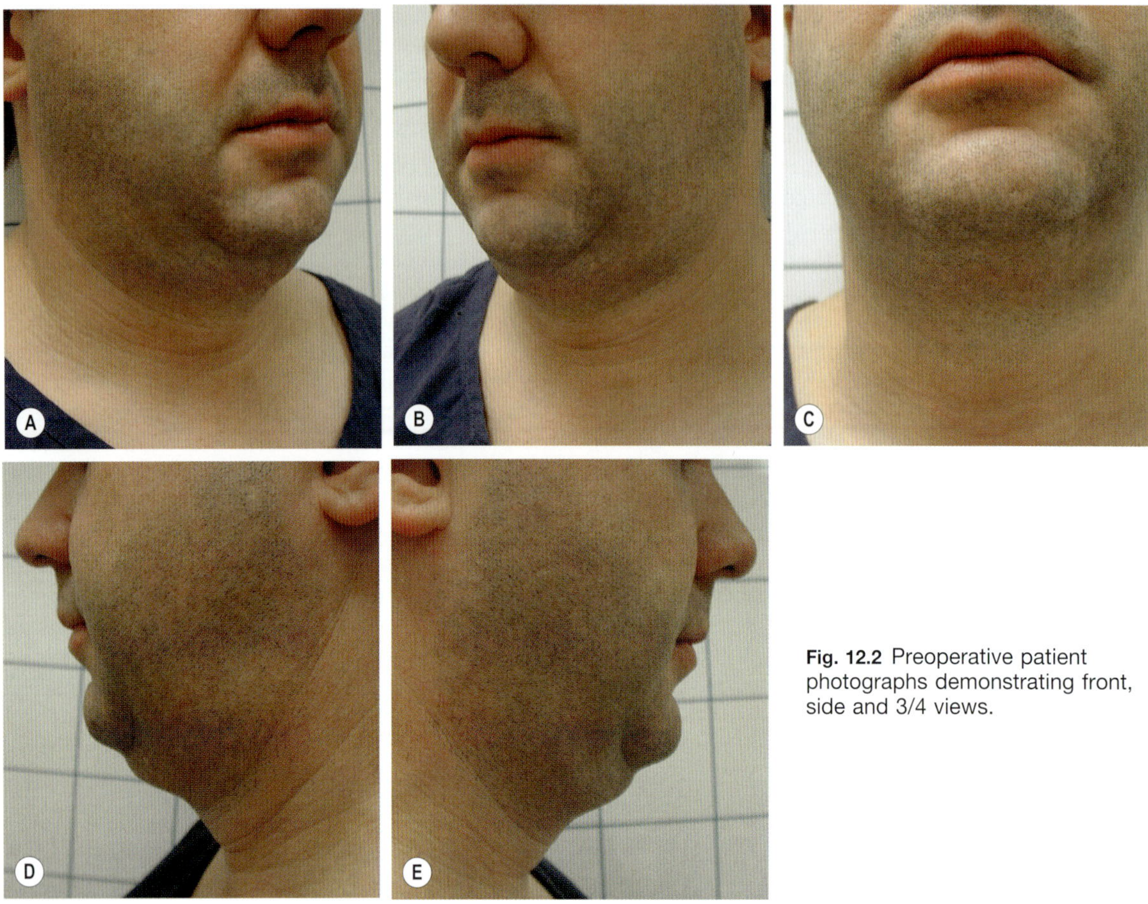

Fig. 12.2 Preoperative patient photographs demonstrating front, side and 3/4 views.

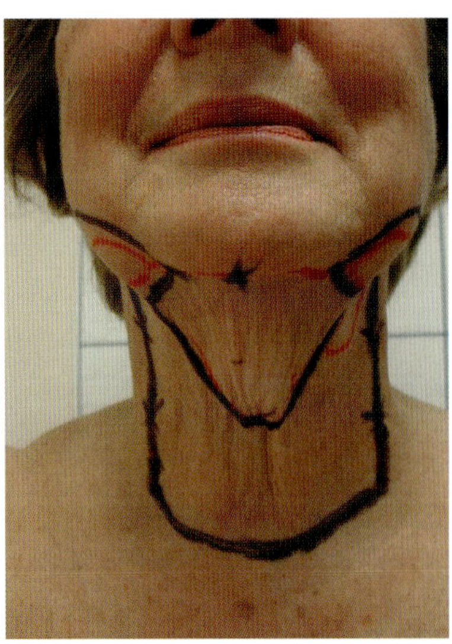

Fig. 12.3 Preoperative surgical markings.

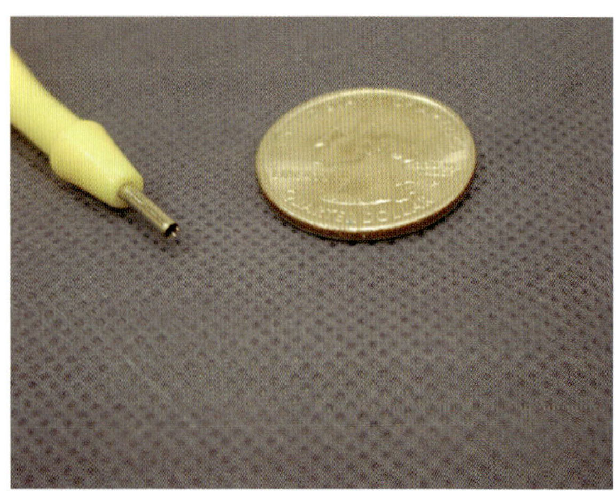

Fig. 12.4 1.5 mm punch for incision sites.

blood and the liquefied fat produced by the laser action. Additionally, because they are so small and are located on concave surfaces, they heal with less noticeable scars than those closed with sutures.

It must be emphasized that virtually all cases of laser lipolysis can be performed with tumescent anesthesia. This is an advantage as multiple studies have documented the superior safety record of tumescent liposuction over liposuction performed under general anesthesia or intravenous sedation. In addition, data illustrate that tumescent liposuction performed in the outpatient setting is safer than any liposuction performed in the hospital inpatient setting.[6]

For the administration of the anesthesia, the patient is positioned supine, with the neck gently extended at the head of the surgical table. Note that when the neck is extended and rotated laterally, the marginal mandibular branch of the facial nerve moves superficially, becoming more susceptible to nerve injury.[7] Extra care should therefore be taken in this area. Local tumescent anesthesia can then be administered via a powered or manual infusion cannula. The authors' preferred cannula size is a 6-inch sprinkler tipped infusion cannula attached to a power infusion pump (Fig. 12.5).

It is prudent, when infusing tumescent anesthesia of the face, submental area and neck, to infuse at a slow rate not to over-infuse, risking potential oral airway compression. The slower rate of infusion also enhances patient comfort during administration. Patient comfort may also be improved by using a warm (40°C) buffered solution. The surgeon should be careful that the liquid anesthesia does not inadvertently wash away the markings made prior to infusing. This can be avoided by carefully placing a 4 × 4 cm gauze over the incision sites to prevent leakage. Between 15 and 45 minutes is adequate time for complete anesthesia. The small size of the laser fiber cannula (1 mm) allows lasing to begin sooner after the administration of anesthesia than with traditional tumescent liposuction.

Patients and medical staff are equipped with protective goggles. The encased laser fiber emitting 1064 nm (Nd:YAG laser system) (Fig. 12.6) is inserted through the incisions and slowly manipulated forward and backward in a criss-cross pattern. As a rough guideline, ten passes per section are made; however, it is important to recognize surgical end points when utilizing laser lipolysis. These end points can be determined by factors such as feel and temperature.

There is a learning curve when becoming comfortable with palpation as an end point. The tissue is continually palpated during cannulation until it feels soft and pliable, contrasting with the preoperative firm, larger, indurated areas. Continue palpation until the density of the treated area is uniform. Specialized cutaneous infrared thermometers can accurately record the surface temperature. In the authors' experience, safe, optimal lipolysis and skin tightening occur at surface temperatures between 35 and 40°C. Finally, additional end points such as the accumulated energy and change in resistance of fiber passage can be employed.

Once lasing is complete, record the total energy utilized. This will assist the surgeon in recognizing the endpoints of future procedures. Continued experience and documentation of previous cases

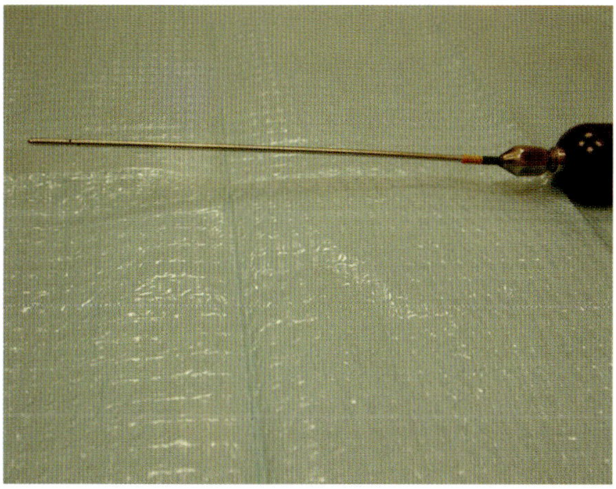

Fig. 12.5 Sprinkler tipped infusion cannula.

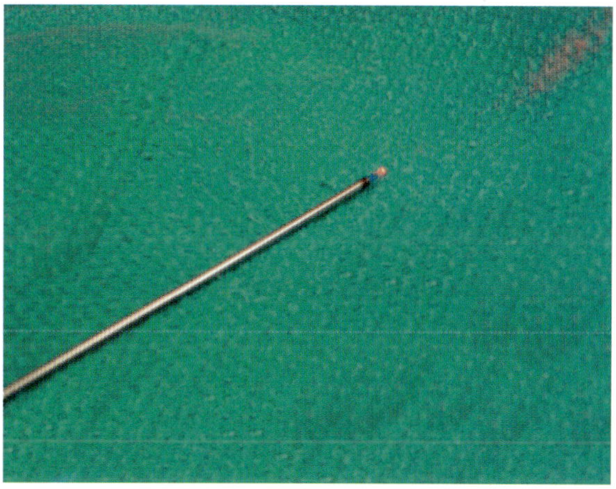

Fig. 12.6 Laser fiber in steel cannula extended 2 mm beyond the tip.

will provide the surgeon with appropriate benchmarks when performing subsequent cases.

OPTIMIZING OUTCOMES

- Proper patient selection.
- Aspiration versus no aspiration.
- Stay deep and pinch skin away from vital structures when operating over marginal mandibular nerve, facial artery, and vein.
- Maximize skin tightening by creating criss-cross tunnels with the laser fiber.

In a previous section, we note that the ideal laser lipolysis patient is one who has localized areas of adiposity and mild-to-moderate skin laxity. Selecting the proper patient is the first step toward optimal outcomes. Again, patients with severe dermatoheliosis or sun damage, or thin skin without noticeable adipose tissue are likely to have less than ideal outcomes and may in fact increase the risk of adverse sequelae.

Controversy does exist surrounding the need for suctioning after lasing. At a 2007 conference of the American Society of Laser Medicine and Surgery, Dr Douglas Key presented his experience using a 1320 nm device comparing lipolysis with aspiration, lipolysis without aspiration and aspiration without lipolysis. He found no clinical difference among the three techniques, suggesting that lipolysis alone was sufficient and safe to achieve optimum results. Doerr also notes that in cases of small areas (usually less than 50 cm^3 of estimated fat) or in patients with mild-to-moderate skin laxity, it is not necessary to aspirate the treated tissue.[8] In the authors' experience, most submental and neck regions do not require suctioning; however, the liquefied fat should be squeezed out through the incisions. Note that larger patients may benefit from minimal suction assistance to optimize results.

Suctioning can be accomplished manually or with a power-assisted device. The syringe method has been evaluated. Some surgeons prefer using a manual suction technique because patients may experience discomfort with the vibratory action associated with a power-assisted device. The authors have not experienced this phenomenon when using a power-assisted device. In fact, they have found more uniform and efficient removal of small, difficult areas with greater ease using a power-assisted device.

To optimize the end results and safety of laser lipolysis of the submental region, it is imperative that the surgeon stays deep in the subcutaneous fat. If the laser is fired too superficially, as with traditional liposuction, irregularities may result. Additionally, the energy from the laser can lead to superficial burns if the operator is too superficial to the skin. Finally, as mentioned earlier, the location of the marginal mandibular branch of the facial nerve is more superficial when the neck of the patient is extended and rotated laterally. Remaining in the proper plane in this location is therefore imperative. These potential risks can best be avoided by continuously pinching the skin away from the underlying structures and ensuring a position that is deep enough to avoid irregularities and burns, but not so deep as to compromise the safety of the marginal mandibular branch of the facial nerve.

An additional method to optimize the shrinking and tightening effect of laser lipolysis is to manipulate the fiber in a series of criss-cross tunnels. As a rough guideline, 10 passes per section are made. This criss-crossing ensures the optimal surface area coverage while preventing overaccumulation of energy in any one particular location.

COMPLICATIONS AND SIDE EFFECTS

With any new technology it is important to understand the associated potential complications and side effects. The potential risks when employing new lasers include burns, purpura, scarring, retinal and corneal damage, hyperpigmentation or hypopigmentation, necrosis and nerve damage. When performing liposuction, risks can be categorized as local or systemic. Local risk factors for liposuction are skin or subcutaneous infection, permanent skin irregularity (dimpling, retraction), seroma, allergic contact dermatitis to tape, skin ulceration or necrosis, permanent sensory nerve damage, unacceptable scars and persistent postoperative edema. The systemic complications include allergic reaction to oral or intramuscular medication, fevers, systemic infection, arrhythmias, anemia, fluid or blood loss requiring a transfusion, pulmonary emboli, fat emboli, shock, bowel or thoracic perforation, seizures, thrombophlebitis and death. When combining lasers with liposuction, the list of potential complications does indeed grow.

Despite these potential local and systemic risk factors and complications, in the authors' experience with over 500 cases actual complications of laser lipolysis have been rare. Out of 537 laser lipolysis cases, one patient developed a localized infection successfully treated with oral antibiotics and four patients developed skin burns.[9] The burns were treated with topical antibacterial ointments and were probably secondary to a rapid accumulation of thermal energy localized to one area. One way to prevent burns is to avoid keeping the laser in one location for too long. To address this complication, one company has developed a built-in safety device referred to as an 'accelerometer.' This device stops lasing when the handpiece is slowed or when the handpiece decelerates to change direction. Another way to prevent inadvertent burns is to monitor the skin with a thermal scanning device that measures cutaneous temperature, being careful not to exceed 40°C.

An additional safety concern is the theoretical possibility of nerve damage. In the 537 cases performed at the authors' center, there were no cases of persistent neuropathy, paresthesias or numbness. Studies by Goldman et al. demonstrated histologically intact nerve fibers with surrounding disintegrated adipose tissue, suggesting a selective thermolytic effect.[10] Despite this histologic finding, take special care when near the marginal mandibular branch of the facial nerve by gently pinching the skin away from the mandible when lasing in this location. Another issue of concern is the possibility of increased serum lipids as a result of lipolyzed adipose tissue. Goldman and colleagues found no significant change in triglycerides and lipid profiles among patients treated with laser lipolysis 1 day, 1 week and 1 month post procedure.

In the authors' experience, laser lipolyis also led to fewer touch-up procedures compared to traditional liposuction. Only 19 touch-up procedures were required in over 500 cases, using laser-assisted lipolysis and the tumescent technique.[7] These 19 patients comprise only 3.5% of the total liposuction cases completed at the center. In contrast, Lawrence and Butterwick studied the number of touch-up procedures at a large liposuction practice and found that over 12% of 954 liposuction cases required a touch-up.[11] The lower touch-up rate associated with laser lipolysis suggests enhanced uniform removal of adipose tissue, thereby contributing to improved physician control and precision of body contouring.

POSTOPERATIVE CARE

Once the procedure is complete, patients are cleaned, bandaged, and assisted into their compression garments. For treatment of the submental region, the garment is worn 24 hours a day for 3 days. Patients should be informed that the day after the procedure they may have minimal normal blood-tinged drainage. Some surgeons have patients return the second day after the procedure, at which time ultrasound, lymphatic drainage, diode laser or defocused Nd:YAG external laser treatment is employed. These treatments, some authors believe, may hasten the healing time.

In the authors' practice, patients return to clinic for reevaluation in 2 weeks, 6 weeks, 3 months and 6 months after the procedure. Patients will note the most rapid improvement 2–3 months after the procedure and will continue to improve up to 6 months after the surgery. To manage patients' expectations, it is important to inform them that maximal skin tightening may take up to 6–8 months. At the 6-month visit, postoperative images are taken and shared with the patient (Fig. 12.7).

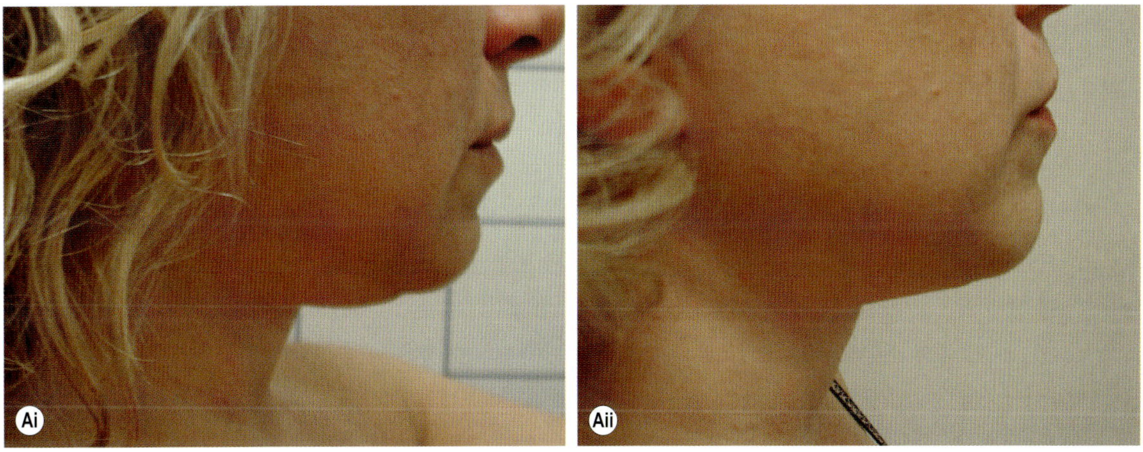

Fig. 12.7 Before and after images for laser-assisted lipolysis (left is preoperative, right is postoperative).

(Continued)

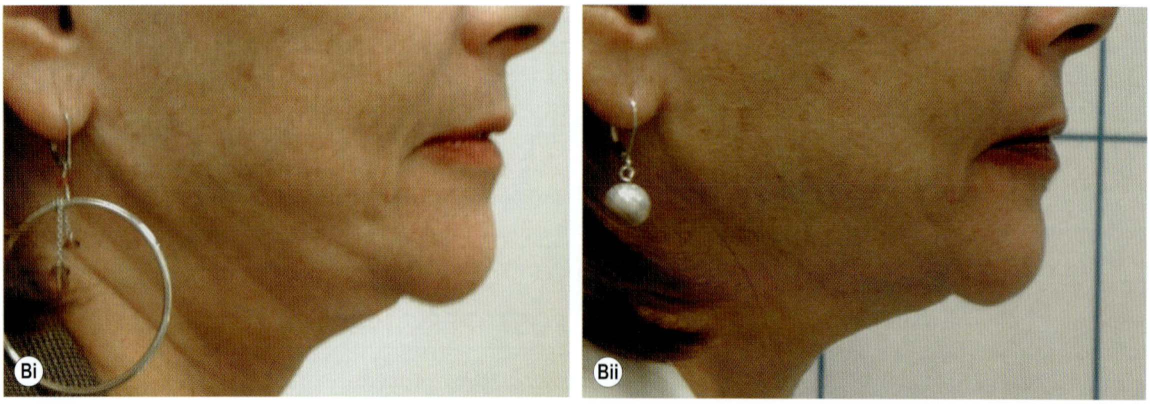

Fig. 12.7— Cont'd

CONCLUSIONS

Laser lipolysis is an exciting new development that efficiently removes fat and tightens skin. The technology continues to improve with various wavelengths and combination systems that promise to improve on original designs. Laser lipolysis of the submental and neck regions is an ideal option for those with small-to-moderate areas of adiposity combined with mild-to-moderate skin laxity. Laser lipolysis is particularly suited to the neck and submental regions due to the inherent contractile nature and, in some patients, may replace neck lifts or platysmaplasties.

REFERENCES

1 *US Food and Drug Administration*. http://www.fda.gov/default.htm 19 March 2009.

2 *American Society for Cosmetic Plastic Surgery*. 11.7m cosmetic procedures in 2007. http://www.surgery.org/public/consumer/trends/cosmetic_procedures_in_2007 19 March 2009.

3 Zins JE, Fardo D. The 'anterior-only' approach to neck rejuvenation: an alternative to face lift surgery. *Plast Reconstr Surg*. 2005;115(6):1761–1768.

4 Lawrence NL, Leonhardt J. Liposuction. In: Robinson JK, Hanke R, Sengelmann R, Siegel DM, eds. *Surgery of the skin: procedural dermatology*. St Louis: Mosby; 2005:13–14.

5 Coleman WP, Glogau RJ, Klein JA, et al. Guidelines of care for liposuction. *J Am Acad Dermatol*. 2001;45:438–447.

6 Hanke WC, Sterling JB, Melton JL, Sattler G. Review of liposuction safety studies. In: Dover J, Hanke CW, Sattler G, eds. *Procedures in cosmetic dermatology: liposuction*. London: Elsevier Saunders; 2005:141.

7 Jacob CI, Berkes BH, Kaminer MS. Liposuction and surgical recontouring of the neck: a retrospective analysis. *Dermatol Surg*. 2000;26:625–632.

8 Doerr TD. Lipoplasty of the face and neck. *Curr Opin Otolaryngol Head Neck Surg*. 2007;15:228–232.

9 Katz BE, McBean JC. Laser assisted lipolysis: a report on complications. *J Cosmet Laser Ther*. 2008;10(4):231–233.

10 Goldman A, Shavelzon D, Blugerman G. Laser lipolysis: Liposuction using and Nd:YAG laser. *Rev Soc Bras Cir Plast. Sao Paulo*. 2002;17(1):17–26.

11 Lawrence L, Butterwick KJ. Immediate and long term post-operative care and touch-ups. In: Narins RS, ed. *Safe Liposuction and Fat Transfer*. New York: Marcel Dekker; 2003: 329–341.

13 Mesotherapy

Alexander Kulick

Included on **DVD**

INTRODUCTION

The term 'mesotherapy' was reputedly first coined by journalists attending a lecture by Dr Michael Pistor, a French physician, in 1958. They mistakenly believed he was referring at the time to the mesoderm, an embryonic layer, and one of the three primary germ cell layers in the very early embryo, as opposed to injections into the dermis, the middle layer of the skin.[1]

Dr Pistor's principles were first enumerated in 1958. His system was at the time primarily used for medical and musculoskeletal disorders, and consisted of the need for:

- correct diagnosis
- the localized application of medications near the target organ
- the use of the smallest dose of pharmaceuticals for effective and localized treatment.
- During his lecture, Dr Pistor used the expression : *" I don't know how, I don't know why but it works."*

There are numerous theories that describe the mechanism of action. Some practioners believe in the reflexive theory, where the mechanism of action is due to the direct mechanical puncture, and chemical (or pharmacological) actions are a result of the action of the injected drugs. An alternative theory is microcirculation stimulation by the local injections close to the vessels damaged by the pathological process. In this theory the applications are made close to arterial paths with 1 or 2 cm in between the punctures. The third theory is Kaplan's interface where molecules with low weight are absorbed by blood vessels and the high molecular weight molecules are absorbed by lymphatic vessels passing through lymphatic nodes.[2]

In 1958 the French Academy of Medicine, endorsed mesotherapy as an integral part of traditional medical standards and in 1996 it was recognized by the National Health Agency of Accreditation and Evaluation in France.

The theory of mesotherapy is simple. The stratum corneum of the skin acts as an effective barrier to most large molecules, hence the paucity of pharmaceutical transdermal patches. In mesotherapy, the integrity of the stratum corneum is pierced, allowing the deposition of small amounts of pharmaceuticals. Numerous studies have demonstrated that molecules deposited in the epithelial dermal layer or the intradermal layer will be found in venous return for up to 8 hours, as opposed to 1 hour for subcutaneous injections. This prolonged exposure at the site of the target lesion leads to a more profound effect.[2]

MATERIALS, NEEDLES AND SYRINGES

Needles

The needles generally used in mesotherapy are 30 g (29 mm) and 27 g (40 mm) with needle lengths ranging from 4 to 13 mm for cosmetic purposes. Generally a 5 cc syringe is used manually or with an injection device.

Injection Devices and Mechanical Syringe Support

In recent years, a large number of mechanical injection devices that can accurately control both the depth and speed of injection have been developed. The most common devices will be described below along with some of the benefits and drawbacks of these devices.[3]

The ideal pistols should fulfill the following criteria:

- All the parts that have direct contact with the patient must be disposable
- The medication does not run inside the pistol but inside the syringe
- Must have mechanisms to calibrate depth of the needle and drug delivery
- Must have energy power or rechargeable battery

- Must be economic
- Must be ergonomic enough to allow injections in deferent angles and positions

Types of devices:

Den-Hub is a simple mechanical pistol fitted with a screw that determines the depth of injection and is activated by a simple trigger. It is an automatic device where a 10 mL syringe is plugged in.

Mesopen – this pistol operates on a lithium battery and both the depth and volume of substance to be delivered can be adjusted.

Mesalyse I – the Mesalyse I is composed of three components: a compressor, a control unit that can be programmed for both speed and depth of the injection and which can be set on a continuous or single injection mode, and a pistol with individual needles. The advantage of this device is that the speed of the injection can be modulated: increasing the speed decreases the patient's discomfort.

U225 – this device is very similar in form and function to the Mesalyse I.

DHN 1, 2, 3 and 4 – offers various degrees of complexity with the DHN 3 being the most complete device. The injection is triggered by pressure of the pistol on the skin and enables injections in continuous mode or single shot.

Piso 4 – this is a battery-operated system that allows the frequency and volume of injection to be adjusted and has one unique feature – *mesoperfusion*. Mesoperfusion allows two to six needles to be fixed to tubing connecting to a device that will perfuse the chosen medication at a low pressure. This allows a large area to be perfused at a low, comfortable pressure, e.g. for cellulite. The disadvantage lies in the need to purge the tubing before each usage and the necessity of replacing the tubing each time, together with a requirement for service and cleaning by the manufacturer every 6 months.

In the hands of a skilled practitioner mesotherapy can be performed manually with a simple syringe and needle. For novices, or if an assistant is to be taught, electronic pistols allow more control since the depth, volume, speed and frequency of the injection can be preset. Many of the devices do not fully retract the needle after penetration, causing superficial lacerations if the injector is 'dragged' across the face or body for continuous injection. This problem is found primarily with the use of needles made in the USA, which have less flexibility than many of the needles manufactured in Europe.

TECHNIQUES AND DEPTHS OF INJECTION

Intraepidermal Injection

Intraepidermal injection involves use of a 13 mm needle, which is is placed horizontally on the skin with the bevel facing upward. A series of injections to 1 mm depth is performed by a vertical flicking of the practitioner's wrist on moving along the desired area. The needle must not be dragged between points of injection or abrasions will result. The product is not injected into the skin but the disruption of the stratum corneum allows for quick localized absorption. The punctures are placed 2–4 mm apart and the movement is sometimes described as a "parkinsonian" type of movement, this technique is referred to in French as *'nappage'*.

Intradermal Superficial Injection

Intradermal superficial injection involves injection with a 6 mm needle at a depth of 1–2 mm. At this depth either point-by-point (PPP), which is a traditional injection technique, or nappage, with a total of 0.1 mL injected approximately at 1–2 mm, can be used. At this depth nappage is frequently described as a 'bouncing' technique, with numerous injections 2 cm apart. Pressure on the plunger is applied when the needle is in contact with the skin.

Deep Intradermal Injections

Deep intradermal injections are administrated at 2–3 mm depth with a volume of 0.5 mL per injection.

Hypodermal Injection

These injections can vary between 4 and 13 mm depending on the pathology being treated. For our purposes, the techniques that will be described are:

- *nappage* at 1 mm for skin rejuvenation (sometimes called mesoglow)
- *nappage* at 2–3 mm for cellulite
- point-by-point at 13 mm for localized fat (lipodissolve injections usually consist of phosphatidylcholine, and are meant for localized fat elimination)
- 'point by point' technique, which may be used to minimize scars.

AESTHETIC MESOTHERAPY

Localized Fat

Adipose tissue has two types of receptors, α and β, that normally interact with epinephrine norephinephrine and glucagon. These receptors may be stimulated by a number of medications that will in turn stimulate or suppress lipolysis. It should be noted that receptors are distributed differently in men and women, but in general there is a higher proportion of alpha receptors in the hip and buttock areas and more beta in the mid and upper torso.[4]

Cellulite

Cellulite refers to dimpling of the skin and most commonly affects the thighs and buttocks. Cellulite is brought about by alternating depressions and protrusions in the upper compartment systems of fatty tissue.

There are three major components in cellulite: hypertrophic adipocytes, thickening of connective tissue and consequently, bad drainage of the intercellular liquid.[4]

The pathophysiology may be attributed to a number of factors:

- genetic, gender and hormone factors
- vascular factors, including venous stasis and decreased lymphatic drainage
- lifestyle factors, such as tobacco, weight gain, and lack of exercise.

On a clinical level (Figs 13.1–13.4) the states can be identified as follows.

- Stage I can be elicited by compressing the skin but is otherwise not visible (Fig. 13.1A & B).
- Stage II is visible only on standing (Fig. 13.2).
- Stage III is visible on standing or lying down (Fig. 13.3).
- Stage IV is visible on both standing and lying down with moderate to severe nodules or pitting (Fig. 13.4).

Histologically, stages I and II are characterized by venous stasis and edema, and stages III and IV by fibrosis, with the eventual encapsulation of adipocytes by collagen fibers, forming micronodules and macronodules that are easily palpated.

Treatment

Treatment of cellulite can be very frustrating for both physician and patient as it often requires a combination of different modalities and an understanding and commitment from the patient to lifestyle changes.

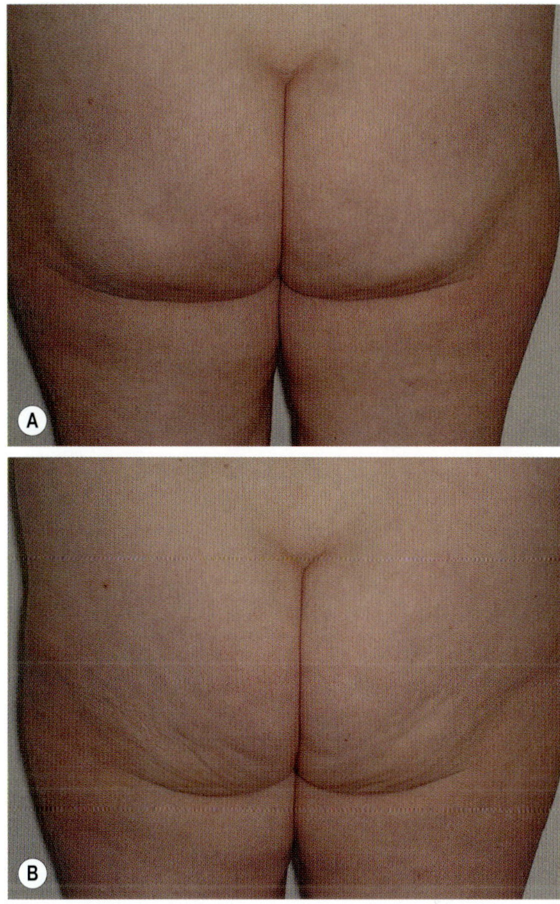

Fig. 13.1 Cellulite, stage I. Courtesy of Dr Eckart Haneke.

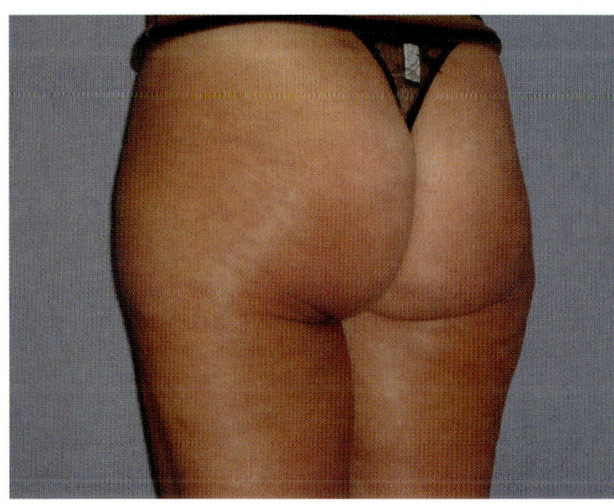

Fig. 13.2 Cellulite, stage II. Courtesy of Dr Eckart Haneke.

In stages I and II the main purpose is to to contract the veins, open the capillaries and decrease the edema to avoid fibrosis in the future. After preparation using an appropriate disinfectant it is

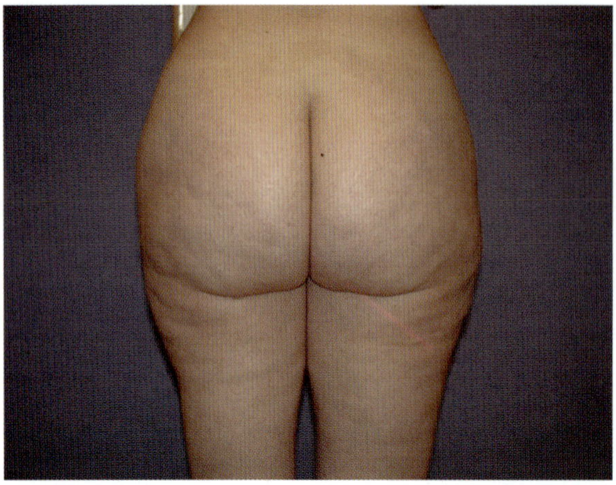

Fig. 13.3 Cellulite, stage III. Courtesy of Dr Eckart Haneke.

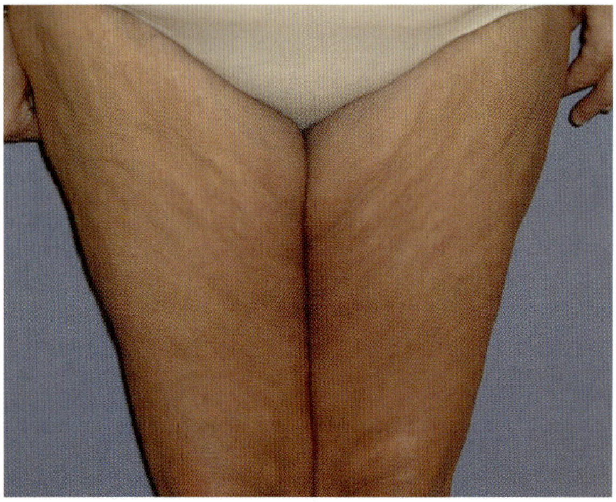

Fig. 13.4 Cellulite, stage IV. Courtesy of Dr Eckart Haneke.

possible to use either point-by-point injections or *nappage* if we wish to avoid bruising. Many combinations are used but in general they include:

- pentoxyphylline (Trental®) and/or phentolamine as a capillary dilator
- dihydroxyergotamine to cause vasoconstriction and reduce edema
- a solution of sodium monomethyltrisilanol orthohydroxybenzoate, associated with a derivative of bioavailable organic silicon and salicylic acid (Conjunctyl®) to increase collagen
- procaine, a potent vasodilator.

In Stages III and IV, phentolamine is always used for dilation. For the fibrosis, Conjunctyl® (monometilsianotriol salicylate) and collagenase may be used sparingly with subcision, to undermine the fibrotic bed of large nodules. Treatments should be weekly for 8 weeks followed by biweekly sessions for 1 month, and then monthly for 2–3 months. Depending on the severity, several other classes of drugs and herbs may be used but we should first briefly discuss the physiology of lipolysis.

Lipolysis

DRUG	ACTION
Aminophylline, Forskolin, caffeine	Phosphodiesterase inhibitors
Isoproterenol	β2 agonists
Yohimbe and phentolamine	Block α2 receptors
Acetyl-L-carnitine	Increases the transport of free fatty acids into the mitochondrion to be metabolized
Artichoke, mellilotus/ rutina	Increase lymphatic drainage and decrease venous stasis

If blood sugar is low or metabolic demands increase, glucagon and epinephrine, respectively, are released. These hormones increase cyclic AMP, which in turn binds to protein kinase and stimulates the lipases. It should be noted that beta-2 receptors increase lipolysis, alpha-2 receptors inhibit it. It is known that if phosphodiesterase is inhibited it will interfere with this process, probably by interfering with the binding of cyclic AMP to protein kinase. Hence inhibiting phosphodiesterase and stimulating the beta receptors (where epinephrine binds) and inhibiting the alpha receptors will all increase lipolysis. Many formulas use these principles.

Localized Fat

Two further treatments are used in the treatment of both cellulite and localized fat. The first is a mixture of phosphatidylcholine 50 mg/mL and deoxycholic acid 4.75 mg/mL, known as PC/DC, which has been used to facilitate lipolysis. Since the injections involved, at 13 mm depth, are into the hypodermis rather than the dermis, many consider this treatment not to be a form of mesotherapy and hence refer to it as 'lipodissolve'. Many practitioners combine PC/DC with the mixture of medication mentioned in the last section for treatment of localized fat and cellulite in Stages III and IV. The technique used is point-by-point PPP, 2 cm apart in the area to be treated. The use of PC/DC will inevitably lead to localized edema, swelling and pain. The pain subsides within 1 day and the swelling within 2–3 days. It is believed that the inflammatory response evoked by the deoxycholic acid causes retraction of the skin after lipolysis. Where a 'cocktail' is used, careful monitoring of the total doses of aminophylline, isoproteronal and yohimbe is required because of the associated cardiovascular effect and aminophylline toxicity. Patients with mitral valve prolapse, coronary artery disease (CAD) or known cardiac arrhythmias should not be injected with isoproterenol or yohimbe. According to Patricia Rittes,[5] the use of PC/DC in pure form, undiluted, has avoided many of the complications associated with the use of the β-agonist, aminophylline, and alpha-2 agonists.

Facial Lipodissolve

Patricia Rittes' protocols involve the use of PC/DC for other localized areas of fat:

- Double chin injections (Fig. 13.5): 0.5 mL of PC/DC in three to four areas and for jowls 0.5–0.6 mL at two points bilaterally.
- Fat pockets in the lower eyelids are treated to a depth of 6 mm with two to three injections of 0.1 mL of product per fat pad.[6]

Any area of the body can be treated with lipodissolve: axillary folds, love handles, saddle bags and abdomen.[7] Generally the abdomen is divided into four quadrants with either the lower or upper abdomen being treated with a maximum of 20 mL of PC/DC in each session. The treatment per area is every 2 weeks for four to six sessions. If results are not achieved, the sessions can be repeated after 2 months, as the PC/DC continues to work for up to 10 weeks.[8] One study on love handles showed histological changes that were primarily inflammatory, with lipolysis and release of free fatty acids and phagocytosis at 10 weeks.[9]

Loose Skin

Attempts have been made to treat loose skin with PC/DC, achieving occasional success in the periumbilical area. The fibrosis necrosis that follows injection into small fat pockets around the umbilicus will occasionally cause retraction and tightening of the lower abdomen.

For the face glutathione and DMAE (dimethylethanolamine) can be applied by *nappage* to a depth of 2 mm to create a mild lifting of the face.

Mesotherapy has not been effective for the tightening of loose skin on the posterior arms and anterior thighs.

Mesoglow/Mesolift

This procedure, shown in Figure 13.6, is used for skin rejuvenation and is not intended to replace Botox® or the various injectables. It is meant to improve the quality of the skin, repair sun damage with antioxidants, and to tighten skin and restore its hydration and shine.

In facial rejuvenation the structures are treated with the following substances:[10]

Fibroblasts:

- DNA stimulates healing and has a profound hydrating effect, as well as acting as a strong antioxidant (Ikeda)
- Conjunctyl® inhibits destruction of collage and elastin, and induces collagen formation
- placental extract (Filatov) controls growth and cellular rejuvenation

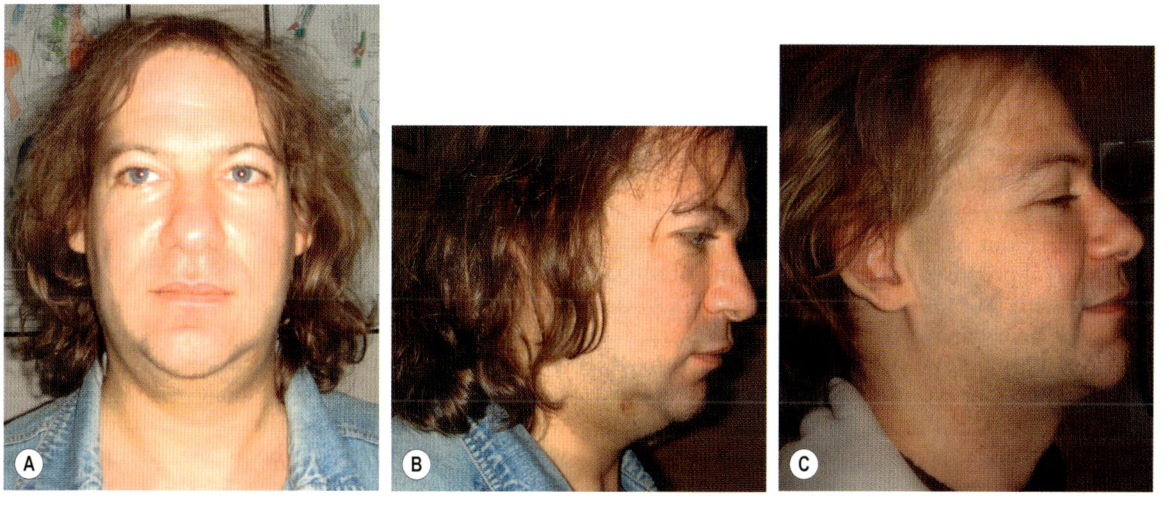

Fig. 13.5 Post-mesotherapy.

actively exercising should be discouraged from having this procedure.
- Although at present there is no literature to support the case, mesotherapy should not be given to patients with history of diabetes type I or type II.
- Patients with autoimmune conditions or extensive skin conditions (such as eczema or psoriasis) should not receive mesotherapy since they may have an increased risk of skin infection and abscess formation.
- Mesotherapy is not recommended in patients with a history of body image distortions, such as body dysmorphic syndrome.

COMPLICATIONS

Most of the undesirable effects are due to bad technique of application. It is important to know the origin of the drugs used, the amount, the number of sessions and the interval between them, and specially avoid the use of more than 4 substances at the same time.[11]

COMPLICATIONS
Pain
Erythema
Mechanical nerve lesion (particularly in superficial nerves)
Hematomas
Cutaneous necrosis
Infection

CONCLUSION

Mesotherapy is a non-invasive procedure and can be a great adjuvant for weight loss, cellulite management, hair growth, and for the delivery of nutrients and antioxidants to achieve healthier skin. Even though most people are potential candidates for mesotherapy, their goals and expectations must be realistic – mesotherapy is not a miracle. In the proper hands, and with the right patient selection, mesotherapy can be of assistance but there are no 'typical results'.

At the moment, there are no double-blind placebo-controlled studies showing average response in a given population group and for this reason the experience of mesotherapy is, for the most part, anecdotal. However, 50 years of mesotherapy treatment, in particular in France, Italy, other European countries and South America, have led to widespread public support for its efficacy. Some doctors report on their websites 'miraculous' results of up to 6 to 13 inches of waist loss. We believe that these types of results will not be consistently achieved and may not be typical; they may depend on the particular treatment that is used by the practitioner. This may contribute to the variability of results seen between different facilities performing mesotherapy. More studies are necessary and data are being collected for future medical presentations. It is a field that is growing rapidly due to the efforts of people like Jorge Silva, Jaque Le Coz, Phillipe Petit and a host of others around the world.

REFERENCES

1 Pistor M. *Un défi Therapeutique: La mesotherapie en pratique veterinaire*. III Congreso Internazionale de Mesotherapia, *Roma*, 1982.
2 Le Coz J. *Mesotherapie en Médicine Génerale*. Paris: Masson; 1993.
3 Rosenbaum R, Hellmer P, et al. An investigation of the morphology and biochemistry of cellulite. *Plast Recon Surg*. 1998;101 (7):34–37.
4 Le Coz J, Fabbi P, Lopez-Barri A. *Mésotherapie et medicine Estetique*. Marseille: Solar Editeurs; 1994.
5 Rittes P. The use of phospatidylcholine for correction of Localized fat deposits. *Aesth Plast Surg*. 2003;27:315–318.
6 Co AC, Abad-Casintahan MF, Espinoza-Thaebtharm A. Submental fat reduction by mesotherapy using phosphatidylcholine alone vs. phosphatidylcholine and organic silicium: a pilot study. *J Cosmet Dermatol*. 2007;6(4):250–257.
7 Duncan D, Rubin JP, Golitz L, et al. Refinement of technique in injection lipolysis based on scientific studies and clinical evaluation. *Clin Plast Surg*. 2009;36(2):195–209 v-vi; discussion 211.
8 Matarasso A, Pfeifer TM. Mesotherapy and injection lipolysis. *Clin Plast Surg*. 2009;36(2):181–92, v; discussion 193.
9 Rose PT, Morgan M. Histological changes associated with mesotherapy for fat dissolution. *J Cosmet Laser Ther*. 2005;7(1):17–19.
10 Iorizzo M, De Padova MP, Tosti A. Biorejuvenation: theory and practice. *Clin Dermatol*. 2008;26(2):177–181.
11 Tennstedt D, Lachapelle JM. Cutaneous adverse effects of mesotherapy. *Ann Dermatol Venereol*. 1997;124(2):192–196.

Skin rejuvenation with platelet-rich plasma

Maria Angelo-Khattar

INTRODUCTION

To date, the various options for skin rejuvenation have included lasers and energy-based devices, such as intense pulsed light and radio frequency, to stimulate neocollagenesis and enhance the skin's microcirculation. Furthermore, restoration of facial volume is currently accomplished by the use of synthetic dermal fillers and autologous fat (Chs 9 and 10, respectively). The therapeutic value of such treatment modalities, particularly with respect to periorbital rejuvenation, including the management of dark circles and under-eye depressions, is rather limited.

The use of autologous platelet-rich plasma (PRP) in cutaneous rejuvenation is a novel treatment strategy that relies on the natural healing capacity of the synergistic cascade of autologous growth factors.

Autologous PRP has been used in clinical practice since the 1990s and has an extremely broad range of healing applications in oral and maxillofacial surgery, cosmetic surgery, cardiovascular surgery, otolaryngology, burns and wound healing.

The latest application of autologous PRP now includes aesthetic treatments to address damaged and aged skin. Platelets, when present in body tissues outside the bloodstream, are activated by various chemicals to release growth factors that attract stem cells to the site of injury. The growth factors stimulate further mitosis of stem cells and differentiation into keratinocytes, fibroblasts and pre-adipocytes. This ultimately results in neovascularization and the production of collagen, elastin and new extracellular matrix. Platelet-rich plasma is a natural and powerful means of delaying as well as reversing cutaneous aging. The significant increase in skin thickness and elasticity, as well as the moderate volumetric effect achieved by both intradermal and subdermal injection of platelets, provides a safe, natural and long-term solution for skin regeneration and, in particular, periorbital rejuvenation. Furthermore, treatments with PRP are well accepted by patients due to the inherent safety of the technique. Because it is an autogenous preparation, PRP is free from transmissible diseases such as HIV, hepatitis and Creutzfeldt–Jacob disease.

PHYSIOLOGICAL ROLE OF PLATELETS IN HEMOSTASIS

Platelets play a central role in the mechanism of hemostasis.

The hemostatic response to injury includes the release of endothelial factors that attract circulating platelets and activate the coagulation process. The platelets aggregate at, and adhere to, the site of injury, where they release granules that contain the various cytokines that initiate coagulation and the formation of fibrin. Moreover, the release of thrombin at the site of injury further enhances the activation of platelets and the formation of a hemostatic plug to arrest bleeding. Both thrombin and the activated platelets are responsible for the initiation of the wound-healing reaction, resulting in tissue proliferation and angiogenesis.[1]

DEFINITION OF PLATELET-RICH PLASMA

Platelet-rich plasma is an autologous concentration of platelets in a small volume of plasma. It is derived from whole blood through the process of gradient density centrifugation. Normal platelet counts in blood average about 200 000 platelets/µl whereas effective preparation of PRP yields concentrations of 1 000 000 platelets/µl. This concentration of platelets in a 5 ml volume of plasma is now recognized as being the working definition of therapeutic enriched PRP.[2]

THERAPEUTIC EFFECT OF PLATELET-RICH PLASMA

The therapeutic effect of autologous PRP is due to mediation of the wound-healing reaction, which is initiated by formation of a fibrin clot and the degranulation of the alpha granules within platelets to release the full complex of growth factors. This action begins within 10 minutes of clot formation. The fibrin clot produced by the cell adhesion proteins in PRP, namely fibrin, fibronectin and vitronectin, serves as a scaffold for the platelets that are entrapped within the fibrin strands. The platelets release growth factors that act as a chemoattractant for stem cells and fibroblasts, which then begin to proliferate. Fibroblasts generate additional cytokines and produce collagen, elastin and glycosaminoglycans. This function of matrix remodelling, initiated by fibroblasts, continues for a period of approximately 300 days. However, the clinical benefit of PRP should last well over a year due to the profound neocollagenesis achieved.

The main fundamental protein growth factors proven to be actively secreted by platelets include the three isomers of platelet-derived growth factor (PDGF αα, PDGF ββ, and PDGF αβ), two of the numerous transforming growth factors β (TGF β1 and TGF β2), vascular endothelial growth factor, insulin-like growth factor and epidermal growth factor. All of these growth factors, with different physiological functions (Table 13.1) have been documented as being present in platelets.[3]

Table 13.1 Growth factors in platelet-rich plasma

Growth factor	Physiological function
Platelet derived growth factor	Stimulates mitosis of connective tissue and other cell types
	Promotes synthesis of collagen and structural proteins
Transforming growth factor	Regulation of cell proliferation, differentiation and apoptosis
Insulin-like growth factor	Regulator of cell metabolism and growth
Vascular endothelial growth factor	Regulates angiogenesis
Epidermal growth factor	Regulates cell proliferation, differentiation and survival

Following the initial release of growth factors, the platelets continue to synthesize and release additional growth factors for their remaining life span of 7 days. Once the platelet is depleted and apoptosis occurs, macrophages invade the area and take over the function of wound healing by further secreting growth factors. An additional source of growth factors is the leucocytes, a high concentration of which is obtained during the PRP preparation process. The presence of the leucocytes also imparts an added antimicrobial effect to the PRP.

The growth factors exert their action by binding to the external surface of cell membranes within the tissues. Studies have shown that adult mesenchymal stem cells, fibroblasts, endothelial cells, osteoblasts and epidermal cells express cell membrane receptors to growth factors in the PRP. These transmembrane receptors in turn activate a protein within the cell, which signals cellular proliferation, matrix formation, osteoid production and collagen synthesis. The significance of this information is to highlight the fact that PRP is not mutagenic and cannot induce tumour formation since it does not enter the cell or its nucleus.[4]

CONTROVERSIES REGARDING PLATELET-RICH PLASMA

There are several critical reports in the literature regarding the clinical efficacy of PRP. Some of these studies have used PRP from donor animals and it must be stated that true PRP is always autologous and not homologous. Furthermore, the success of the procedure is highly contingent upon the PRP preparation process. The centrifugation process must be sterile and the system used must allow for the sequestration of platelets in high concentration without damaging them in the process. Studies suggesting that there is no benefit from PRP can therefore be traced to poor quality PRP preparation by inadequate devices.

A positive cellular response in terms of fibroblast proliferation and type I collagen production may only be achieved by optimal platelet concentrations of four to five times baseline value.[5] Investigators using US Food and Drug Administration (FDA) and Certification Europe (CE) approved kits that allow for sufficient enrichment of plasma have reported significant enhancement of bone and soft tissue healing in face-lift surgeries[6], cosmetic dermal fat grafts,[7] mandibular bone grafts[8] and a multitude of other indications. However, to date there have been no clinical studies published on the use of PRP for cosmetic indications in skin rejuvenation.

PREPARATION OF PLATELET-RICH PLASMA AND INJECTION TECHNIQUE

Several platelet enrichment kits are available but the one used by the authors was the Regen PRP-Kit® by ReGen Lab (Mollens, Switzerland). This class IIa medical device, cleared by Certification Europe (CE), is a quick in-office procedure that requires less than 30 minutes of preparation time.

Preparation Procedure

- Blood (8.5 ml) is aspirated into a RegenTHT® (thrombocytes harvesting tube) containing citrate anticoagulant and a gel separator.
- The RegenTHT® tube is centrifuged for 8 minutes at 3100 rpm, which results in fractionation of the blood, with the erythrocytes being separated from the platelets, leucocytes and plasma by the gel separator.
- This yields on average 5 ml of plasma. To further enrich the preparation, 20% of the volume of the plasma is aspirated prior to resuspension of the platelets and leucocytes by tipping the tube several times.
- The tube is allowed to stand for 10 minutes prior to injection.
- The plasma is then aspirated into a 3 ml syringe containing 0.3 ml of 10% calcium chloride, which serves to activate the platelets.

Injection Technique

The activated platelets must be injected within 10 minutes of preparation; otherwise the fibrin clot will form inside the syringe. The PRP must then be injected very superficially, such that small blebs are obtained on the surface of the skin. Multiple injections are performed at almost every centimeter of the treatment area, akin to the 'coup par coup' technique of mesotherapy. Alternatively, for treatment of fine lines and wrinkles, PRP may be injected into the deep dermis and sub cutis, in the same manner as a dermal filler. Typical average injection volumes are: 1.5 ml per eyelid, 5 ml per cheek, 4 ml for the forehead, 7 ml for the neck and 8 ml for the back of each hand.

Pain management during injection may be achieved with either topical anesthetic cream or infiltration anesthesia, as required.

AESTHETIC INDICATIONS AND CONTRAINDICATIONS OF PLATELET-RICH PLASMA

Aesthetic indications

Skin aging, resulting from the progressive decrease in dermal collagen and elastin, manifests as early as the late 20s, due to both chronological and, most significantly, environmental factors. PRP can therefore be used for the prophylaxis of cutaneous aging, as of the early 30s. In older individuals where there is a need for rejuvenation and the reversal of the aging process, PRP can be used to fill out fine lines and wrinkles as well as to improve general skin tone and elasticity. Figure 13.8 shows the results of two PRP treatments on the full face of a 63-year-old patient. Figure A is the baseline photo and Figure B was taken two months after the second treatment. Typically

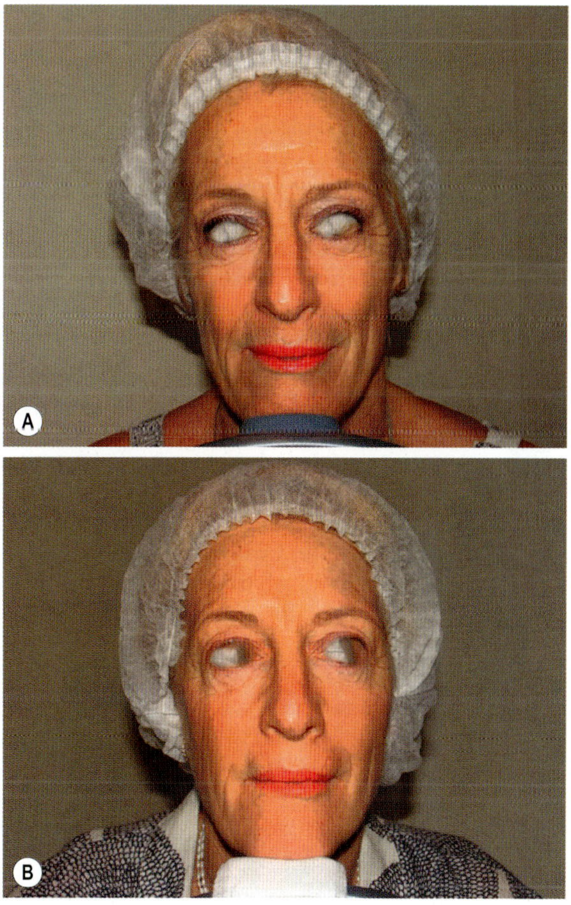

Fig. 13.8 A 63-year-old female patient before (*A*) and two months after (*B*) two treatments of the whole face with platelet-rich plasma.

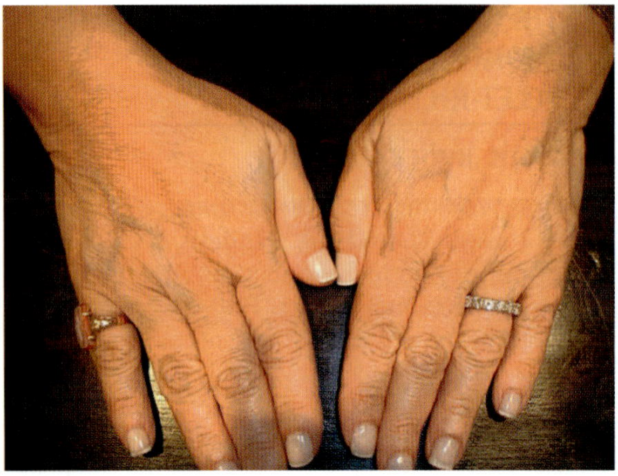

Fig. 13.9 Hands of a 57-year-old female patient taken 2 months after two treatments of the back of the left hand, with the right hand serving as a control.

PRP is injected in facial skin but is also beneficial for the restoration of skin on the neck, décolleté and back of the hands. Figure 13.9 shows the increase in skin thickness and elasticity 2 months after two PRP treatments on the left hand of a 57-year-old subject, with the right hand serving as a control.

Platelet-rich plasma is also a very effective treatment for saucerized acne scars, in particular when performed subsequent to ablative fractional laser resurfacing. In Figures 13.10 and 13.11 two patients with atrophic acne scars were treated with PRP alone. The figures exhibit a decrease in the depth of the scars 1 month after a single treatment.

One of the most impressive outcomes of PRP is in periorbital rejuvenation. Platelet-rich plasma results in a decrease in fine lines and wrinkles as well as a significant reduction in dark under-eye circles and depression such as the tear trough and nasojugal groove. Both the upper and lower eyelids of the patient shown in Figure 13.12 were treated twice with PRP at an interval of 6 weeks. There was a significant reduction in both under-eye depressions and skin laxity 1 month post treatment. Figure 13.13 shows the results obtained 1 month after a single treatment of the lower eyelids.

Dark circles affect individuals of all ages, both genders and all races. They give the person a tired and sad appearance. Although infraorbital darkening is attributed to multiple etiologic factors, the most commonly implicated factor is the superficial location of the vasculature, which is further exacerbated by skin laxity. The fact that infraorbital circles are seen in several members of the same family suggests a hereditary basis.[9] The increase in skin thickness and elasticity achieved with PRP yields a very natural and long-lasting solution to the rejuvenation of the lower eyelids. Improvement in skin texture of the upper eyelids is also achieved with PRP, in particular post-blepharoplasty since it is possible to increase skin thickness and thus camouflage the telengiastasia often seen after eyelid surgery.

The aesthetic indications for PRP can be summarized as follows:

- reduction of fine lines and wrinkles on the face and neck;
- improvement of skin elasticity on face, neck, décolleté and hands;
- treatment of post-acne atrophic scars;
- treatment of infraorbital dark circles and hollows;
- treatment of upper eyelids.

Contraindications of platelet-rich plasma

The contraindications of PRP are few and basically include clotting abnormalities and treatment with anticoagulant drugs. The only minor complication of PRP thus far encountered has been bruising due to needle trauma. However, as with any dermal filler or even autologous fat, there is a potential risk of intravascular injection or nerve trauma. Post treatment, patients are advised not to take any steroids or

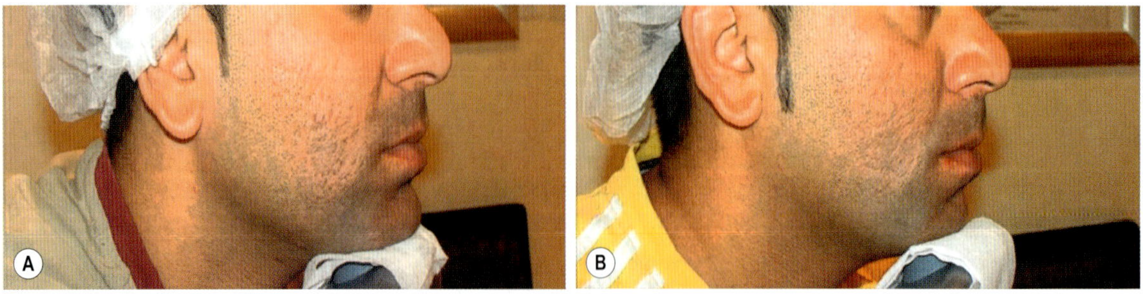

Fig. 13.10 A 34-year-old male patient before (*A*) and 1 month after (*B*) a single treatment for acne scars.

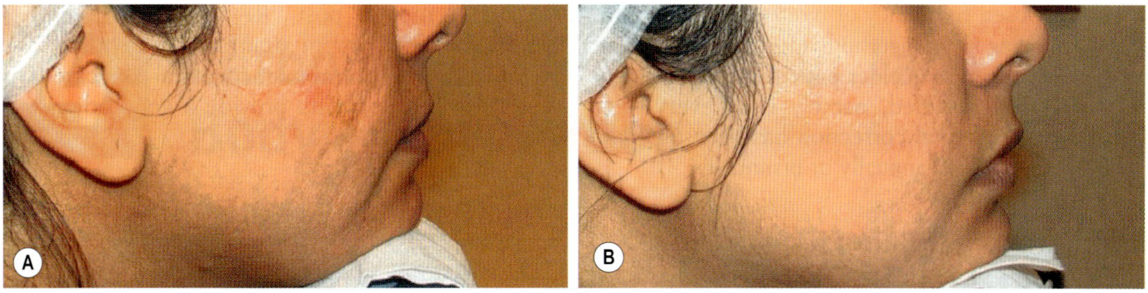

Fig. 13.11 A 29-year-old female patient before (*A*) and 1 month after (*B*) a single treatment for acne scars.

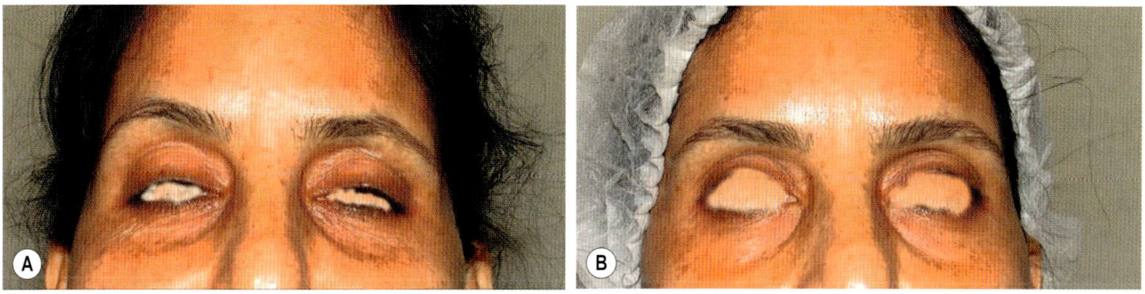

Fig. 13.12 A 56-year-old female before (*A*) and 1 month after (*B*) two treatments of the lower and upper eyelids.

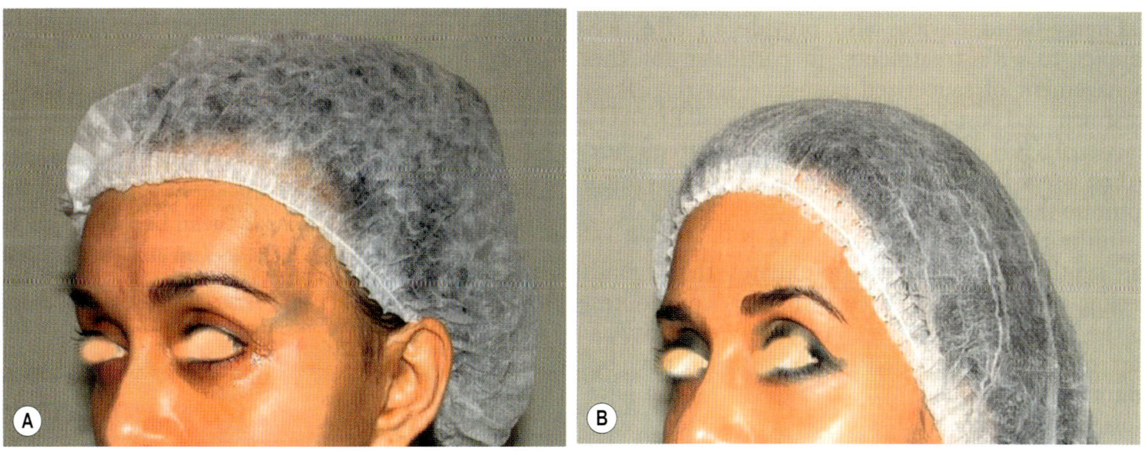

Fig. 13.13 A 45-year-old female before (*A*) and 1 month after (*B*) a single treatment of the lower eyelids.

non-steroidal anti-inflammatory drugs (NSAIDs), as this would suppress the immune response, which is integral to the wound healing reaction.

The contraindications to PRP can be summarized as follows:

- platelet abnormalities such as low platelet count;
- infection in the area of proposed treatment;
- febrile illness;
- chronic liver disease;
- anticoagulation therapy (warfarin or heparin).

Post-treatment

The patient should be maintained on a daily regimen of 3000 mg of Vitamin C orally for optimum collagen synthesis as well as the use of topical dermocosmeceutical products rich in vitamin C, vitamin A, idebenone or alphalipoic acid. The patient should also be cautioned against the ingestion of non-steroidal anti inflammatory agents since these might suppress the wound healing response, which is integral to the success of the treatment.

- old stretch marks
- hair loss
- recent scars and acne scars
- psoriasis.

EFFECTS OF CO_2 INJECTIONS ON THE BODY

Transcutaneous or injected CO_2 produces various effects on the body.

Vasodilatation

One of the first effects to be noticed following CO_2 injection is a strong vasodilatation and blood flow increase as well as a higher pO_2.[2,3]

The Bohr Effect

Local oxygen release is improved because of the Bohr effect. The Bohr effect describes the tendency of hemoglobin to have less affinity for oxygen when the blood concentration of CO_2 is increased. This lower affinity leads the hemoglobin to better release the oxygen in superficial tissues and muscles. This effect facilitates the transport of oxygen from the lungs to the tissues which need it. In the lungs, the oxygen binds to the hemoglobin and is transported to the tissues. When a tissue metabolic rate increases, the CO_2 production also increases. CO_2 is quickly converted to bicarbonates and H^+ acid in presence of the carbonic anhydrase enzyme.

$$CO_2 + H_2O \rightarrow H^+ + HCO_3^-$$

This reaction causes the tissue's pH to decrease (become more acidic). A lower pH increases the dissociation of O_2 from hemoglobin, allowing the tissue to become more oxygenated (Fig 14.1).

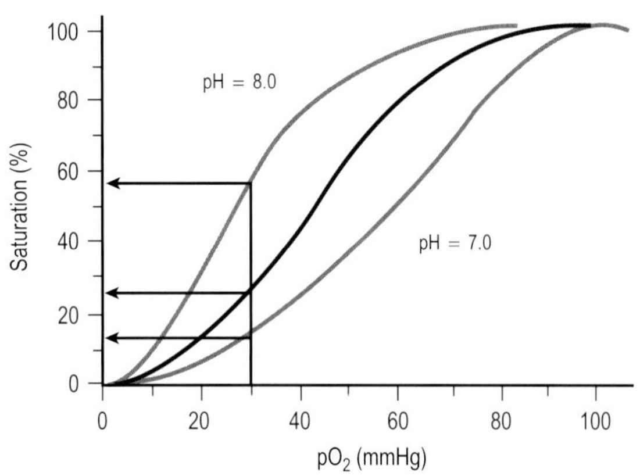

Fig. 14.1 The Bohr effect.

Stimulation of Collagen Synthesis

A 2008 Brazilian study on rats showed a visible compacting of collagen fibers following an intradermal injection of CO_2.[4] It was demonstrated that the CO_2 increases the collagen turnover. We tend to compare this improvement to the improvement from laser remodeling. Initiating a trauma to the dermis launches a healing process with collagen synthesis.

CO_2 has two other interesting properties to enhance healing. First, it increases neovascularization so more healing substances and factors will be on site. Second, it releases more oxygen around and in the healing area, improving the recovery phase. We feel studies on combined therapies associating CO_2 injections, remodeling lasers (1064–1550 nm), LED stimulations, radiofrequency(RF) and infrared skin tightening devices may improve results further.

Neo-angiogenesis Effect

Besides the increase of blood flow, CO_2 injections are capable of stimulating neoangiogenesis with the development of new capillaries.

Suspected Melanocyte Pigment Synthesis Stimulation

Although there are no studies concerning this effect, we have observed that CO_2 injections tend to improve the melanocyte metabolism, therefore increasing the production of melanin. Further studies need to be undertaken.

Receptor Activation and Lipolysis Improvement

There are various differences between the morphology of fat tissue and normal tissue, i.e. their blood circulation, lymphatic drainage and biochemistry.

The effect of CDT on the microcirculation leads to a higher blood flow and therefore to more oxygen being released, which produces a more oxidative lipolytic effect.

The pressure receptors in the Golgi apparatus work in synergy with Pacinian corpuscles pressure receptors. When stimulated by pressure, trauma or pain, they lead to a synthesis or release of bradykinin, histamine, serotonin and catecholamine. These mediators activate beta-adrenergic receptors and tissue cyclic AMP, leading to stimulation of lipase enzymes. These cascading reactions improve the lipolysis process in injected areas.

EQUIPMENT

Almost all CDT machines are based on the same architecture. They contain the following parts (Fig. 14.2):

- CO_2 tank
- pressure regulator
- 0.22 µm filter
- electromechanical valves
- embedded central processing unit board and human/machine interface
- gas heater
- tubes/terminal, 0.22 µm filter, 30G needle

CO_2 Tank

A CO_2 tank is normally purchased or rented from a medical gas supplier. It contains medical grade CO_2, which is the same as the gas used for abdominal surgery that is found in most hospitals. The tank's size varies from one country to another and there are different sizes on the market. Care is required to ensure that the CDT machine is compatible with the tank. Most of the time an adaptor/regulator is delivered with the machine when it is installed.

There are several precautions necessary when manipulating gases. The tank should be delivered with a safety sheet covering most of the points of which practitioners should be aware.

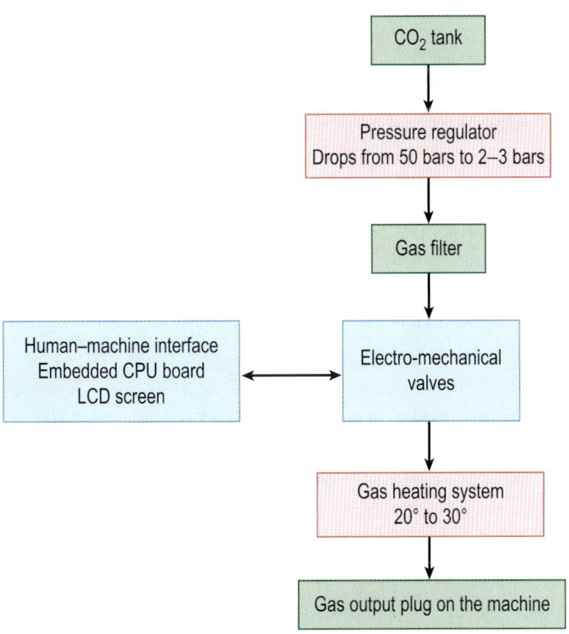

Fig. 14.2 Components of a CDT machine.

- Keep oil and other lipids away from the tank as pressure and fat may cause an explosion.
- Use the CDT machine in a ventilated room to avoid accumulation of CO_2, which could potentially cause breathing difficulties.
- Control the temperature of the room where the equipment is operated.
- Verify that tubes are properly attached and locked in place to avoid leaks. A leak could empty a tank in a few hours and could also lead to unstable output pressure, compromising the treatment.

Pressure Regulator

Almost all medical gases are stored in tanks at very high pressure. CO_2 tanks are usually at 50–60 bars. For CDT, we lower the pressure to 2–3 bars. The gas regulator should adjust the pressure and stabilize it. Most of the time the output pressure can be manually adjusted according to treatment needs. A suggested output pressure is 3 bars. Most pressure regulators have two manometers: one for input pressure (typically 50 bars) and one for the output pressure (treatment pressure) (Fig. 14.3). Although it should only be necessary to adjust the pressure when the tank is opened, it is not a bad idea to check manometers from time to time during the day as gas bottles can empty or need adjusting.

First Filter

The first filter, typically 0.22 µm, may be optional in some machines. The filter (Fig. 14.4) is provided in order to block viruses, bacteria and impurities so that a pure, filtered gas enters the CDT machine.

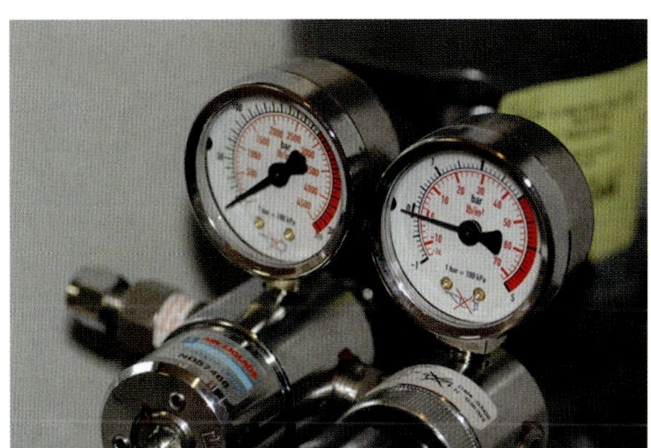

Fig. 14.3 Pressure regulator: most CO_2 tanks are at 50 bar. The regulator lowers the pressure to 2–3 bars (30–40 psi).

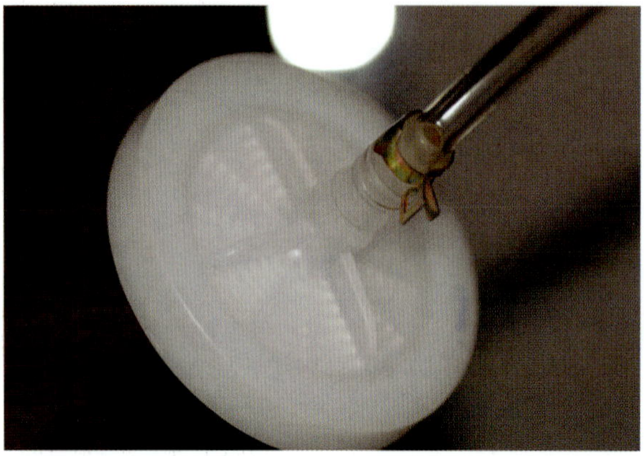

Fig. 14.4 A 0.22 μm filter, which is inserted between CO_2 tank and CO_2 equipment in most machines. It prevents contamination and dust from entering the system.

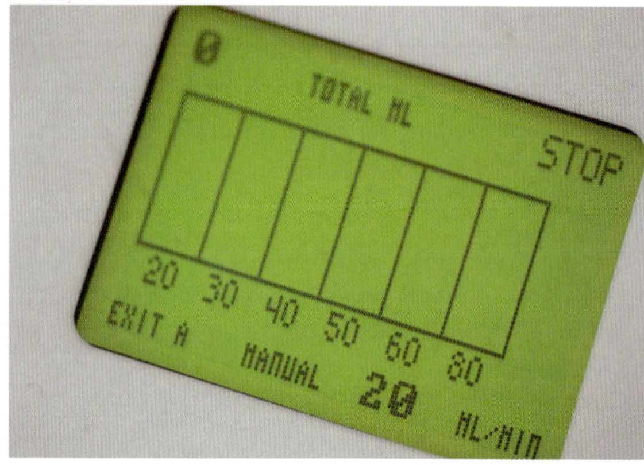

Fig. 14.5 Front liquid crystal display of a CO_2 insufflation machine. The most important parameters are flow value, total amount of CO_2 delivered, heated or non-heated mode.

The filter should usually be changed every 3 months to maintain its efficacy. After some time the membrane could be affected and may allow dust, particles, bacteria and viruses to pass through. If this is the case, the risk of bacterial colonization of the inside of the machine is increased.

Electro-mechanical Valve Compartment

The heart of any CDT system is the electro-mechanical valve compartment. Once the gas pressure has been set to 3 bars, the total amount of delivered CO_2 has to be controlled at a constant volume per minute (cc/min). To achieve this goal, each machine has a set of electronically monitored valves, which open or close to maintain a precise flow and CO_2 quantity.

Computerized Area

Valves should deliver a precise amount of CO_2 at a predetermined flow. For this reason, they are driven by an embedded electronic computer. This computer reads values from a flow meter and is capable of controlling the positions of all the valves. Timer functions are used by the computer to stop the injection when a precise amount of gas has been delivered to the skin.

In most machines, the CPU board also accepts the operator's commands through a digital touch liquid crystal display interface (Fig. 14.5). The physician is able to select a flow and duration, and sometimes a specific injection mode.

Gas Heater

It has been demonstrated that warm CO_2 is better than cold as it gives more vasodilation and an increased Bohr effect with better oxygen release. Frozen, decompressed gas also gives a higher level of pain when it is injected into the dermis or into subcutaneous skin layers. New generations of CDT machines are all able to deliver heated gas.

Tubes, End Filter and Needles

Tubes, filter and needles are the consumables attached to the CDT machine. They are sterile, for obvious reasons, and are changed for each patient. These parts are not much different from the tubes used in traditional intravenous injections of drugs.

The plastic tube should resist the 3 bars pressure and should be long enough to let the operator work easily. A minimum length of 1 m is required.

The tube is attached to a bacteria/virus filter which lets the CO_2 gas pass through. It is a 0.22 μm membrane. This filter receives a 30 G mesotherapy needle. The shape of the filter is designed to let the operator manipulate the needle with precision (Fig. 14.6).

INDICATIONS AND CONTRAINDICATIONS

CDT has various indications. Most publications cover vascular disease and localized fat where protocols and indications are relatively clear.

We can split indications into two groups: medical vascular diseases and aesthetic procedures. The first group is the best documented, with a large number of publications since 1930.

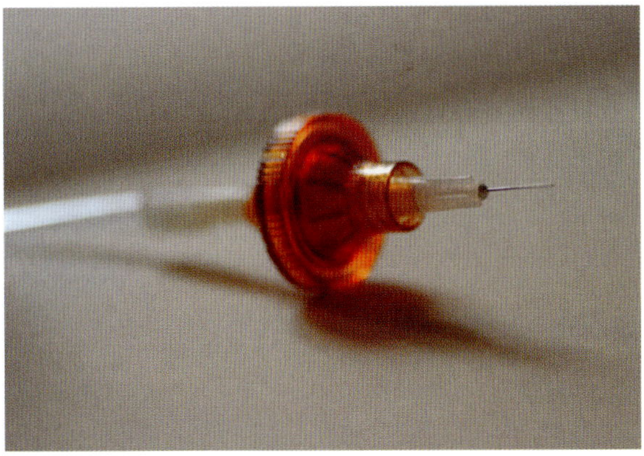

Fig. 14.6 The CO_2 end filter and 30 G mesotherapy needle. The filter is held by the operator's fingers. It is a 0.22 μm filter, which will prevent most bacterial or viral infections.

CDT Indications

Vascular

- Raynaud's phenomenon
- Lower limb arterial diseases and ischemia
- Erectile dysfunction with micro-vascularization disorders

Aesthetic

- Localized fat
- Acne scars
- Surgical scars
- Traumatic scars
- Stretch marks
- Eye wrinkles, fat deposits and under-eye dark circles
- Rejuvenation of the hands, décolletage, neck
- Psoriasis
- Nasogenian folds and peri-oral wrinkles

It should be noted that some South American physicians, although not published, use CDT prior to surgery to lower scarring complications. Some operators also use CDT to treat skin grafts and burnt skin.

Vascular Indications

Raynaud's Phenomenon

Raynaud's phenomenon is a vasospastic disorder of the extremities causing discoloration of fingers and toes, and pain. It is an inappropriate vasomotor response to cold and/or emotional stress, with sympathetic system hyper-activation, which leads to strong vasoconstriction of the peripheral blood vessels, causing tissue hypoxia. Chronic Raynaud's phenomenon may lead to skin atrophy.

CDT has blood flow increase properties, especially targeting microcirculation of the superficial tissues. In addition, the Bohr effect has strong anti-ischemic properties. CDT may therefore be a complementary treatment for this condition.

Lower Limb Vascular Diseases with Ischemic Symptoms

CDT has been widely used in France's Royat Spa since the beginning of the 20th century to treat arterial diseases of the legs. There are now better treatments available such as bypasses and vessel grafts. CDT should only be seen as a complementary procedure for lower limb ischemic arteriopathy.

Ulcers (Arterial and Venous)

Ulcers are related to venal or arterial insufficiency. Consequently, the healing process may be improved by intradermal CO_2 injections. Although particularly painful, CDT sessions to treat ulcers require very low flows until complete re-epithelialization.

Aesthetic Indications

Localized Fat

Since its publication at the University of Siena, the use of CDT for localized fat has been among the best known indications for the technique.[3]

Direct pressure causes trauma to the adiposities and, although this is unproven, seems to weaken them. Blood flow increase and the Bohr effect bring more oxygen to the adiposities leading to an optimized physiological lipolysis.

CDT can be used alone for localized fat or combined with liposuction for even better results. It can also be used to improve the 'wave effect', which may be seen after a liposuction, especially in areas which were either not treated or not treated effectively. Physicians should be aware that liposuction may create septations, preventing the gas from diffusing normally and requiring multiple CO_2 punctures.

Acne Scars

CDT works in various ways for acne scars. It has been demonstrated that CO_2 injections stimulate the synthesis of collagen. This property is used to improve atrophic scars by increasing the quantity of collagen below the atrophy. Nd–YAG (1064 nm) or erbium–glass (1320–1550 nm) lasers produce the same effect. The use of CDT is adapted to imperfections and mild acne scarring.

Some CDT procedures may also be of use in a way which can be compared to subcision. Some physicians use high flows of CO_2 to simulate the effect of a needle. This technique aims to break fibrous septae which pull the scar below the skin surface. As yet, no stabilized protocol has been published but before/after photographs show interesting results.

Surgical Scars

CDT is also used to improve post-surgery scars. CO_2 may restore skin laxity and color, and speeds up the wound-healing process. It is an interesting procedure for white thyroidectomy, caesarean, appendectomy scars and other scars in general.

Some physicians also use CDT in a presurgical procedure to prepare the skin for the healing phase before the surgical incision.

Traumatic Scars

Recent trauma may benefit from the healing properties of CO_2. The improvement of oxygen concentration and the neo-vascularization induced by subcutaneous injections shortens skin restoration times. CO_2 may prevent hypocromic scars, especially with dark phototypes.

Stretch Marks

Stretch marks are very common among women and are a good indication for CDT. While recent marks may benefit from pulsed dye laser or potassium-titanyl-phosphate (KTP) laser sessions, old white marks still remain a problem for the physicians. Some authors have stimulated pigmentation using excimer lasers or UV-B narrow-band lamps. Others are using collagen remodeling lasers such as with Nd–YAG, erbium–glass and fractional lasers. All these approaches have a non-negligible level of patient dissatisfaction. CDT is a relatively new indication for old white stretch marks. It works in three different ways:

- neo-angiogenesis below the mark, which adds a pink color
- melanin stimulation caused by increased oxygen in the tissues
- collagen synthesis, which reduces the creased appearance.

Eye Wrinkles, Lower Lid Fat Deposits and Under-eye Circles

Because it stimulates collagen synthesis and has a local lipolytic action, CO_2 injection may be an indication for eye rejuvenation and fat deposits. The procedure is easy, fast and produces virtually no pain.

There are several possible causes of dark under-eye circles:

- Deposition of pigments and melanin after the lower lid has been exposed to allergy and chronic irritation/inflammation can be compared to post-inflammatory hyperpigmentation. This is not a good CDT indication. Physicians would probably use peelings and/or lasers (KTP, Q-switched).
- Vascular pooling with congestion of the lower eye lid capillary network results in a bluish appearance that can be seen through the skin. CDT is a good indication for this condition: better oxygenation and higher flow will convert the blue color to red, decreasing the dark circle appearance.
- The depression beneath the lower eyelids known as 'tear trough deformity' is not a good indication for CDT. Patients need fillers to restore volume.
- Fat accumulation in the lower part of the lower lid, known as 'fatty prolapse' is a good indication for CDT sessions as the procedure has lipolytic properties. Extreme care should be taken in this area because the skin is fragile and thin. Low flow values should be used.

Rejuvenation of the Hands, Décolletage and Neck

Carbon dioxide injections are also good for skin laxity and therefore skin rejuvenation, in all the exposed areas.

The dorsal side of the hands may be treated using intradermal injections. The expected effect is skin tightening after four or more sessions. CDT will have no effects on lentigos, which will require other treatment modalities such as nitrogen, KTP laser, Alexandrite laser or Q-switched laser.

Neck and décolletage rejevenation are very good indications for CDT.

Psoriasis

Some physicians use CDT for psoriasis treatment. There do not appear to be any protocols or published studies about this indication, which should be considered experimental.

Nasogenian Folds and Peri-oral Wrinkles

CDT is an alternative to fillers in some cases. Patients with contraindications to fillers or who do not want filler injections may be treated with CO_2 injections. Physicians and patients should be informed that several sessions are necessary with CO_2, with progressive improvement, whereas fillers have immediate results.

CDT CONTRAINDICATIONS

CDT contraindications are limited and very similar to those for mesotherapy. There are general contraindications, local skin contraindications and temporary ones.

General Contraindications

The general contraindications for CDT are:
- needle phobia
- stress, with history of vagal unconsciousness event
- severe heart failure, congestive heart disease
- recent heart infarction or instable angina pectoris
- restrictive pulmonary disease, chronic obstructive lung diseases
- sleep apnea
- renal failure, dialysis
- recent cerebrovascular accident
- uncontrolled blood pressure
- epilepsy
- recent phlebitis or pulmonary embolism
- uncontrolled diabetes
- immunosuppression or deficiency
- chemotherapy, cancer (healing disorders)
- patients with impaired healing
- connective tissue disorders or diseases
- bleeding diseases: Willebrand's disorder, hemophilia.

Local Contraindications

There are also a series of local contraindications:
- bacterial infection: dermatitis, cellulitis
- foreign body in the area to be treated (jewellery implants and so on)
- herpes simplex in acute phase and other acute skin viral infection
- skin disease with abnormally increased local circulation
- facial rosacea
- poikiloderma of Civatte
- red necks and red décolletage.

Temporary Contraindications

Temporary contraindications include:
- pregnancy (precautionary principle)
- lactation (precautionary principle)
- anticoagulation, recent aspirin or antiinflammatory drugs intake
- acute skin infection (wait until it is cured)
- other aesthetic procedure or skin traumatism less than 15 days prior to CDT.

SKIN LAYERS AND CDT CONCERNS

CDT indications require different planes of injection, depending on the effect desired. We can schematize two different injections: subcutaneous and intradermal; each one giving different effects.

Skin Layers

Mesotherapy 30 G needles for CDT have an approximate length of 11 mm. This size is ideal for targeting the two different layers of the skin. Although the subcutaneous layer is easy to inject, intradermal injections may be hard for novices to administer precisely, a problem similar to that encountered by medical students trying to administer intradermal reaction tests for tuberculosis vaccinations. Carboxytherapists should proceed in the same way in order to target intradermal layers (Fig. 14.7).

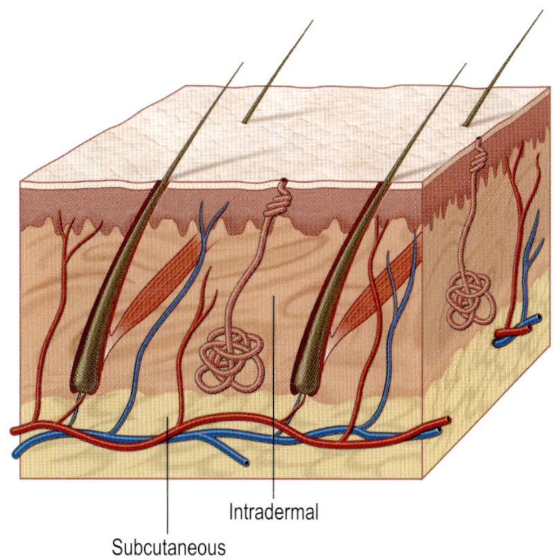

Fig. 14.7 Different CO_2 injection layers.

Subcutaneous Injections

Subcutaneous CDT injections are administered to reach the localized fat area, activate lipolysis and improve blood flow (Figs 14.8–14.11).

Subcutaneous injections require a 30 G mesotherapy needle with a length of 11 mm mounted on the 0.22 µm filter. The skin is disinfected at least 1 minute before injecting CO_2.

The needle should point at an angle of 35–45° to the skin. It is possible to pinch the skin to ease the penetration of the needle. In traditional mesotherapy, it is necessary to make multiple injections as the liquid drug does not diffuse much. CDT, on the other hand, injects a gas, which is able to diffuse, sometimes very far from the puncture. Because the gas diffuses both along the surface and to greater depths, it is not necessary to place the needle too deep to get a good effect. Moreover, placing the needle too deep will prevent the operator seeing and controling the end point. Making a superficial subcutaneous injection will therefore let the operator monitor the CO_2 below the skin. Usually, a good subcutaneous injection will produce a 15–18 cm red circle on the skin surface. This circle has a granite-like appearance. For an optimized session, it is necessary to move the needle for each injection by 15–18 cm, with no overlapping, to cover the fat areas. While pain is limited in thick areas of fat, it may be higher in areas when the fat layer is thin.

In CDT, it is important to be aware that after the first session the gas will not diffuse too far from the injection point. In the subsequent sessions (around five to eight), the CO_2 gas will tend to diffuse great distances from the needle. This phenomenon is normal and permits fewer injections/treatment sessions to be required. Patients also report less pain from one session to another as the skin layers get used to be separated.

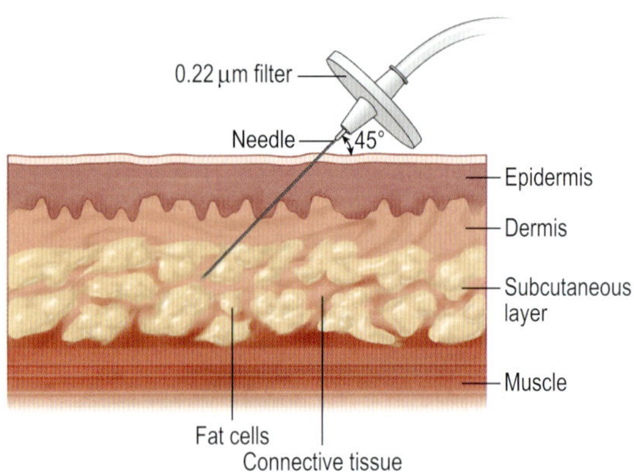

Fig. 14.8 Subcutaneous injections require a 45° angle to target fat cell areas.

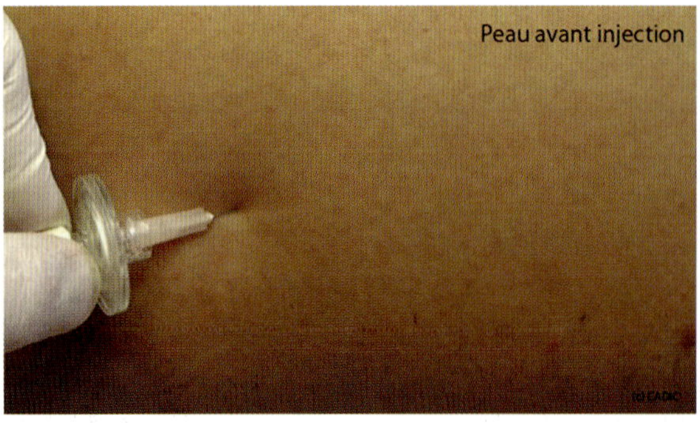

Fig. 14.9 Beginning of a subcutaneous injection.

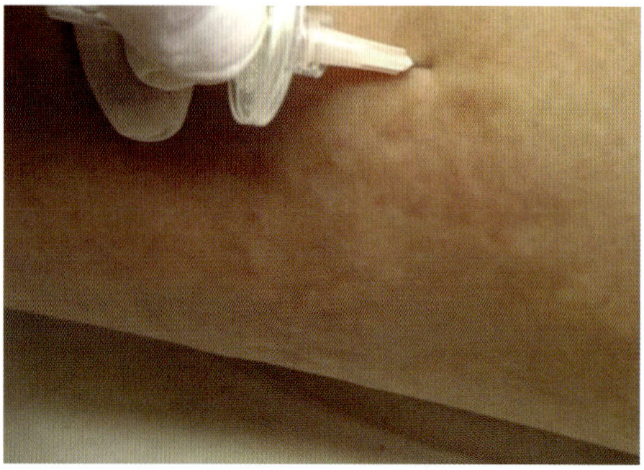

Fig. 14.10 End of injection and skin appearance after 2 minutes.

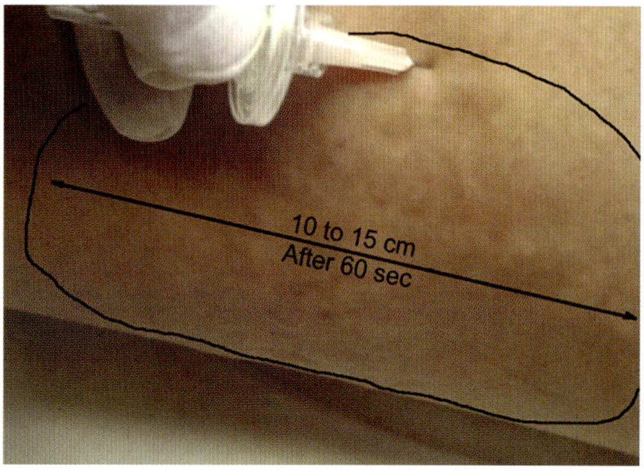

Fig. 14.11 In the first sessions, the gas diffuses to create a 10–15 cm circle where the skin appearance is modified.

Intradermal Injections

Intradermal injections (Fig. 14.12) are performed in most CDT procedures. The goal is to stimulate the dermis to collagen synthesis. As with deep-penetration lasers, we are aiming to get a remodeling effect.

The intradermal injection is made with a 30 G mesotherapy needle mounted on the 0.22 µm filter. The skin is disinfected at least one minute prior to puncturing the skin.

The injection is made at an angle of less than 15°, needle bevel up or with an extremely small rotation angle. The operator should not push the needle too far. If properly positioned, there is a short skin whitening appearance before immediate inflation. The whitening indicates a good intradermal position.

Most intradermal injections will produce a 1.5–2 cm red disk with a granite-like skin appearance. In some cases, a very superficial skin detachment may also be seen, producing the appearance of fern leaves. To cover the full area, the needle should be moved by 2 cm each time, with no overlapping. The endpoint of the treatment is when redness (erythema) affects the skin.

If there are any remaining white areas, these indicate untreated areas and should be injected immediately.

Using intradermal injections for the décolletage (Figs 14.13 and 14.14) may be uncomfortable for the operator as getting a proper injection angle – lower than 15° – is sometimes hard with large surfaces. It is possible to bend the needle to maintain a low puncture angle.

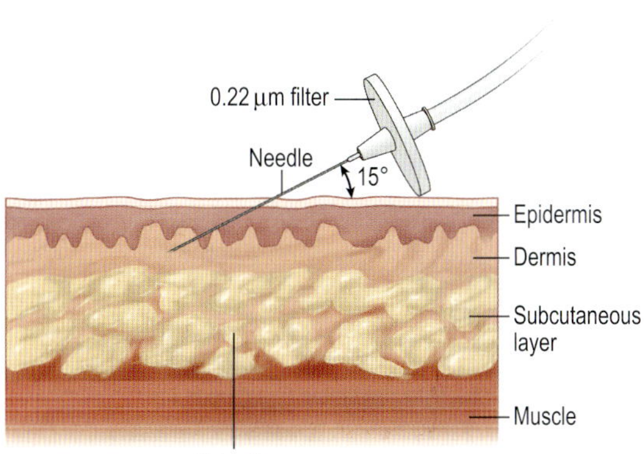

Fig. 14.12 Intradermal injections require very low needle angle to treat the dermis.

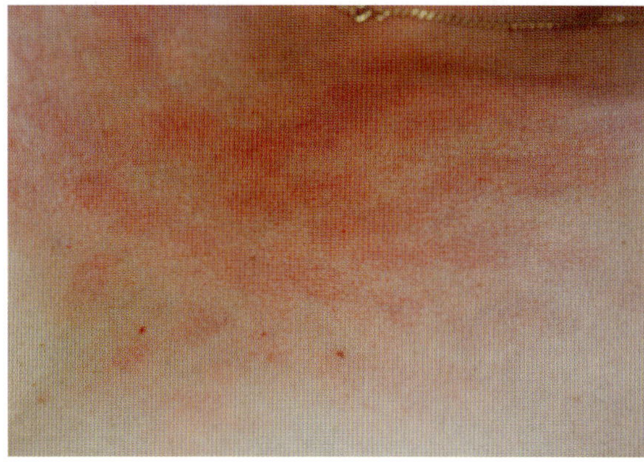

Fig. 14.13 Example of a décolletage area, 3 minutes after CO_2 therapy.

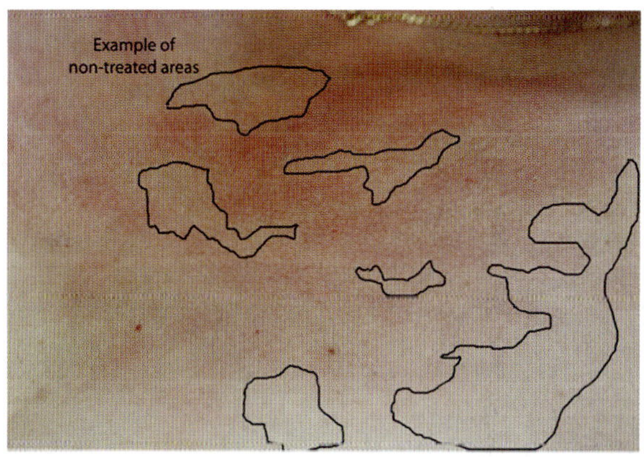

Fig. 14.14 Example of a décolletage area, 3 minutes after CO_2 therapy with treated areas marked.

OPERATIVE APPROACH

This section of the chapter is intended to be a tool for the operator or physician, therefore all the operative approaches are presented as a practical checklist for everyday use. These are tools act as aides-memoires and are particularly useful for novices. Plastic-wrapped photocopies attached to the machine are a simple way of using these in practice.

RAYNAUD'S PHENOMENON

Principle

Improve micro-circulation of the fingers. Increase blood flow and oxygen release in the superficial skin layers of the fingers. Stimulate neovascularization.

Indication

Any form of Raynaud's phenomenon, after diagnosis has been established.

Protocol

Subcutaneous layer

1 injection per day for 15–20 days (Fig. 14.15).

Flow: 50–80 cc/min

Technique

Inject CO_2 into the distal interphalanx spaces. Pull up the skin to limit the risk of pinching vascular or nerve structures. After each injection, remove the needle and use the finger to apply a proximal to distal massage, which will push the gas into the fingers (Fig. 14.16). As the strategy is to let the gas diffuse down to the fingers, use the hand that is not injecting to prevent the gas from going the wrong direction. During the insufflation apply gentle pressure to the dorsal side of the hand to stop the gas.

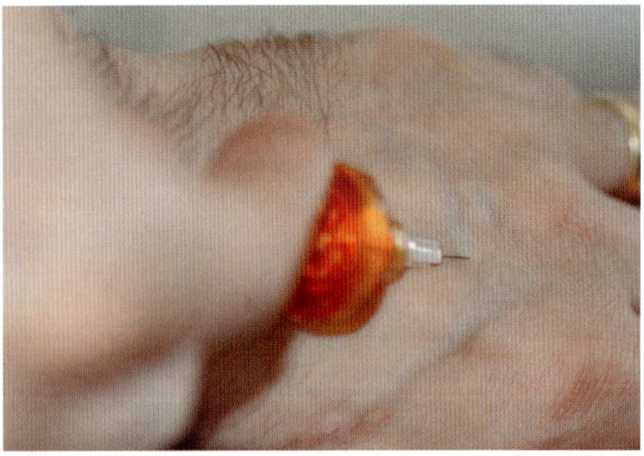

Fig. 14.15 Subcutaneous injection (Raynaud's phenomenon).

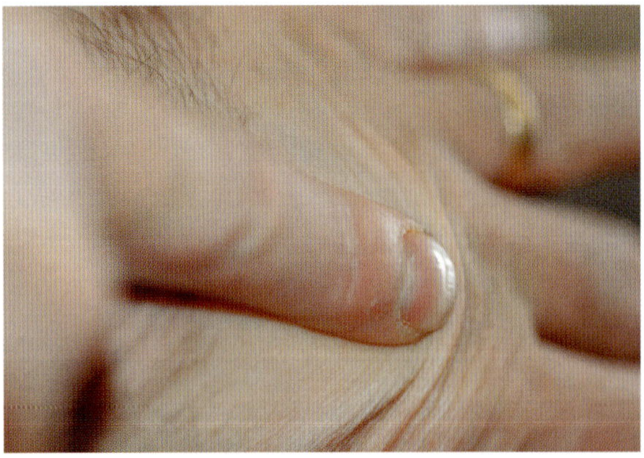

Fig. 14.16 Raynaud's phenomenon: the CO_2 gas is pushed down to the fingers with massage.

Injection Points

Interphalanx spaces

Endpoint

Subcutaneous spaces will inflate. The skin attains a crepe paper appearance. Gas will climb up to the dorsal side of the hand.

Post-treatment Care

No postinjection treatment is necessary.

Pain Management

To limit pain, start the first sessions with low flow values and increase them from session to session.

Results

Reduction of the pain and duration of spastic phases.

Reinforcement Sessions

Each year, before winter.

General Advice

Patient should continue to protect hands against the cold, wear gloves and so on.

LOCALIZED FAT

Refer to Figures 14.17 and 14.18.

Principle

Stimulate blood flow and activate receptors involved in the natural lipolysis of the body.

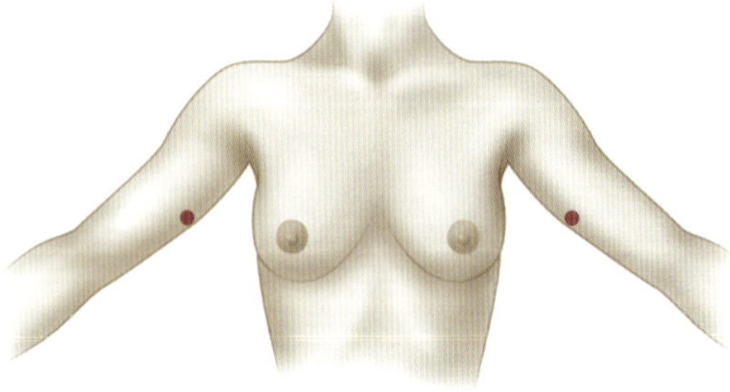

Fig. 14.17 Arm injection points.

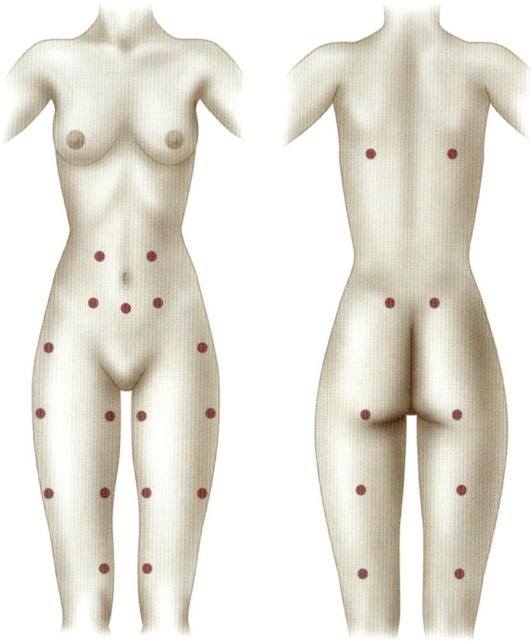

Fig. 14.18 Body injection points.

Indication

Any kind of localized fat or skin irregularity after liposuction. Also a complementary treatment to liposuction.

Protocol

Subcutaneous layer
- 1 session per day to 1 per week
- Flow: 1–2 cc/kg/min (50–80 cc/min)
- Approximately 2 minutes per injection
- Punctures spaced 15–20 cm apart
- Number of sessions: 10–20
- Progressive flow (automatic mode) available with some machines

Submentonian area: deep dermis (and/or subcutaneous)
- Flow: 1–2 cc/kg/min (50–80 cc/min)
- Approximately 30–60 seconds (until onset of erythema or pain)
- Usually three punctures.

Technique

Pinch and pull the skin between thumb and index finger and inject the pinched skin in its subcutaneous layers.

Injection Points

Injection points should be made in the area where localized fat resides. There are variations between men and women.

Men: abdomen, lumbar area, chest, submentonian area
Women: hips, abdomen, thighs, buttocks, submentonian area, back

Endpoint

Subcutaneous injection will let the gas diffuse and create a 15–20 cm diameter disk. Skin has a granite-like appearance and shows erythema. Move the needle 15–20 cm away from the previous injection point (no overlapping) to treat the entire fat area. Note that the 15–20 cm circle occurs only during the first sessions. After several sessions, typically five to six, the skin offers less resistance to the gas diffusion and one or two injection points may then be enough to treat all the cellulite area.

Post-treatment Care

None.

Pain Management

Pain can be reduced with a 'piano' massage during the injection. Pain is more frequent during the first sessions: CO_2 flow can be reduced in the first sessions and progressively increased from session to session. If too much pain is reported, change the injection point and reduce the treatment time, giving more, shorter injections. Some CDT machines have a progressive flow mode, which starts the injection at a low flow and increases it progressively during the course of the injection.

Results

Most patients report improvement after six to eight sessions. Treatment is usually delivered for up to a maximum of 20 sessions.

Maximizing Results

CO_2 procedures may benefit from combined treatments such as RF, Cellu-M6®, Velasmooth®, manual lymphatic drainage massage and so on. Some nutritional advice and the maintenance of a steady body weight are recommended.

Reinforcement Sessions

Patients are usually advised to renew the treatment at least once each year in order to maintain the effect.

Remarks

After liposuction, fat areas may be compartmentalized and this will require multiple punctures to be made, as the gas will not diffuse evenly. Ultrasound imaging with high frequency probes may help.

Submentonian Fat Tightening

Refer to Figure 14.19.

CELLULITE/ORANGE PEEL SKIN

Principle

Stimulate blood flow and activate receptors involved in the natural lipolysis of the body. Improve skin tightening to reduce orange peel skin. Fibrous cellulite treatments will require mechanical disruption of fibrous septae with high CO_2 flows.

Indication

All types of cellulite from grade I–II to grade III–IV. Subcutaneous irregularities after liposuction. Complementary treatment to liposuction, which does not have any efficacy on cellulite.

Protocol

There are various protocols derived from the Royat Spa, the use of which depends on the patient' availability for treatments. At least one session per week up to one session daily.

Cellulite grade I or II
- Combination of subcutaneous and intradermal injection
- One session per day to one per week
- Flow: 1–2 cc/kg/min – approximately 2 minutes per subcutaneous injection
- Punctures: 15–20 cm spaced, no overlapping
- Number of sessions: 10–20
- Progressive flow (automatic mode) available with some machines

Cellulite grade III or IV
- Combination of subcutaneous and intradermal injection
- One session per day to one per week

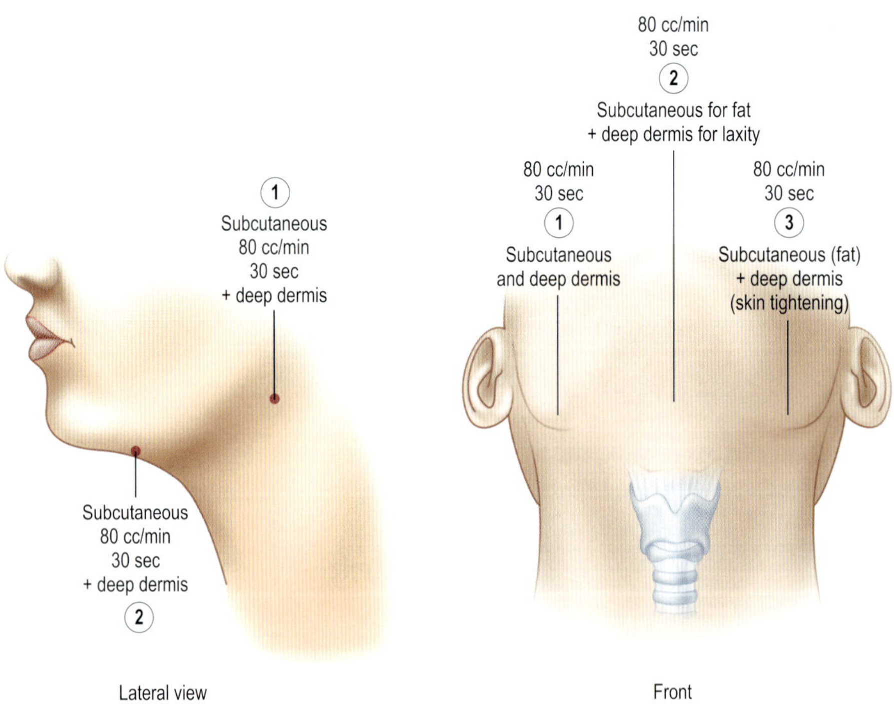

Fig. 14.19 Submentonian: areas and parameters.

Flow: >2 cc/kg/min
Punctures: 15–20 cm spaced, no overlapping
Number of sessions: 10–20
Progressive flow (automatic mode) available with some machines

Technique

The operator's hand movement should target both the subcutaneous layer and the intradermal layer as both lipolysis and collagen synthesis for skin toning need to be improved. Start by injecting the dermis and, when done, push the needle further/deeper to inject the subcutaneous layers. This appears to be the easier approach, although injecting the subcutaneous layers first still appears to work.

Injection Points

Injections points should be made in the area where cellulite resides. It is almost always in the hips and thighs (Fig. 14.20).

Endpoint

Subcutaneous injection will let the gas diffuse and create a 15–20 cm diameter disk. The skin has a granite-like appearance and shows erythema. Move the needle 15–20 cm away from the previous injection point (no overlapping) to treat the entire cellulite surface. Note that the 15–20 cm circle occurs during the first sessions. After several sessions, typically five to six, the skin offers less resistance to the gas diffusion, one or two injection points may then be enough to treat the cellulite area.

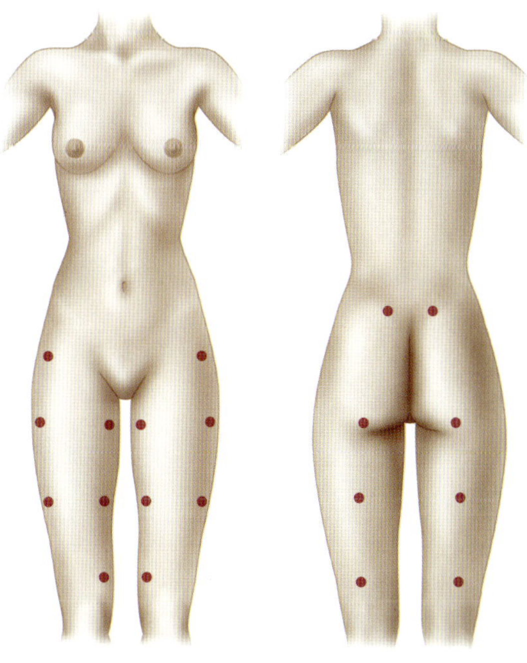

Fig. 14.20 Cellulite injection points.

Post-treatment Care

No post-injection care is necessary. Advise the patient not to take long warm baths during the following 24 hours, nor to perform active sports for 24–48 hours and to avoid new skin trauma or bleeding.

Pain Management

Pain can be reduced with a 'piano' massage during the injection. Pain is more frequent in the first sessions: CO_2 can be reduced in the first sessions and progressively increased from session to session. If too much pain is reported, change the injection point and reduce the treatment time, giving more, shorter injections. Some machines have a progressive flow mode which starts the injection at a low flow and increases it progressively during the course of the injection.

Results

Most patients report improvement after six to eight sessions. Treatment is usually delivered for up to a maximum of 20 sessions.

Maximizing Results

CDT may benefit from combination with such treatments as RF, Cellu-M6®, Velasmooth® and manual lymphatic massage. Dietetic advice should be given to help the patient maintain a stable weight.

Reinforcement Sessions

Patients are usually advised to renew the treatment at least once a year in order to maintain the effect.

ACNE AND SURGICAL SCARS

Principle

Same effect as needle subcision. Improve blood flow, vascularization and collagen synthesis.

Indications

Recent scars treated during the healing phase, atrophic scars, white scars. Thyroidectomy scars, caesarean scars, post-traumatic scars and postsurgical scars. Narrow atrophic scars.

Protocol

It is important to evaluate the scar hardness. The harder the scar is, the higher the required CO_2 flow.

Depressed scars
- Combined subcutaneous and intradermal injection
- One session per week
- Flow: 80 cc/min
- Punctures inside the scar
- Number of sessions: four to six
- Deeper injections are more painful for patients with adhesions
- Multiple injections in deep layers as CO_2 does not diffuse well

Narrow scars, non depressed scars
- Intradermal injection only
- One session per week
- Flow: 30–40 cc/min for soft scars
- Punctures inside the scar (as per stretch marks)
- Number of sessions: four to six

Acne scars (face)
- Combined subcutaneous and intradermal injection
- One session per week
- Flow: 30–40 cc/min for minor scars (soft), >80–90 cc/min (subcutaneous) to get a subcision-like effect on retracted acne scars and hard scars.
- Punctures inside the scar
- Number of sessions: four to six
- Deeper injections are more painful for patients with adhesions
- If adhesions are suspected: multiple injections in the deep layers as CO_2 does not diffuse well

Technique

Hand movement should target both the subcutaneous layer and the intradermal layer for depressed scars. If adhesions are suspected, multiple subcutaneous injections are required. The dermal plane is usually injected first and then the needle is pushed further, into the subcutaneous plane, in a second movement. For small scars or scars that are not depressed, only intradermal injections should be necessary.

Injection Points

Directly into the scar.

Endpoints

Erythema (subcutaneous injections); popcorn effect or fast inflation (intradermal injections).

Post-treatment Care

No post-treatment care is required. If treatment is to the face, a sun protection cream and a moisturizer are usually provided.

Pain Management

Emla® if too painful (this cream may lower the Bohr effect, because vasoconstriction may reduce blood flow); lower flow will reduce pain (but may reduce efficacy in breaking septae).

Note 1: A few physicians use CDT for the treatment of keloids, applying higher flows (first session around 50 cc/min, then usually 90–100 cc/min) as scars are tough. Results are apparently very variable. We have no personal experience of treating these scars.

Note 2: Patients with acne and acne scars may benefit from combined treatments:
- traditional acne drugs and carboxytherapy
- erbium-glass/Nd-YAG laser and CDT (not during the same session but 15 days apart)
- fractional laser and CDT.

STRETCH MARKS

Refer to Figures 14.21–14.23.

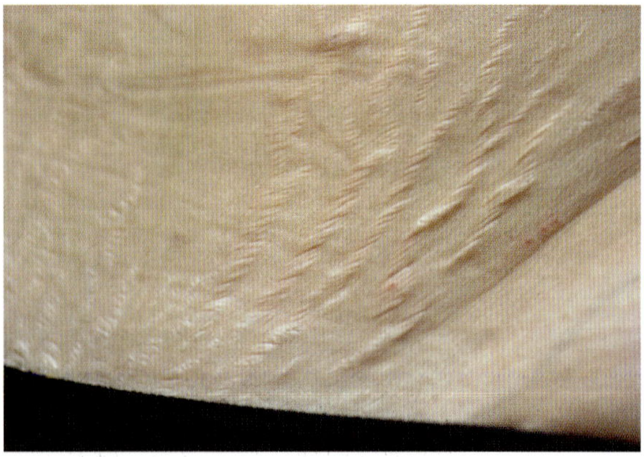

Fig. 14.21 Stretch marks before injection.

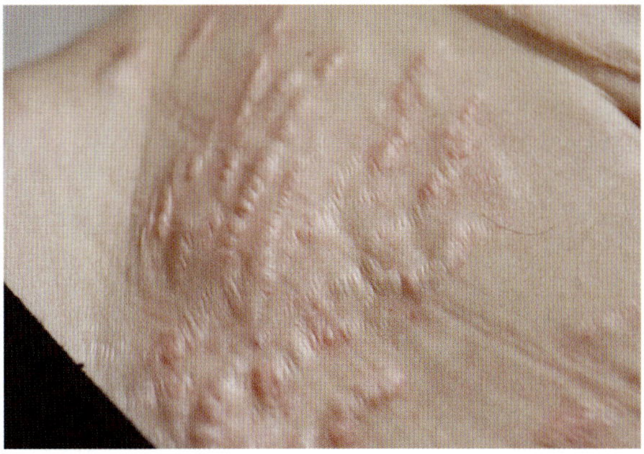

Fig. 14.22 Stretch marks 3 minutes post injection: intradermal: 150 cc/min.

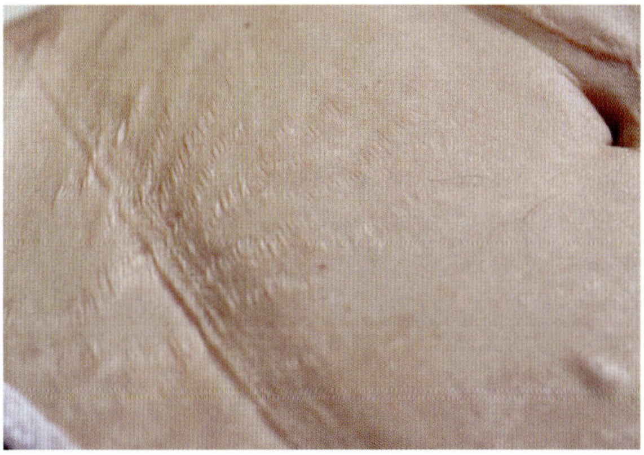

Fig. 14.23 Stretch marks 1 month after three sessions.

Principle

Improve neovascularization and blood flow (red color seen via skin transparency will appear pink, close to the natural skin color), improve melanocyte pigment production to darken white stretch marks. Improve collagen synthesis to reduce the wave appearance of old stretch marks.

Indications

Old white stretch marks, deep depressed stretch marks, irregular old stretch marks are the main indications. For young pink/red stretch marks, laser treatment is preferred: KTP or pulsed dye laser, one to three sessions, 1 month apart.

Protocol

Combined intradermal and subcutaneous injections
One session per month
Flow: 80–150 cc/min
Puncture inside the mark
Number of sessions: four to ten

Technique

It is preferable to start injecting the dermis and when done push the needle further to inject the subcutaneous layers. This appears to be the easiest approach.

Endpoints

Popcorn appearance (inflated stretch marks) for 1 or 2 minutes then erythema.

Injection Points

Follow each stretch mark and inject each 1–2 cm.

Post-treatment Care

No post injection care is required. Sun protection is advisable.

Pain Management

Injecting stretch marks is often painful. Patients describe a burning sensation. Although flow greater than 100 cc/min is recommended, it is sometimes impossible to maintain these values because of the pain. Lowering flows to 70–80 cc/min may make the patient more comfortable.

EYE PROCEDURES

Principle

Increase blood flow, stimulate collagen production, reduce fatty prolapse in some cases (lipolytic effect).

Indications

Fatty prolapse, eye wrinkles, under-eye dark circles.

Protocol

Eye wrinkles
Combined intradermal and subcutaneous injections
One session per month

Flow: 20–40 cc/min
Four to five punctures around the lower orbit bones
Number of sessions: three to six

Under-eye dark circles
Intradermal injections
One session per month
Flow: 20–40 cc/min
Four to five punctures around the lower orbit bones
Number of sessions: three to six

Fatty prolapse (see Fig. 14.24)
Subcutaneous and intradermal injections (Fig. 14.25)
One session per month
Flow: 20–40 cc/min
Puncture in the fatty area
Number of sessions: three to six

Technique

Very few injections are required to treat the eye. For eye wrinkles and fatty prolapse both intradermal and subcutaneous injections can be used. The needle's angle is less than 15°. Under-eye dark circles will require superficial dermis intradermal injections.

Injection Points

Refer to Figure 14.26. Fatty prolapse will receive two to four quick punctures in the area where the fat resides. Eye wrinkles and dark circles require from four to six punctures, 1 or 2 cm spaced, 1 or 2 seconds each, made all along the external inferior border of the eye orbit, next to the orbit bones (zygomatic bone) (Fig. 14.27). The free hand may

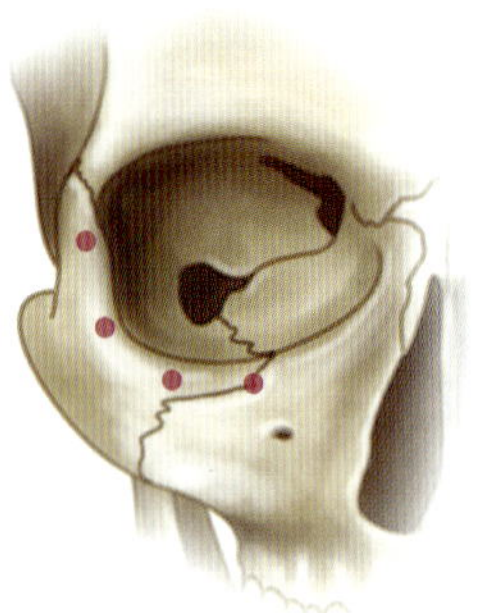

Fig. 14.24 Eye treatment follows the bone's border.

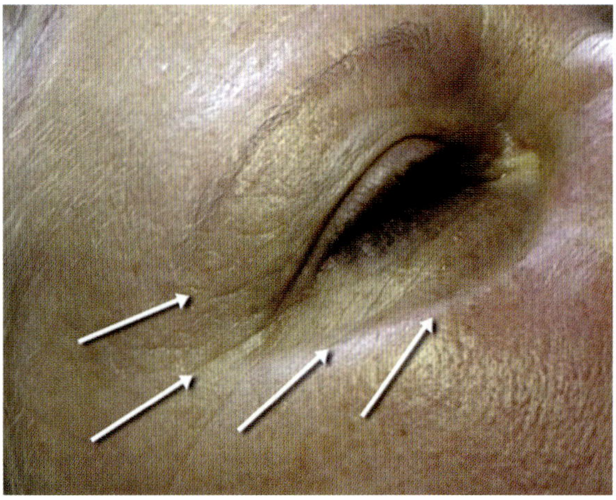

Fig. 14.26 CDT rejuvenation of the eye: injection points.

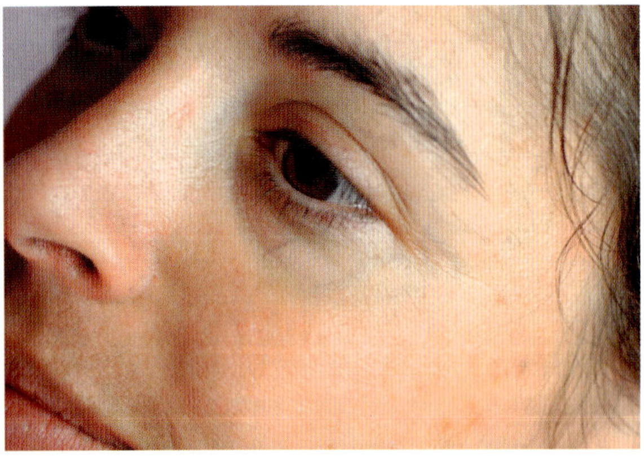

Fig. 14.25 After one session at 40 cc/min: subcutaneous and intradermal injection.

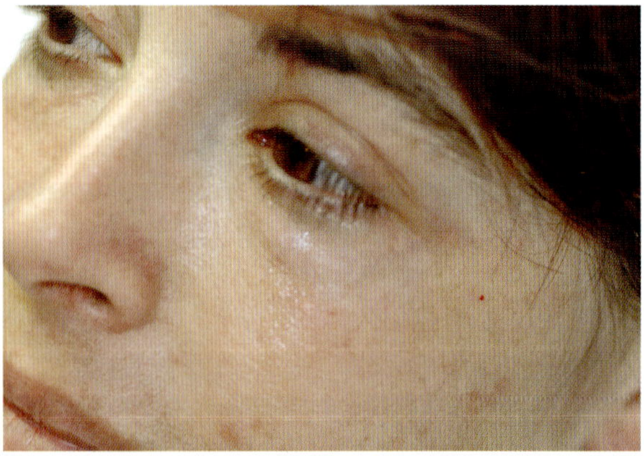

Fig. 14.27 Before carboxytherapy treatment.

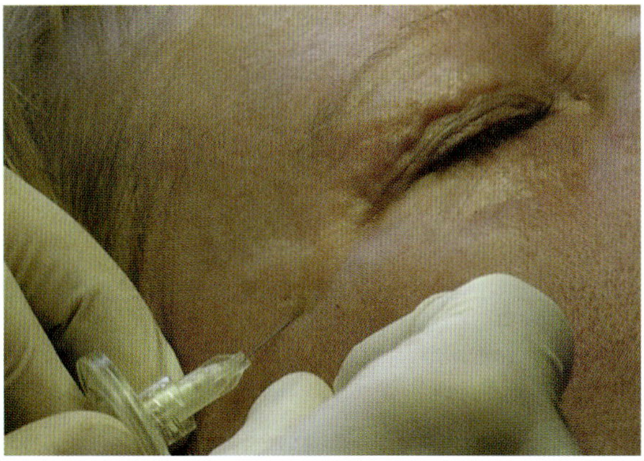

Fig. 14.28 End point after injection.

be used to gently maintain the patient's head in position that avoids any unwanted movement.

Endpoints

Eye lid becomes distended and inflated. Upper eye lid distention may be important (Fig. 14.28). Fatty prolapses are inflated and red. The eye returns to normal appearance within 2 or 3 minutes.

Post-treatment Care

No post-treatment care is required. Sun protection is advisable.

Pain Management

Emla® if treatment is too painful (this cream may lower the Bohr effect, because vasoconstriction may reduce blood flow); lower the flow and increase the number of punctures to limit pain.

Caution

One of the major CO_2 side effects and complications is pertinent to the eyelid procedure. It is important to purge and remove any trace of oxygen/air in the tubes and needle. O_2 injection into the eye lid leads to a strong inflammatory reaction which lasts 4 or 5 days, with redness, edema, closed eye and pain.

CDT Rejuvenation

See Figures 14.29–14.31.

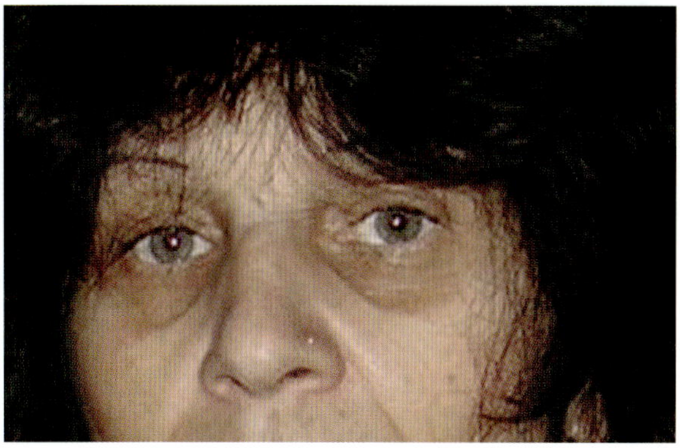

Fig. 14.29 CDT rejuvenation of the eye: 1 year before CDT.

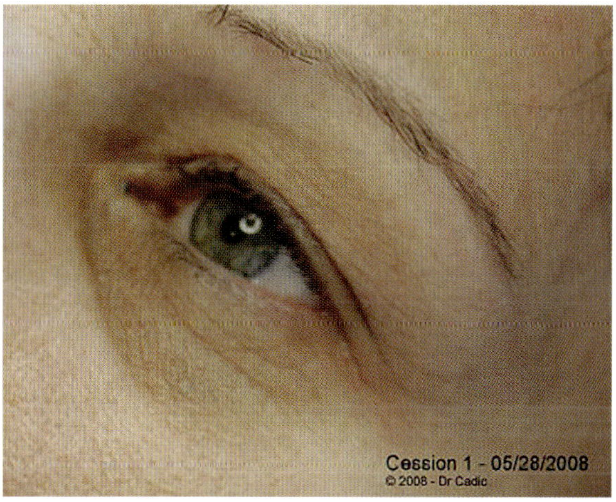

Fig. 14.30 CDT rejuvenation of the eye: after one session.

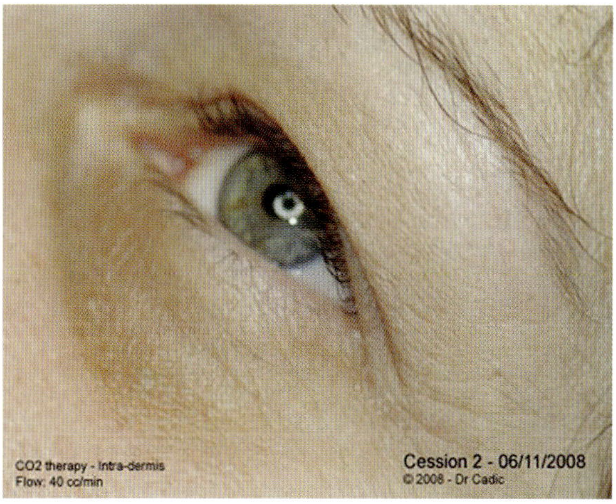

Fig. 14.31 CDT rejuvenation of the eye: after two sessions.

NASOGENIAN FOLDS, PERI-ORAL WRINKLES AND CROW'S FEET LINES

Refer to Figure 14.32. Nasogenian folds and peri-oral wrinkles may be improved with carboxytherapy too. Unlike fillers or Botox®, CO_2 should be injected close to the wrinkle line but not into the line or the walls. Injecting into the walls may produce a deeper wrinkle.

Principle

Stimulate the synthesis of collagen.

Indication

Thin to mild wrinkles.

Protocol

Nasogenian folds
- Intradermal injections
- One session per month
- Flow 20–40 cc/min
- Punctures each 1 or 2 cm all along the nasogenian fold (do not inject into the wrinkle or onto its walls)
- Number of sessions: three to six

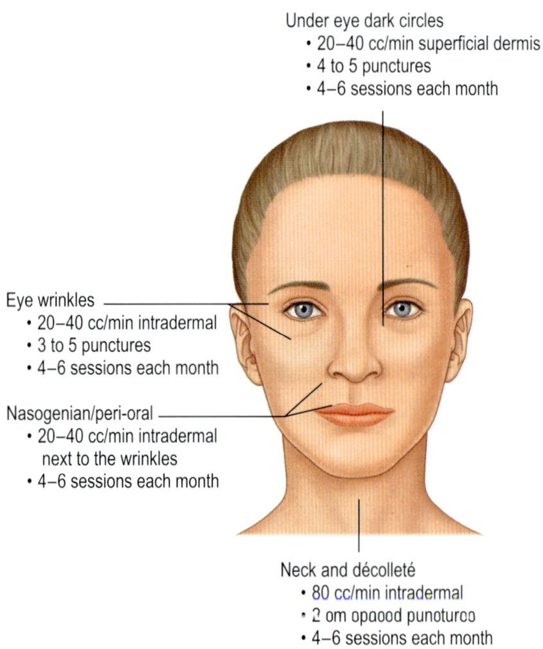

Fig. 14.32 Strategy to rejuvenate the face with CDT.

Peri-oral wrinkles
- Intradermal injections
- One session per month
- Flow at 20 cc/min. (These injections are usually painful and may require numbing cream). Punctures should be near the wrinkles (do not inject into the wrinkle or onto its walls). Punctures spaced 1 or 2 cm apart.
- Number of sessions: three to six
- Emla® is almost always required because this treatment is painful.

Post-treatment Care

None required.

Pain Management

Peri-oral wrinkle injections are painful. Multiple punctures with a low flow may lower the pain level. Emla® may be necessary. Avoid cold chillers as they give a vasoconstriction effect limiting the effect of the CO_2. Emla® may also cause a vasoconstriction and therefore a limited Bohr effect.

HANDS, NECK AND DÉCOLLETAGE REJUVENATION

Principle

This rejuvenation procedure aims to stimulate collagen synthesis and skin elasticity.

Indication

Neck skin laxity, neck laces, neck wrinkles, hand rejuvenation, décolletage skin laxity (lentigo and other pigmented lesions are not good indications for CDT).

Protocol

Intradermal injections
One session per month
Flow at 80 cc/min
Punctures spaced 1 or 2 cm until the full surface is covered.
Number of sessions: three to six sessions

Technique and Injection Points

Refer to Figures 14.33–14.35.

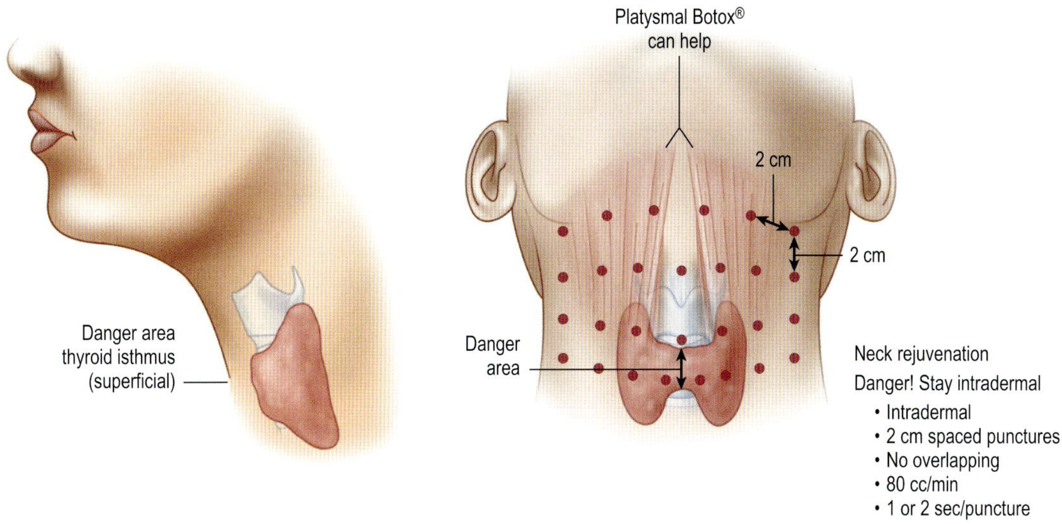

Fig. 14.33 CDT injection points for neck rejuvenation.

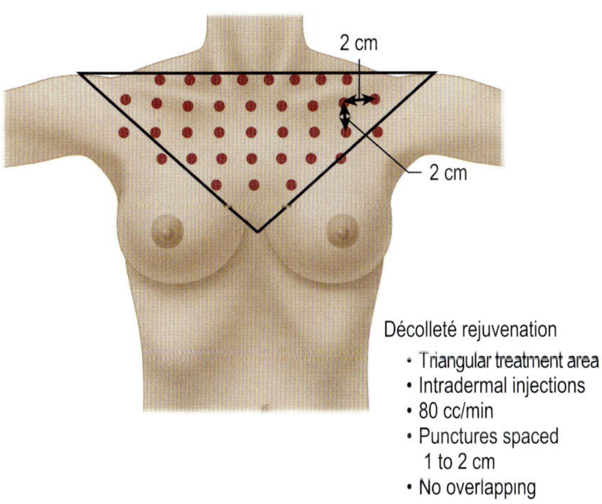

Fig. 14.34 CDT rejuvenation of the décolletage.

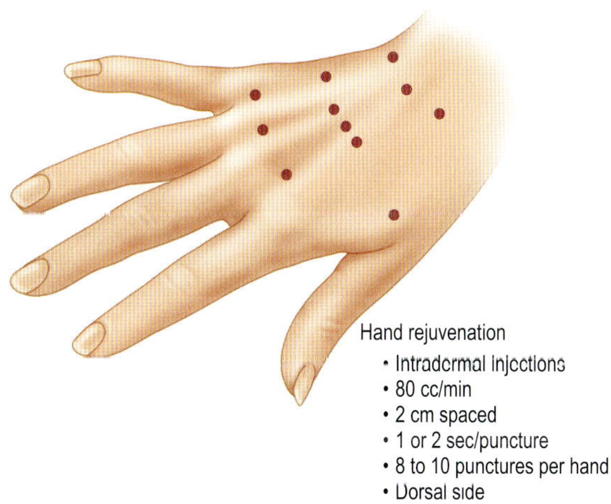

Fig. 14.35 CDT rejuvenation of the hands.

Neck: cover the full surface with punctures 1–2 cm apart
Hands: cover the full surface with punctures 1–2 cm apart

Décolletage: cover the full surface with punctures 1–2 cm apart. The needle may be bent to ease the tangential puncture of the décolletage.

No overlapping should occur. A well-treated area appears red. Any white disks remaining are untreated zones, which the operator needs to correct. When treating the hands, it is necessary to pinch the skin and pull it so as to avoid nerves or blood vessels when injecting.

Endpoint

A circle of skin 1–2 mm wide whitens momentarily when the needle is intradermal. Then, almost immediately, the skin detaches, remaining detached for 1 or 2 minutes, after which there is redness for 15 minutes.

Post-treatment Care

No post-treatment care is necessary.

Pain Management

If pain is experienced, lower the flow or make multiple punctures instead of a few.

OPTIMIZING OUTCOMES

Avoid cold compresses or topical gel application since it could compromise vasodilation and the Bohr effect.

Localized Fat Procedure

Sessions should be frequent: up to five per week, if the patient can tolerate this many. It is medically acceptable.

Manual massage during injections to lower pain and optimize CO_2 diffusion.

Combine with Endermology®, Velasmooth®, Velashape®, Lipotron® or any RF device available.

Rejuvenation

Combine with amino-acid mesotherapy or mesolift.

Combine with lasers and injectables (not in the same session). Wait at least 15 days until the skin recovers from the initial trauma.

Maximizing Results After a CDT Session

Do not use cold compresses or cold gel to lower pain as this leads to vasoconstriction that lowers the effect of CDT.

Advise patients not to take too long, hot baths or saunas, or to take part in active sports in the hours following CDT.

Massage during injection or immediately after puncture may improve gas diffusion and lower the number of punctures necessary. During subcutaneous injection this is a good way to lower the sensation of pain. An efficient massage lowers 'under-skin pressure' during injection. One useful technique is a 'piano' CDT massage, the four fingers of a hand pressing alternately, in the manner in which a pianist would play the A, B, C and D keys (Fig. 14.36).

A Cellu-M6® session, between CDT sessions or immediately after a CO_2 injection, is known to optimize results. Endermology® is also a non-surgical approach that increases circulation, optimizing natural lipolysis. We assume CO_2 and Endermology® to have a synergistic effect.

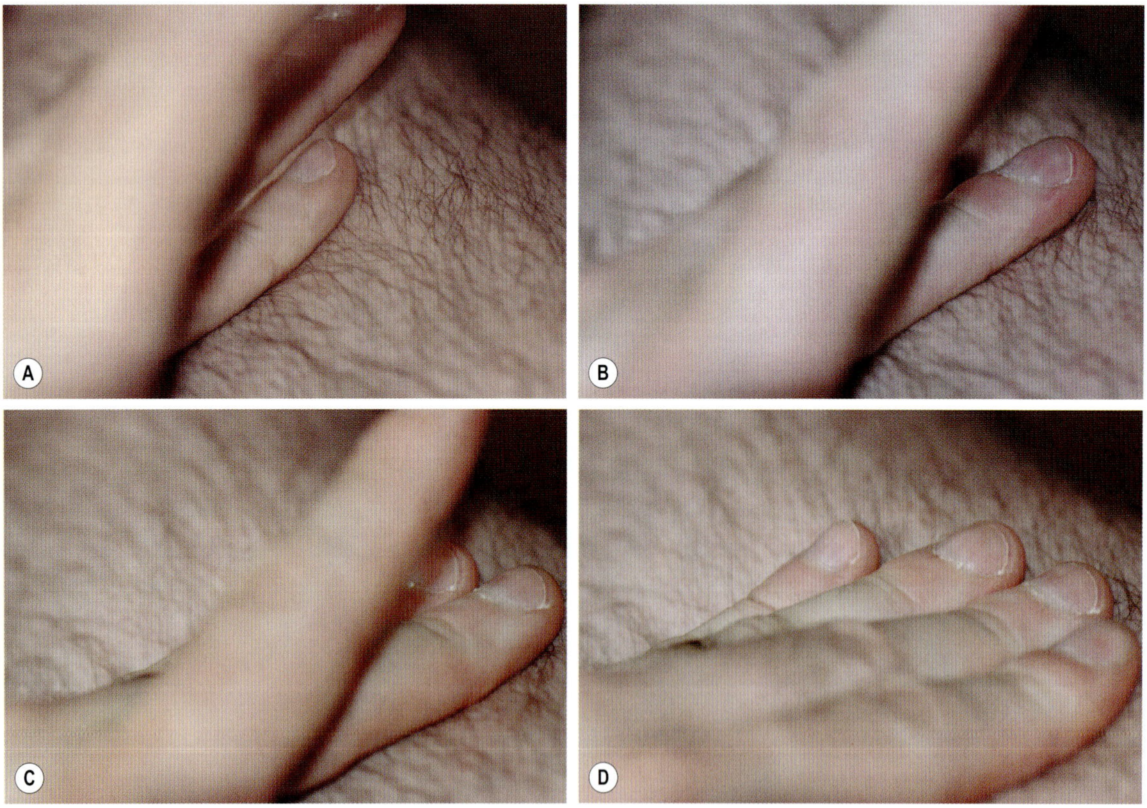

Fig. 14.36 The piano technique to lower pressure and decrease pain.

Some authors are experimenting with combined treatments including:

- CDT and monopolar or bipolar RF
- CDT and lipolysis laser
- CDT and remodeling laser
- CDT and mesotherapy.

These studies have yet to be published, however. Combination therapy is likely to offer significant improvements over single treatments.

Note: CDT is often used after liposuction. Where compartmentalization occurs, CO_2 will not diffuse well and it will be necessary to make multiple punctures.

COMPLICATIONS AND SIDE EFFECTS

Vagal Reaction, Vaso-vagal Syndrome and Syncope

Vagal reactions may be seen in any procedure with the use of needles and though rare may lead to syncope. The occurrence can probably be limited with good patient education and patients can be assured of the low morbidity of the treatment. It may not be a good idea to perform CDT immediately after a meal.

A vagal reaction can be dealt with in the same way as with any other emergency. A scope is a plus but blood pressure can be monitored manually and heart frequency checked. Depending on the level of the incident, the legs can be raised to move blood into the general circulation system. Atropin 0.25 mg subcutaneous may be used in severe vagal reactions.

Heavy Arm, Limbs and a Sensation of Anesthesia

A majority of patients report a sensation of anesthesia below the injection area (distal anesthesia). In most cases this sensation occurs in the lower limbs and arms. It seems to be more frequent in arm procedures (cellulite, skin laxity and localized fat procedures). Patients often report a 'dead hand'. This sensation is short and lasts around 2 to 3 minutes maximum.

Heart or Respiratory Disease Unmasking

Because of blood flow increase and the modification of gas exchange in the body, CDT might unmask an unstable respiratory system or heart disease, although this is rare. Precautions should be taken and CDT procedures should be avoided for patients with severe heart pathologies or respiratory insufficiency.

Epilepsy Triggering

There is very little information concerning CDT and epilepsy. One article mentions the possibility but with no clear explanation. It is not illogical to think that a temporary hypoxemia may lead to a crisis. Further studies are necessary.

Infection

Infection is most likely to be caused by poor skin disinfection measures. CDT is similar to mesotherapy, sharing the same low level of risk. Disinfection of the skin 1 or 2 minutes before injection is required. It can be performed with alcohol or quaternary ammonium, for instance, and a compress tissue.

Protocol for Disinfection

Hand wash with liquid soap and hydro-alcoholic solution between each patient. If no handwash is available, the minimum is hydroalcoholic handwash.

The operator should wear non-sterile hypoallergenic gloves and these should be changed between patients.

Skin disinfection with a compress and alcohol 70% or quaternary ammonium at least 1 minute before injection. Skin is cleaned in centrifugal circles.

Leave 1 minute for the disinfectant to dry. During this time, the operator may prepare needles, apply machine settings and so on.

Care should be taken with periocular disinfection since alcohol fumes may burn the cornea and conjunctiva. Eyes should be kept closed until the disinfectant evaporates from the skin.

Herpes Simplex Reactivation

Herpes simplex can be reactivated because of the trauma to the skin. As with laser procedures, if there is previous history a prophylactic treatment with an antiviral drug a few days prior to the session is recommended, maintained for 5 days after the session. This pre-treatment is efficient in lowering the risk of triggering.

Bruises and Bleeding

Patients with a history of bleeding should be treated carefully. Bleeding and bruises are found in 20% of patients, including those with no known history. Anticoagulatory drugs, aspirin and antiinflammatory drugs may also increase the risk.

Lower Lid Wound or Tear due to Movement During Injections

Injecting the eye area with CO_2 has the same risk level as doing so with fillers or Botox. Some patients may be nervous and might move their heads by accident or because of pain. A fast and unwanted movement while the needle is in the dermis may lead to a trauma and/or bleeding. Immobilizing the patient's head with the free hand can prevent the patient from moving too much.

Corneal or Conjunctival Wound During Injection

Eyelid injection points are usually far from the cornea and therefore puncture of the cornea is rare. Usually it is due to an unwanted movement by the physician or the patient. The head of the patient should be gently immobilized.

Persistent Eyelid Insufflation (Oxygen/Air Injected by Accident)

Refer to Figure 14.37. It is extremely important to properly purge the needle line/tubing before making any injection into the eyelids. Only CO_2 should be injected. Oxygen or air injected by accident lead to major inflammation, sometimes preventing the patient from opening the eye. They experience major lid edema and erythema. This reaction lasts approximately 3–5 days, but the healing process may be shortened using antiinflammatory drugs or ice-packs.

Pain (Puncture of a Local Terminal Nerve)

Pain is frequently reported by patients during CDT sessions. Some procedures may be painful while some others are well tolerated.

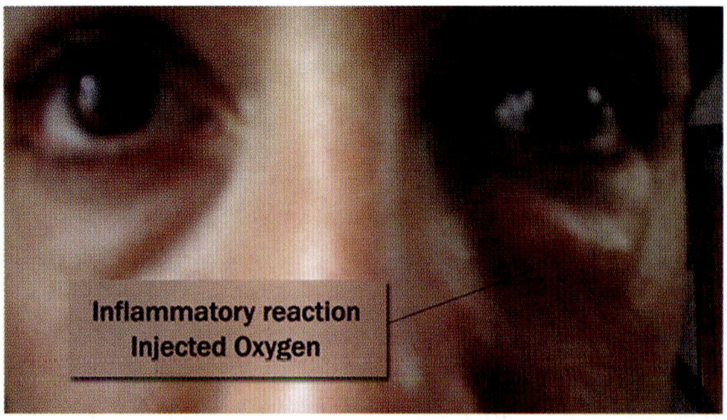

Fig. 14.37 Complications caused by oxygen injection during a CDT session.

Types of pain in CDT include:

- sensation of burn during the injection
- sensation of too much compressive pressure.

It is important to let patients understand the difference between pain and gas spreading feelings, which are:

- sensation of water spreading below the skin
- sensation of insects creeping below the skin.

Flow Rates and Pain

Logically, the higher the flow the higher the pain risk. This is certainly true in the treatment of localized fat, especially during the first sessions when the skin is not used to gas diffusion. It may be necessary to start with lower flow values and increase them from session to session. The operator normally stops and changes the point of injection when the patient reports pain. The flow is lowered by 20–30% if the patient remains uncomfortable. Note that some machines have an automatic mode. This mode can begin the injection with a very low flow and increase it progressively up to the optimal level, leaving time for the skin to adapt.

It is also known that injecting around the periphery of fat is more painful than injecting in the center, especially in the thighs (external and internal sides).

The experience of pain during stretch mark procedures is known to be very sensitive to flow parameters. A normal 120–100 cc/min flow may be uncomfortable for some patients, with a significant burning sensation. Lowering the flow value to under 90 cc/min solves the problem.

For facial wrinkles, pain may also be related to flow values. The strategy is to reduce the flow rate until pain is no longer experienced, before making further injections.

Skin Layers and Pain

Experience shows that subcutaneous injections are less painful than intradermal injections. The depth of subcutaneous injections does not seem to make a difference to pain levels. Superficial subcutaneous injections give visual control on how far the gas is diffusing.

Procedures and Pain

Some procedures are more painful than others. A listing by level of pain is given in Figure 14.38. A true evaluation of pain with using the Visual Analogic Pain scale is currently being developed by the authors.

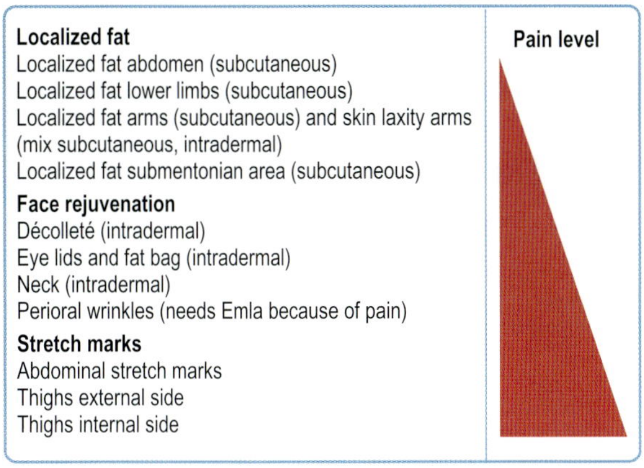

Fig. 14.38 Listing of pain levels.

Injection Areas and Pain

Patients may experience different levels of pain for a given procedure, depending on the area treated. Flow values may be lowered and/or the number of injections increased.

- Localized fat: abdomen is usually painless. Internal sides of thighs are usually more painful than external sides. Peripheral injections of fat area are usually more painful than in the center. Lower ends of thighs and arms are usually more painful than the proximal ends.
- Cellulite: pain levels are similar to localized fat.
- Stretch marks: although having a high level of patient satisfaction, CDT for stretch marks is almost always painful with a sensation of burning. Intradermal injection with very high flow over 100 cc/min is used. Upper parts of the abdomen are less sensitive than lower parts and pubis. Concerning the thighs, the internal areas are more painful than the external ones. Treatment of marks on chests and arms are usually tolerated with a low level of pain by most patients.
- Wrinkles: facial wrinkles are usually treated with gentle flows (20–40 cc/min) and therefore with low pain levels reported. Anesthesia is rarely used for face and eye rejuvenation exception for peri-oral wrinkles, for which the level of pain is extremely high. We use Emla® or an equivalent (one application 1 hour before treatment, a second application 30 minutes before treatment).
- Ulcers: arterial and venous ulcers, although treated with extremely low flows (20–40 cc/min) are known to be very painful. The onset of pain is the endpoint.

Lowering Pain

Cold packs and pulsed cryogenic sprays are very good for lowering pain during laser sessions but they may lead to vasoconstriction. Vasoconstriction increases distal vascular resistance leading to a slower blood flow, which is the opposite of the effect sought. It is then illogical on one hand to optimize blood flow with CDT and, on the other hand, to reduce it with cryogen anesthesia.

Use of Emla® cream should be limited as much as possible, since it may give vasoactive effects in the superficial layers of the skin.

Accidental Thyroid Puncture (in Neck Rejuvenation)

CDT is a technique with low risks. However, there is an area where the procedure should be undertaken with extreme care: the thyroid isthmus zone. Women with long thin necks have a very superficial isthmus, which could be injured if the needle goes deeper than the dermal plane. To avoid such accidents, it is necessary for the needle to remain intradermal.

Accidental Fragmentation of the Needle Below the Skin

This is extremely rare, most incidences occurring with intra-muscular injections.

Increased Telangiectasias or Rosacea

Telangiectasia and rosacea are capillary disorders caused by a permanently high blood flow. Using CDT on skin with signs of hyper-vascularization is not a good indication as it can worsen the disease.

Sensation of Warmth in the Injected Area

This sensation is the most commonly reported complication of CDT. Any CO_2 injection will lead to vasodilatation and blood flow increase. When these reactions occur, the patient feels warmth. This feeling is generally reported between the first few minutes and 1 hour after the start of treatment.

CONCLUSIONS

CDT is an old French technique for treatment of vascular diseases. It has found new application in the rejuvenation and anti-aging market with interesting results, especially for face rejuvenation around the eye and stretch marks. It is a simple technique to learn, with very few known side effects, all of which are well controlled.

The procedures involved in CDT are simple and easy to implement in a medical practice, either surgical or clinical, due to its many clinical applications. In most countries, a nurse can legally make CO_2 treatment under a physician's supervision.

Among aesthetic CDT procedures, some are more popular than the others because they are easy to perform, with quick results in a few sessions, and within a reasonable patient budget, for example:

- stretch marks
- scar revision
- eyelid rejuvenation.

Although often used on their own for aesthetic purposes, we believe that CDT should be used more often as part of combination therapies with, for example, fillers, Botox®, lasers, peeling, surgery, radiofrequency treatment and mesotherapy.

While this chapter has been based around our own work with CO_2 in rejuvenation indications, CDT is also used by South American and Central European doctors for reconstructive purposes with promising results.

REFERENCES

1 Tavares Ferreira JC, Haddad A, Navarro Tavares SA. Increase in collagen turnover induced by intradermal injection of carbon dioxide in rats. *J Drugs Dermatol.* 2008;7(3):201–206.

2 Brandi C, D'Aniello C, Grimaldi L, et al. Carbon dioxide therapy in the treatment of localized adiposities: clinical study and histopathological correlations. *Aesthetic Plast Surg.* 2001;25(3):170–174.

3 Komoto Y, Nakao T, Sunakawa M, et al. Elevation of tissue pO_2 with improvement of tissue perfusion by topically applied CO_2. *Adv Exp Med Biol.* 1985;222:637–645.

4 Savin E, Bailliart O, Bonnin P, et al. Vasomotor effects of transcutaneous CO_2 in stage II peripheral occlusive arterial disease. *Angiology.* 1995;46:785–791.

5 Cadic P. *Carboxytherapy.* Available: http://www.carboxyworld.com; 6 March 2009.

6 Cadic P, Cantisano-Zilkha M. CO_2 insufflation for stretch marks – revamping an ancillary technique. 29th Annual Meeting of the International Society for Dermatologic Surgery, October 2–5, 2008, Las Vegas/USA. Available: http://www.youtube.com/watch?v=DID4EwXsEY4&feature=channel_page31; March 2009 and http://www.carboxyworld.com/isds2008stretchmarks.pdf31; March 2009.

15 Cosmetic Dentistry of the Perioral Area — The Odontological Point of View

Luiz Gustavo Nascimento de Melo,
Marcelo Pereira Nunes, Marcelo Wolff Fernandes,
Luciane Magalhães Antonini, Maria Beatriz RG de Oliveira

INTRODUCTION

'The complete dental solution is a holistic approach that recognizes as a significant factor the psychological well-being of the patient and provides a healthy appearance as well as functional restoration. Aesthetics is an inseparable part of today's dental treatment.'[1] From a purely cosmetic standpoint, the value of the appearance of one's teeth has taken on a greater importance in our society. The public places an increasing priority on a healthy and attractive smile. The dental profession's traditional domain, centered around the eradication of disease, now finds itself on the threshold of uncharted territory: the enhancement of appearance. Yet, foundations of health, proper function, and sound scientific principles with consistency of results, reliability of treatment modalities and long-term prognosis also must prevail.[2]

The essentials of an aesthetic smile involve the relationships between the teeth, the lip framework and the gingival scaffold.[3]

THE LIPS

Garber and Salama[3] stated that the lips form the frame of a smile and, as such, define the aesthetic zone. Liplines have classically been defined as being high, medium or low. In the typical low lipline, only a portion of the teeth is exposed below the inferior border of the upper lip. The high lipline shows a large expanse of gingiva extending from the inferior border of the upper lip to the free gingival margin. The medium lipline shows a nominal exposure of 1–3 mm of gingiva from the most apical extent of the free gingival margin to the inferior border of the upper lip. Thus, the teeth in their entirety are on display, as well as the interdental gingival tissue and the border of free gingiva around the cervical area of the tooth (Fig. 15.1).

THE GINGIVAL CONTOUR

An irregular gingival arrangement, despite being healthy, may strike a discordant note, and it may become desirable to establish a certain harmony and continuity of form to the gingival margin.[3] One significant feature of gingival morphology is the gingival line, which is defined as a line joining the tangents of the gingival zeniths of the central incisor and canine. The gingival zenith is the most apical aspect of the free gingival margin.[4] It is commonly accepted that the gingival zenith of the two central incisors should be at the same level. The gingival zenith of the lateral incisors, however, should be slightly above (coronally) the central incisor's zenith (<1 mm). The canines, in turn, would have the free gingival margin at the same level of the central incisors and matching one another (Fig. 15.2,*A*). Extending distally, the tissues on the premolars would be somewhat coronally positioned.[5] However, a recent study[5] observed, on analyzing maxillary casts of 103 young adults, that the gingival zenith is, in fact, apical to the gingival zenith of the incisors, and the gingival zenith of the lateral incisors is below (81.1%) or on (15%) the gingival line when the head is oriented in the axis orbital plane. Periodontic plastic procedures, such as the basic gingivectomy, soft tissue grafting or the apically positioned flap, may be used to change the silhouette form of teeth and their relative proportion.

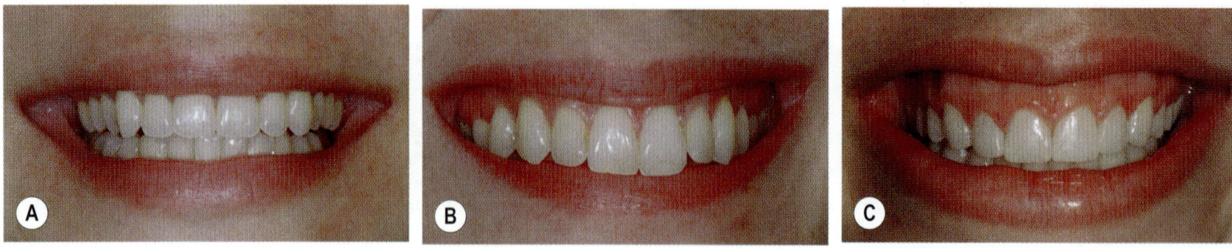

Fig. 15.1 *A*, Low lipline, *B*, medium lipline, *C*, high lipline.

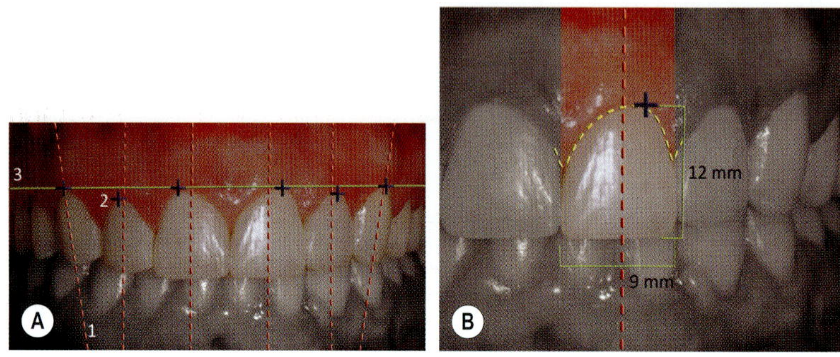

Fig. 15.2 *A*, The aesthetic gingival contour: 1, midline of the teeth; 2, gingival zenith; 3, gingival line. *B*, The tooth ideal height-to-width contour.

THE TEETH

The dentist is concerned with the color, position and shape or silhouette form of teeth. The advent of adhesive dentistry has allowed a literally instantaneous change in the color, shape and position of teeth via bonding techniques such as porcelain-laminated veneers and direct composite bonding.[3] It is possible to establish the appropriate height of the six maxillary anterior teeth, changing the aspect ratio of teeth for an improved aesthetic appearance. The tooth's aspect ratio, or height-to-width contour, for the six maxillary anterior teeth is generally considered to be optimal when the tooth is 75% as wide as it is tall[6] (Fig. 15.2,*B*).

GEOMETRIC PARAMETERS OF HARMONY

Elements of the aesthetically pleasing, well-balanced smile have been extensively reviewed.[3,6–8] It is commonly accepted that the maxillary anterior teeth should be completely displayed during a full smile, with a maximum of 3 mm of gingiva revealed above the central incisors. According to Garber and Salama,[3] within the confines of the lipline, the remaining two components of the smile, the gingival scaffold and teeth, need to be arranged in such a way as to develop a certain continuity of form, harmony and balance. Classically, the level of the gingival margins of the maxillary teeth parallels the form of the upper lip. The incisal edges of these maxillary teeth tend to follow the form of the lower lip. In a transverse dimension, the teeth should extend progressively posteriorly and laterally to fill the vestibule, extending to the corners of the smile (Fig. 15.3).

Continuity of linear horizontal form between the gingival expanse, the teeth and the upper lip is critical. Any asymmetry in this parallelism disturbs the sense of balance in the composition, disturbing the flow, and results in an unaesthetic smile.[3] By this definition, a high lipline in itself may not be unaesthetic if these basic rules are followed. However, in today's mass media-influenced culture, many people consider even the slightest excessive display of gingival tissue, the 'gummy smile,' unattractive.[3] The

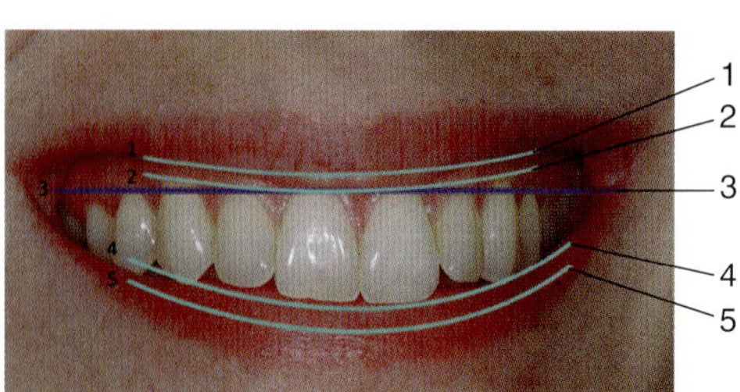

Fig. 15.3 Smile with various components in harmony. The gingival line (3) is in proximity with the inferior border of the upper lip. The line joining the zeniths of the six anterior teeth (2) follows the form of the upper lip (1). The teeth's incisal edge line (4) follows the form of the lower lip (5).

gummy smile or high lipline case with an expanse of soft tissue can result from two problems: (1) altered passive eruption and (2) vertical maxillary excess.

ALTERED PASSIVE ERUPTION

In a person with healthy dentition, each tooth and its alveolus actively emerges from its crypt.[9,10] The teeth continue to erupt through the gingiva until they make occlusal contact with the teeth in the opposing arch. This stage is followed by passive eruption or the exposure of the teeth by apical migration of the gingiva. Altered or delayed passive eruption is the failure of the gingival tissue to adequately recede to the proper level to the tooth's cementoenamel junction (CEJ). The consequence of this is short crowns and gingival excess.[11] Coslet et al.[12] classified altered passive eruption into two categories for differential diagnosis and appropriate treatment.

In type I, there is typically an excessive amount of gingiva, as measured from the free gingival margin to the mucogingival junction.

In type II, there is a normal dimension of gingiva when measured from the free gingival margin to the mucogingival junction. Although these might appear to be clinically similar in that there is tissue extended over the coronal portion of the tooth, therapeutically the diagnosis between the two types is essential to determine the appropriate treatment modality.

Type I can further be subdivided on an anatomical histological basis into subcategories A and B. This subclassification depends on the relationship of the osseous crest to the CEJ of the tooth.

In subcategory A, the dimension between the level of the CEJ and the osseous crest is greater than 1 mm, which is sufficient for the insertion of the connective tissue fibrous attachment component of the biological width.

In subcategory B, detected by the process of bone sounding via the sulcus, the osseous crest occurs in close proximity to the CEJ, thereby diminishing the space for the insertion of the connective tissue of the biological width.

The term 'biological width' refers to a length that includes:

- the epithelial attachment, known as the junctional epithelium, which rests on the root's cemental surface
- the connective tissue fibers that insert on the root's cemental surface and which are located below the junctional epithelium.[13]

Based on necropsy studies conducted by Gargiulo et al.,[14] the average dimensions of the biological width were considered to be approximately 2.7 mm: about 1 mm for the junctional epithelium, 1 mm for the connective tissue attachment and 1 mm for the sulcus. In clinical practice, the authors have found this to be a more varied dimension, often exceeding the 3 mm average.

VERTICAL MAXILLARY EXCESS

According to Garber and Salama,[3] the gummy smile frequently results from a skeletal dysplasia such as a hyperplastic growth of the maxillary skeletal base. This results in the teeth being positioned farther away from the skeletal maxillary base and a display of gingiva below the inferior border of the upper lip. Diagnosis in the high lipline case involving a vertical maxillary excess requires ruling out the case due to a superimposition of altered passive eruption in combination with maxillary hyperplasia. Garber and Salama proposed a classification for vertical maxillary excess.[3] The classification was developed to help determine the most appropriate treatment modality. The diagnosis relative to the degree of severity is predicted on first treating the altered gingival display (removing the altered passive eruption component) to develop a normal tooth form (crown form). Degrees of severity I (2–4 mm of remaining gingival display), II (4–8 mm of remaining gingival display) and III (more than 8 mm of remaining gingival display) are then determined by the amount of gingival display. The treatment modalities range from orthodontic intrusion alone through complex treatments involving orthognathic surgery, orthodontics, restorative components and periodontal plastic procedures.

TREATMENTS FOR ALTERED PASSIVE ERUPTION AND VERTICAL MAXILLARY EXCESS: INDICATIONS AND CONTRAINDICATIONS

Treatment of Type I A Altered Passive Eruption

The typical case of altered passive eruption type I A exhibits short, square-looking teeth and an expanse of gingiva below the inferior border of the upper lip. A gingivectomy using scalpel, electrosurgery or carbon dioxide laser is indicated and will readily remove this tissue. This procedure will result in a revised silhouette form for the tooth that is more

Table 15.1 Treatments for altered passive eruption and vertical maxillary excess: indications and contraindications

Condition	Indications	Contraindications
Altered passive eruption type I A (>1.5–2.0 mm of attached gingiva)	Gingivectomy	Osseous resection
Altered passive eruption type I B (> 1.5–2.0 mm of attached gingiva)	Gingivectomy Apically positioned flap with osseous resection	–
Altered passive eruption type II A (≤ 1.5–2.0 mm of attached gingiva)	Apically positioned flap with osseous resection	Gingivectomy
Altered passive eruption type II B (≤ 1.5–2.0 mm of attached gingiva)	Apically positioned flap with osseous resection	Gingivectomy
Vertical maxillary excess – degree 1	Orthodontics Orthodontics and periodontics Periodontics Periodontics and restorative dentistry Lip repositioning	Orthognathic surgery
Vertical maxillary excess – degree 2	Periodontics and restorative dentistry Orthognathic surgery Lip repositioning	–
Vertical maxillary excess – degree 3	Orthognathic surgery plus Periodontics and restorative dentistry where necessary	Lip repositioning

Adapted from reference 3

elliptical and attractive, and will resolve the unwarranted excessive display of gingiva apparent during smiling[3] (Table 15.1). When the amount of attached gingiva is normal or minimum (= 1.5–2.0 mm of attached gingiva), gingivectomy is contraindicated.

Treatment of Type I B Altered Passive Eruption

The clinical appearance of Type I B altered is similar to type I A altered passive eruption, with an excessive amount of gingiva from the free gingival margin to the mucogingival junction readily shown during smiling. On bone sounding via the sulcus, however, it would appear that the osseous crest is at the same level as the CEJ. This would seem to be contrary to the concept of the biological width, as the connective tissue fibrous attachment cannot insert into the enamel and yet must be present. The proximity of the osseous crest to the CEJ requires surgical relocation of the soft tissue apically via reduction of the osseous crest to allow for insertion of these fibers in a more coronal position, followed by a concomitant apical positioning of the junctional epithelium and the sulcus. This ultimately results in the free gingival margin being positioned right at the CEJ.[3] When the amount of attached gingiva is normal or minimum (= 1.5–2.0 mm of attached gingiva), gingivectomy is contraindicated (Table 15.1).

Treatment of Vertical Maxillary Excess

The combined case (altered passive eruption with vertical maxillary excess) requires for optimal treatment a multidisciplinary approach to treatment planning involving an orthodontist, a periodontist, an orthognathic surgeon and a restorative dentist. Orthognathic surgery for gummy smile treatment has been described previously.[15,16] Clinical examination and radiographic interpretation of cephalograms generally permit the clinician to correctly diagnose vertical maxillary excess. Dolt and Robbins[17] recommended that, if the clinical crowns of the teeth are short as a result of altered passive eruption, clinical crown lengthening should be performed before orthognathic surgery. However, Garber and Salama[3] have suggested a two-phase approach: initial gingival surgery before the orthognathic procedure (to create an attractive silhouette form for the teeth developing normal anatomical form and give the surgeon a definitive guideline as to the potential lip-to-tooth relationships and the amount of impaction necessary), with a second possible alteration of gingival display following orthognathic surgery (Table 15.1).

As orthognathic surgery is frequently associated with significant morbidity and requires hospitalization, an alternative method, called lip repositioning, has been recently recommended for vertical maxillary excess treatment.[18] The lip-repositioning technique is accomplished by removing a strip of mucosa from the maxillary buccal vestibule, then suturing the lip mucosa to the mucogingival line. This results in a narrower vestibule and restricted muscle pull, thereby reducing gingival display during smiling.[18]

CASE 1 – PREOPERATIVE HISTORY AND CONSIDERATIONS

A 26-year-old female patient was referred from the Division of Esthetic Dentistry of School of Professional Improvement (EAPGOIÁS) with a complaint of an excessive gingival display. The preoperative view of the smile showed an excessive display of gingiva and a significant alteration of the basic shape of the teeth (Fig. 15.4). They appeared to be short and squat, meaning that the vertical dimension appears too short compared with the horizontal dimension. After clinical and radiographic examination, a diagnosis of altered passive eruption was determined (Fig. 15.5). Her treatment goal was to minimize gingival display in her smile. The treatment plan for this patient included the aesthetic anterior teeth crown lengthening associated with the lip-repositioning technique to reduce the amount of gingival display and raise the height of the anterior teeth, along with raising the incisal length of the incisors, canines and premolars with porcelain-laminated veneers to follow the contours of the lower lips.

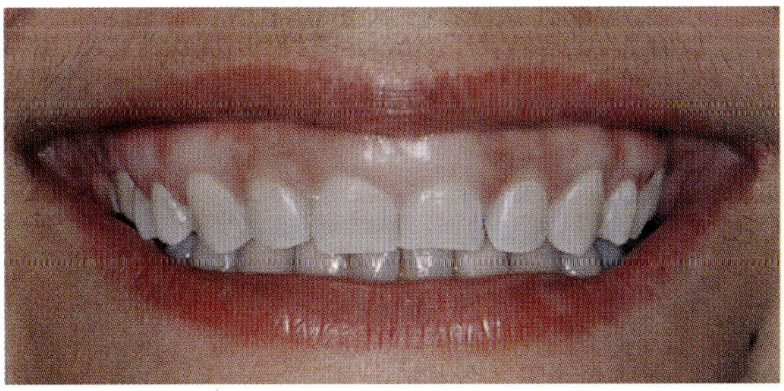

Fig. 15.4 Preoperative smile.

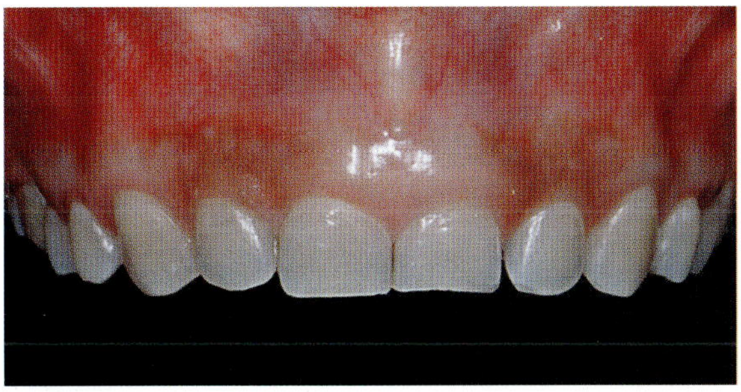

Fig. 15.5 This condition was diagnosed as an altered passive eruption.

Operative Approach

Mucoperiosteal flap reflection from the buccal aspect revealed alveolar bone to the level of the CEJs. Osseous recontouring was performed on the buccal aspect, from the right first molar to the left first molar, to locate the alveolar crest 3 mm apical to the CEJ (Fig. 15.6). This allowed the dentogingival junction to heal with the gingival margin at the level of the CEJ. A stable, aesthetic result was seen at 3 months following the crown-lengthening procedure, and the silhouette form of teeth became more attractive (Fig. 15.7,*A*). After the crown-lengthening procedure, the passive eruption component from the case was removed, leaving only the vertical maxillary excess evident (Fig. 15.7,*B*). A second surgical

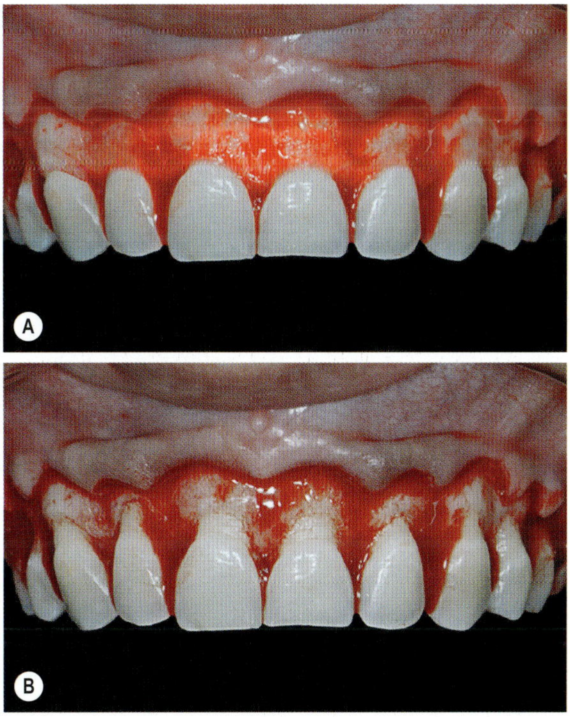

Fig. 15.6 *A*, The crestal bone was at the level of the cementoenamel junctions. *B*, This was subsequently recontoured to permit healing of the dentogingival junction with an optimum display of the clinical crowns.

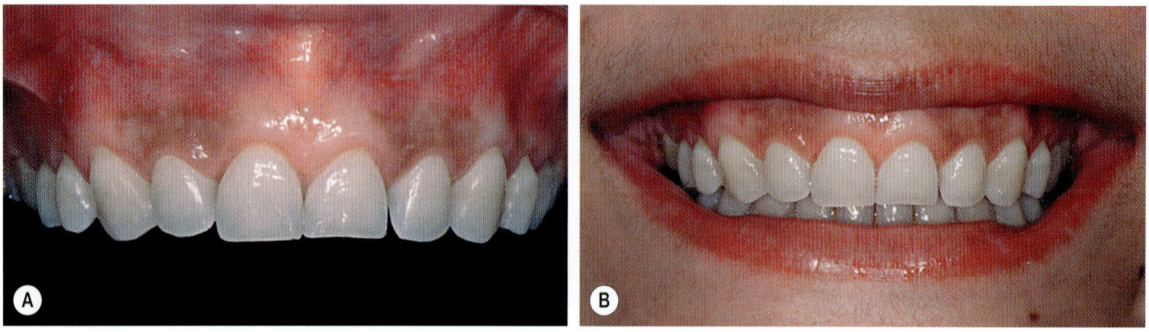

Fig. 15.7 *A*, A stable, aesthetic result is seen intraorally, 3 months following the crown-lengthening procedure. *B*, A residual excessive gingival display is still evident extraorally after the crown-lengthening procedure.

procedure was therefore proposed to minimize the residual excessive gingival display.

The technique proposed was the 'lip-repositioning' related by Rosenblatt and Simon.[18] Local anesthetic (mepivacaine 2% with epinephrine, 1:1 000 000) was administered in the vestibular mucosa and lip from maxillary right to left first molar. A partial-thickness incision was made at the mucogingival junction from the mesial line angle of the first molar to the mesial line angle of the left first molar. A second partial-thickness incision, parallel to the first, was made in the labial mucosa, 10–12 mm apical to the mucogingival junction (Fig. 15.8). The incisions were connected at each first molar, creating an elliptical outline. The epithelium was removed within the outline of the incisions, leaving the underlying connective tissue exposed (Fig. 15.9). The parallel incision lines were approximated with interrupted stabilization sutures (Vycril 6.0) at the midline and other locations along the borders of the incision to ensure proper

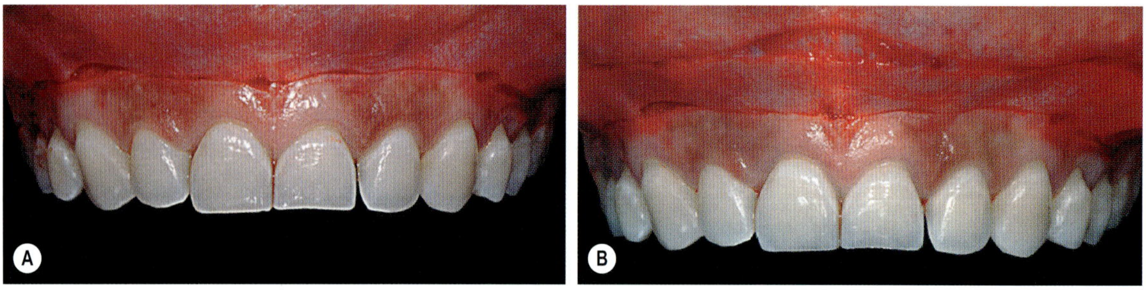

Fig. 15.8 *A*, First partial thickness incision made at the mucogingival junction. *B*, A second partial thickness incision.

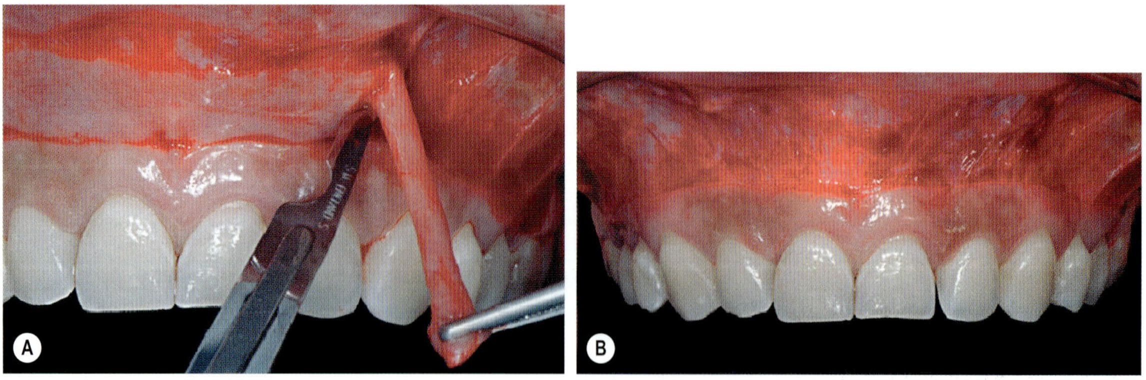

Fig. 15.9 *A*, The epithelial layer is removed. *B*, A partial-thickness flap exposes the underlying connective tissue.

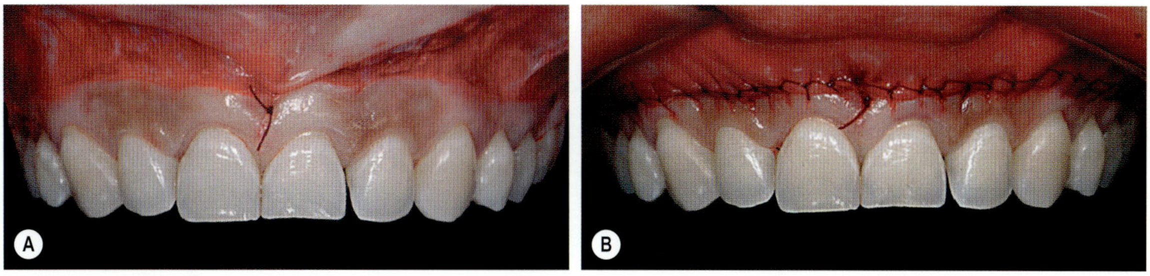

Fig. 15.10 *A*, Initial interrupted suture at the midline is applied to stabilize the desired line of closure. *B*, The wound is sutured continuously.

alignment of the lip midline with the midline of the teeth. Then, a continuous interlocking suture was used to approximate both flap ends (Fig. 15.10). Sutures were removed 2 weeks later. A follow-up examination 2 months later showed a reduction in the patient's excessive gingival display (Fig. 15.11). The laminated porcelain veneers were placed 6 weeks after the aesthetic crown lengthening.[19] An image of the patient's smile line at the placement of the veneers demonstrates that the contours of the gingival margins, and the length and incisal plane of the teeth are closer to ideal (Fig. 15.12).

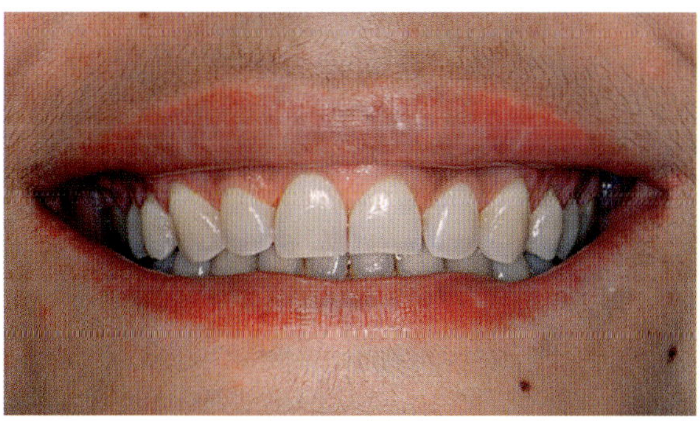

Fig. 15.11 Postoperative smile.

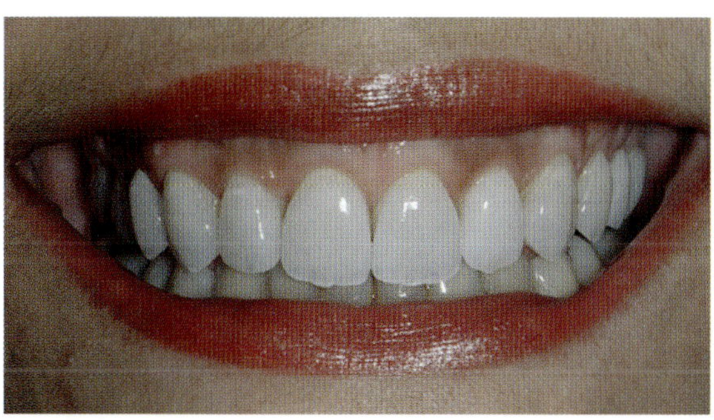

Fig. 15.12 Smile after 6 weeks with porcelain veneers laminated.

Optimizing Outcomes

In aesthetic crown lengthening, neither palatal nor interdental soft tissue should be reflected to ensure maintenance of interdental papillae.

Complications and Side Effects

In the lip-repositioning technique, during the epithelium removal, care must be taken to avoid damage to any minor salivary glands in the submucosa.

Postoperative Care

The suture line healed in the form of a scar that was not apparent when the patient smiled because it was concealed in the upper lip mucosa. A follow-up examination 2 months later showed a reduction in the patient's excessive gingival display (Fig. 15.11).

CASE 2 – PREOPERATIVE HISTORY AND CONSIDERATIONS

A 25-year-old female patient was referred from EAPGOIÁS with a complaint of a 'gummy smile' (Fig. 15.13). However, during the clinical examination, a hypertrophied, broad, thick labial frenum

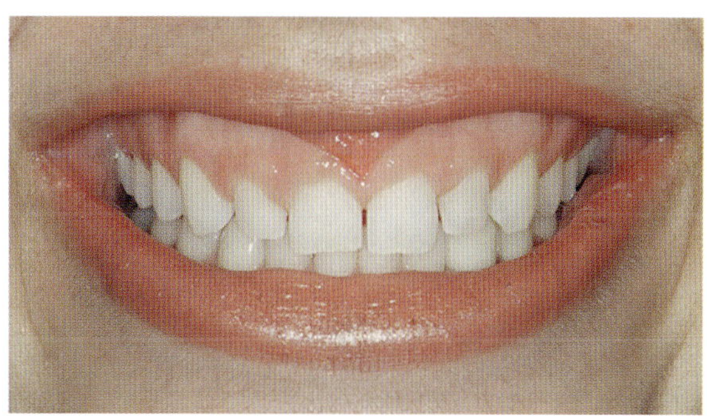

Fig. 15.13 Preoperative smile.

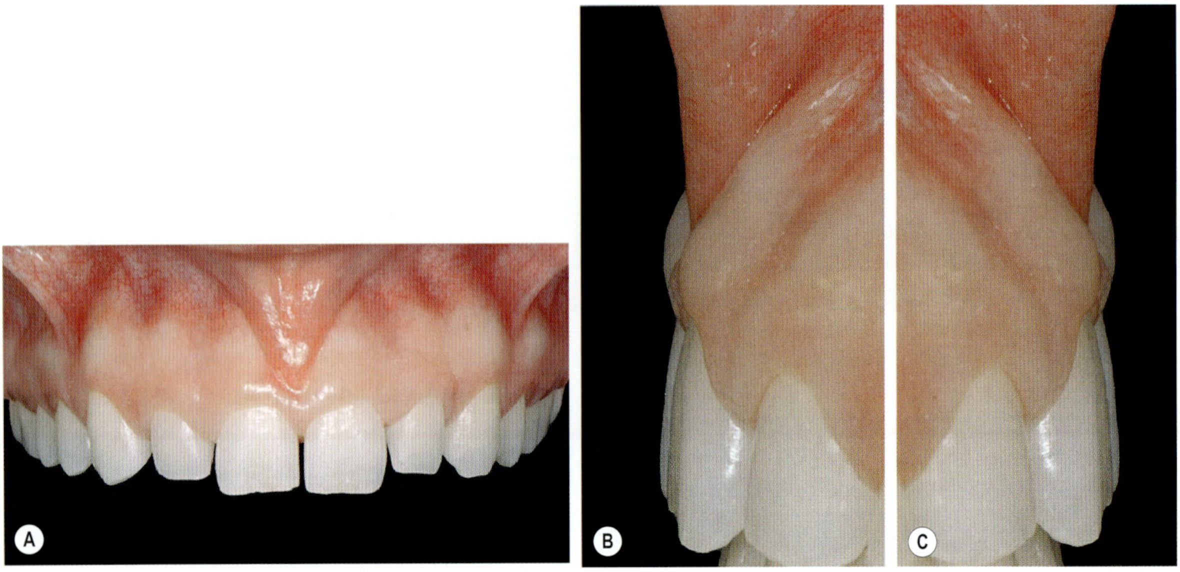

Fig. 15.14 *A*, Preoperative smile, with a hypertrophied, broad, thick labial frenum from the right (*B*) and from the left (*C*).

was also observed (Fig. 15.14). Her treatment goal was to minimize excessive gingival display in her smile. The treatment plan for this patient included aesthetic anterior teeth crown lengthening to reduce the amount of gingival display and raising the anterior teeth, along with raising the incisal length of the incisors, canines and premolars with resin composite.

Operative Approach

A modern technique of frenectomy was planned considering the patient's concern for aesthetics and the wide, thick hypertrophied frenum with abnormal attachment, which can leave a wide defect after excision by traditional techniques, leading to scar formation.

The maxillary anterior region was anesthetized (mepivacaine 2% with epinephrine, 1:1 000 000), by local infiltration on the buccal and palatal aspects. The frenum was immobilized with a pair of hemostats. A V-shaped oblique partial incision was placed at the gingival base of the frenal attachment with an external bevel. Fibrous tissue attached to the lip was dissected with scissors, and undermining of the labial mucosa was done. In association with frenectomy and for an improved surgical and cosmetic result, a triangular-shaped gingival graft, harvested from palate, was sutured in place (Fig. 15.15).

In addition, an aesthetic crown-lengthening including the molars to reduce the amount of gingival display was proposed. To accomplish this, the initial surgical incision was mapped out by measuring the length of the maxillary teeth and using a periodontal probe to create a bleeding point at the height of contour before making the incision. After the initial incision, a second intrasulcular incision was made and the collar of gingiva was removed (Fig. 15.16).

After a healing period of 30 days, the incisal length of the incisors, canines and premolars was raised and widened with resin composite. A stable, aesthetic result was seen following the cosmetic

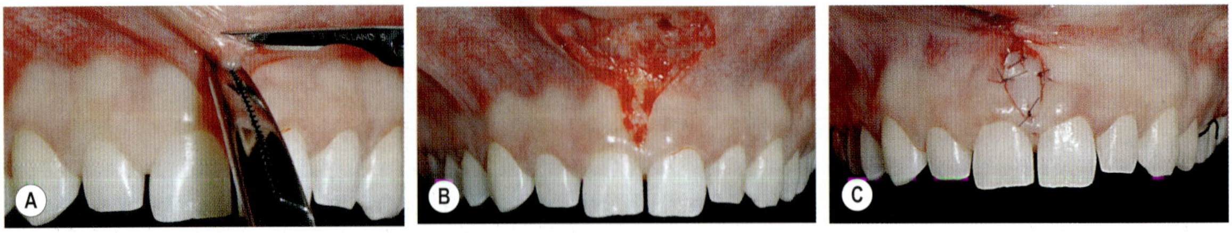

Fig. 15.15 *A*, Frenum immobilized with a pair of hemostats. *B*, Partial thickness dissection of fibrous tissue attached to the lip. *C*, Triangular-shaped free gingival graft sutured.

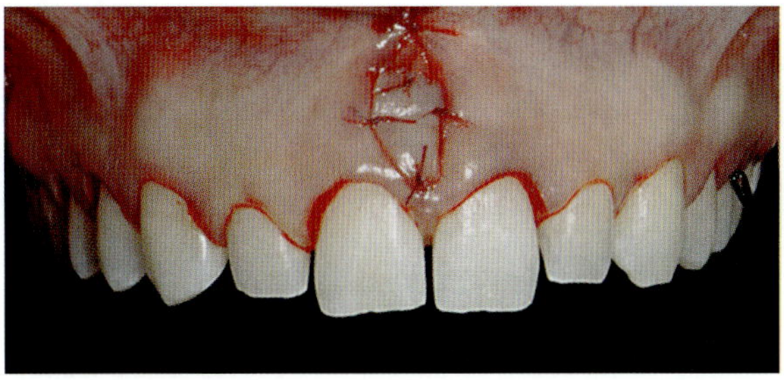

Fig. 15.16 Aesthetic crown lengthening performed with gingivectomy.

dentistry procedure, and the silhouette form of teeth became more attractive (Fig. 15.17). After the crown-lengthening and cosmetic dentistry procedures, the vertical maxillary excess was still evident (Fig. 15.18). A lip-repositioning procedure was therefore proposed to minimize the residual excessive gingival display (Fig. 15.19). A follow-up examination one month later showed a reduction in the patient's excessive gingival display (Fig. 15.20).

Optimizing Outcomes

In aesthetic crown lengthening, during the initial incision, it is important to observe that the height of the gingival contour is not a symmetrical arch

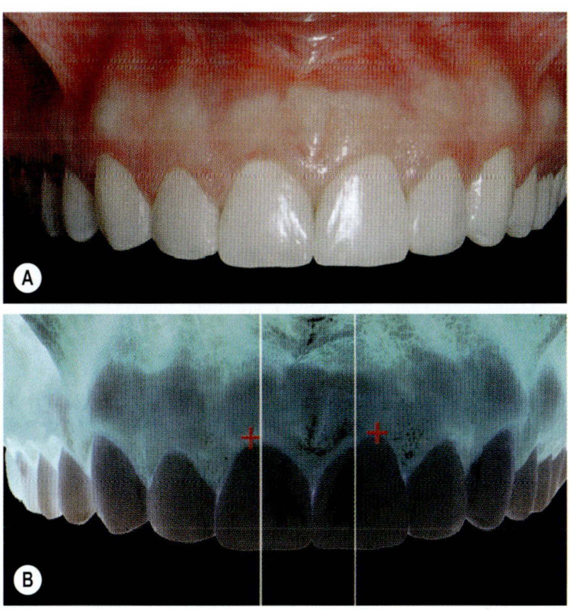

Fig. 15.17 *A*, Stable aesthetic result following the cosmetic dentistry with a more attractive silhouette form of teeth. *B*, Negative view of the final restorations indicating the harmony of gingival contour with the correct height and localization of the central incisor's zenith.

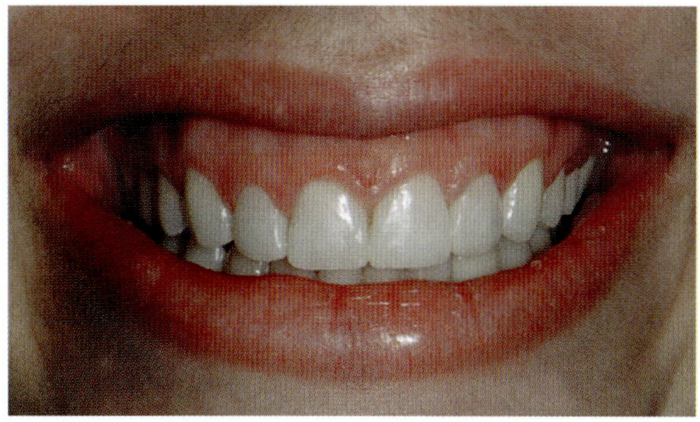

Fig. 15.18 A residual excessive gingival display is still evident extraorally after the crown-lengthening procedure.

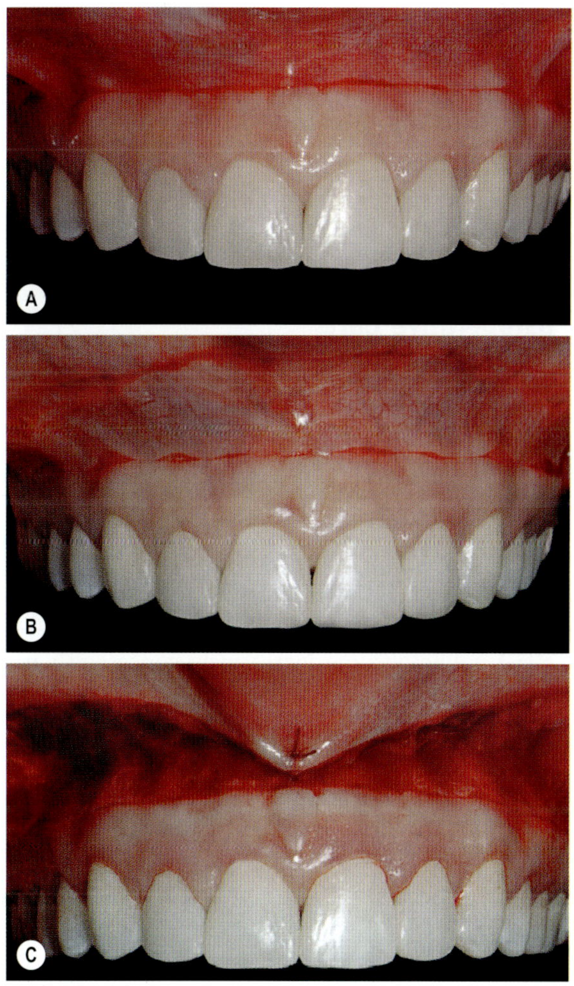

Fig. 15.19 The lip-repositioning procedure. *A*, First partial thickness incision made at the mucogingival junction. *B*, A second partial thickness incision. *C*, Initial interrupted suture at the midline.

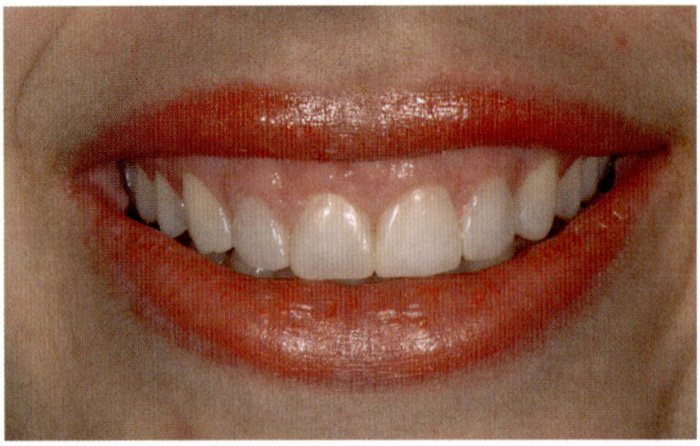

Fig. 15.20 Postoperative smile after 30 days of follow-up.

on the maxillary central incisors; it actually is at the distal one-third of the tooth on the incisors and follows the natural distal inclination of the roots of the incisors (Fig. 15.17).

Complications and Side Effects

In the lip-repositioning technique, according to Simon,[18] the sutures must be left in for a few months (using maxon 6/0 sutures) to prevent relapse of the lip position.

Postoperative Care

The suture line healed in the form of a scar that was not apparent when the patient smiled because it was concealed in the upper lip mucosa. A follow-up examination 1 month later showed a reduction in the patient's excessive gingival display (Fig. 15.20).

CONCLUSIONS

As the public become increasingly concerned with looking younger and healthier, aesthetic considerations will become increasingly more relevant in dental treatment planning. As such, dentists must define the basic tenets of an aesthetic smile – extending that vision beyond simply 'pretty teeth' to a concept whereby total dentofacial harmony is developed. Aesthetics is not simply a matter for restorative dentists; it uses restorative dentistry as one of the disciplines, but it is about beauty. The same rules that apply for a denture are, therefore, pertinent for crown and bridge and/or implants, and must be applied in all aesthetic endeavors.[3]

REFERENCES

1 Nowzari H. Aesthetic periodontal therapy: introduction. *Periodontol 2000*. 2001;27:8–28.

2 Morley J. The role of cosmetic dentistry in restoring a youthful appearance. *J Am Dent Assoc*. 1999;130:1166–1172.

3 Garber DA, Salama MA. The aesthetic smile: diagnosis and treatment. *Periodontol 1996*. 2000;11:18–28.

4 Charruel S, Perez C, Foti B, Camps J, Monnet-Corti V. Gingival contour assessment: clinical parameters useful for esthetic diagnosis and treatment. *J Periodontol*. 2008;79(5):795–801.

5 Allen EP. Use of mucogingival surgical procedures to enhance esthetics. *Dent Clin North Am*. 1988;32(2):307–330.

6 Chiche GJ, Pinault A. *Esthetics of Anterior-Fixed Prosthodontics*. Chicago: Quintessence Publishing Company, Inc; 1994.

7 Cohen ES. *Atlas of Cosmetic and Reconstructive Periodontal Surgery*. Lewiston, NY: BC Decker Inc; 2007.

8 Morley J, Eubank J. Macroesthetic elements of smile design. *J Am Dent Assoc*. 2001;132:39–45.

9 Evian CI, Cutler SA, Rosenberg ES, Shah RK. Altered passive eruption: the undiagnosed entity. *J Am Dent Assoc*. 1993;124 (10):107–110.

10 Wolffe GN, van der Weijden FA, Spanauf AJ, de Quincey GN. Lengthening clinical crowns – a solution for specific periodontal, restorative, and esthetic problems. *Quintessence Int*. 1994;25(2): 81–88.

11 Kao RT, Dault S, Frangadakis K, Salehieh JJ. Esthetic crown lengthening: appropriate diagnosis for achieving gingival balance. *J Calif Dent Assoc*. 2008;36(3):187–191.

12 Coslet JG, Vanarsdall R, Weisgold A. Diagnosis and classification of delayed passive eruption of the dentogingival junction in the adult. *Alpha Omegan*. 1977;70(3):24–28.

13 Cohen DW. *Periodontal preparation of the mouth for restorative dentistry*. Presented at the Walter Reed Army Medical Center, Washington, June 1962.

14 Gargiulo AW, Wentz FM, Orban B. Dimensions and relations of the dentogingival junction in human. *J Periodontol*. 1961;32: 261–267.

15 Arnett GW, Kreashko RG, Jelic JS. Correcting vertically altered faces: orthodontics and orthognathic surgery. *Int J Adult Orthodon Orthognath Surg*. 1998;13(4):267–276.

16 Sarver DM, Weissman SM. Long-term soft tissue response to Lefort I maxillary superior repositioning. *Angle Orthod*. 1991; 61(4):267–276.

17 Dolt 3rd AH, Robbins JW. Altered passive eruption: an etiology of short clinical crowns. *Quintessence Int*. 1997;28(6):363–372.

18 Rosenblatt A, Simon Z. Lip repositioning for reduction of excessive gingival display: a clinical report. *Int J Periodontics Restorative Dent*. 2006;26(5):433–437.

19 Kois JC. Altering gingival levels: The restorative connection. Part I: Biologic variables. *J Esthet Dent*. 1994;6:3–9.

16 The Importance of the Aesthetician in a Cosmetic Practice

Susanne S Warfield

INTRODUCTION

Cosmetic practices have a growing need to associate additional specialized services, including those offered by aestheticians. From the physician's perspective, the influx of managed care, reduced insurance reimbursements and rising malpractice insurance premiums have severely impacted on revenues and the costs of doing business. Physicians have an unavoidable need to adapt to this changing marketplace.

At the same time, baby boomers are becoming more focused on achieving or maintaining a younger, more vibrant appearance, and expectations have opened the door for many professionals to enter the aesthetic arena and for consumers to seek out their services.

For the physician looking to develop an aesthetic healthcare niche, there are a number of obstacles to overcome, including lack of time to develop the expertise and knowledge about the issues surrounding their new endeavor. Here is where the aesthetician can step in to provide many services of benefit to both the physician and the patient.

WHAT IS IN IT FOR YOU, THE PHYSICIAN?

'How much time do you presently spend with your patient?' If the answer to this question has you pausing for reflection, that is intended. The patients of today have high expectations for medical care and, with the high cost of their medical insurance premiums, patients are demanding a right to quality time with the physician and staff. The physician must offer the cosmetic patient a complete informative consultation, including a medical evaluation, treatment plan and statement of costs involved. Once the physician has completed the initial phase of a medical evaluation, the aesthetician can work with the patient for a skincare evaluation and treatment. The time allotted for this session may vary depending on the procedure and/or diagnosis, but by having the professionals working to supplement one another's roles, the patient is generally the beneficiary.

The aesthetician is an integral member of the healthcare team in a cosmetic medical practice. The aesthetician helps both the physician and the consumer by reinforcing the proper usage of pre- and post-operative medications and home-care instructions.

Acting as a liaison between the patient and physician, the aesthetician is in a position to educate the patient and reinforce compliance to pre- and post-operative instructions and care.

Women, being social animals by nature, confide and trust their aesthetician and like to discuss with them anything and everything. It is only natural that the physician's aesthetician is privy to information not heard by the doctor, including their dissatisfactions and happiness with treatments and outcomes. This becomes an extremely relevant tool, not only in educating patients and preparing them for the different treatments and possibilities and their post-operative care, but also in guiding the physician in changes of proposed plans and goals during the patient's treatment. It is important for the physician to carefully assess patients seeking cosmetic surgery to be sure that they are good candidates for the procedures, both physically and psychologically. The aesthetician can contribute to this assessment by communicating with the physician about any additional information that may impact on the patient's care. When such communication between physician and aesthetician is open and ongoing, the patient is ultimately the beneficiary.

ARE THEY PATIENTS OR CLIENTS?

As some traditional medical practices strive to achieve a more cosmetic practice environment, a new breed, the medi-spa, emerges, offering all sorts of cosmetic services. In such an environment, the line between patient and client begins to get blurred. A patient, as described in dictionary terms, is '... one who is suffering an ailment, disease or is a victim'. The use of the word 'client', on the other hand, is described as '... a future customer, buyer, purchaser, service user'. Based on dictionary definitions, the use of the word 'client' better suits what today's cosmetic patient is all about. As the lines become blurred, the dilemmas and ethical considerations seem to spawn. Some physicians believe that those they treat are still patients, as they come seeking sound advice from a qualified physician who holds a medical degree. Others think the changing face of medicine and infiltration of managed care have forced them into taking a hard stand against the traditional views and have adopted client terminology instead.

It is this author's belief that they are still patients even though we do market to them as future consumers or clients of cosmetic services. The bottom line is that, regardless of the approach to obtaining each client (i.e. marketing), the care they receive must be of equal quality, regardless of patient/client terminology.

THE WORK OF AN AESTHETICIAN IN A MEDICAL PRACTICE

This chapter is not a textbook of medical aesthetics, but it is appropriate to outline in broad terms what procedures the aesthetician working in a medical practice is likely to carry out. The work can be divided into two broad categories:

1. preparation of the skin for cosmetic or medical procedures
2. postoperative care of the skin, for example lymphatic drainage to assist in reduction of bruising and swelling, camouflaging cosmetics to cover scars postoperatively, micropigmentation for reconstruction or cosmetic purposes, electrolysis or laser light sources for unwanted hair removal, and more.

SKINCARE SERVICES BENEFICIAL IN A COSMETIC SURGICAL SETTING

Preoperative Care

The care given by the aesthetician 4–6 weeks prior to cosmetic surgery may consist of a deep cleansing facial, which may include a chemical exfoliation using a variety of different products that essentially exfoliate the skin. The surgeon prepares the skin by prescribing to the patient a tretinoin or glycolic preparation. The aesthetician performs treatments that can optimize the surgical outcome through procedures such as removal of comedones and hydration of the skin.

One aspect of these treatment visits that is often overlooked is the ability of the aesthetician to monitor the state of the patient through the preoperative phase. Patient compliance to the proper use of topical medications and starting the prophylactics phase of treatment with the antiviral or antifungal medication can also be monitored. The patient who may be experiencing second thoughts about the procedure may express those concerns to the aesthetician, and they can be immediately brought to the physician's attention.

Chemical Exfoliation

There are two purposes for the use of the word 'exfoliation' as opposed to 'chemical peel'. The first is to clarify the fact that aestheticians are not physicians performing 'peels'. The second purpose is to ward off problems with proposed legislation by the Food and Drug Administration concerning the use of alpha-hydroxy acids (AHAs) by aestheticians for professional use.

The National Coalition of Estheticians, Manufacturers/Distributors & Association (www.NCEA.tv) is a coalition of active skincare associations, companies and individuals who have united to establish standards and best practices, and provide political representation for the profession to state legislators and licensing boards. They have taken the position that appropriately trained aestheticians, who have completed a mandated course including theoretical and practical applications, be allowed to perform chemical exfoliation procedures.

The NCEA recommends that aestheticians abide by federal, state and local regulations. There are risks involved with using higher percentages of AHAs that require the skill of a properly trained physician. There is not one state of which this author is aware that allows the aesthetician to:

(a) use treatments that go below the stratum corneum, or
(b) perform invasive procedures.

Tissue Hydration

The hydration of the skin is a primary focus of aesthetic treatments and is one of the considerations to look for in a skincare evaluation.

Comedone Extraction

The extraction of comedones has long been a part of the 'facial' treatment process. Some state aesthetician boards do not allow the invasive use of implements, therefore the aesthetician is taught to 'prepare' the skin for extractions using exfoliants or preparation masks, galvanic desincrustation and steaming (the most widely used procedure).

Lymphatic Drainage

Manual lymphatic drainage massage is a hands-on technique that enhances the movement of lymph and connective tissue fluids in the body and promotes the normal, healthy functioning of the lymphatic system. A highly specialized set of massage techniques designed to promote the movement of lymphatic fluids was developed in the early 1930s by Emil and Estrid Vodder. This technique came to be known as Dr Vodders' manual lymph drainage (MLD). While there are several forms of lymphatic drainage massage in the world today, all owe their origins to the work of the Vodders. MLD has been widely employed in Europe, where the technique is practiced in hospitals and clinics. It is recognized by the Austrian and German government health insurance plans. Only recently has the technique become more widely known and practiced in the USA.

Mechanical methods of lymph drainage work on a similar premise of manual, but a machine with either a pulsating suction or a constant flow is used to accomplish similar goals. The Lymphobiology® system developed by Catherine Atzen, San Jose, CA, is one popular device among practitioners of lymphatic drainage.

Cosmetic Camouflage Makeup

The use of cosmetics for camouflaging redness and swelling has become a necessary part of the physician's cosmetic practice. The patients of today require a 'quick-fix' in order to return in a timely fashion to their daily chores and routines. Also of importance are the thousands of people who use this technique on a daily basis to simply cover burn scars or other injuries that require more opaque make-up coverage than standard cosmetics offer.

Within the medical setting, this type of service is essential, especially with the postlaser resurfacing patient, who may have prolonged erythema. The camouflage make-up manufacturers offer a wide range of purchasing options for the physician and aesthetician wanting to incorporate this service into their practice and business. The dilemma, however, is whether to charge the cosmetic surgery patient for this 'extra service.' The response to this is 'no.' Another important point is to know that most aesthetic schools do not teach camouflage make-up as part of the standard curriculum. Training can be received at postgraduate facilities and from manufacturers of these products.

Dermal Micropigmentation/Permanent Cosmetics

Implanting pigment into the upper dermis is also known as permanent cosmetics, microstipling and tattooing. The enhancement of eyeliner, lips lines and brows are only a few of the cosmetic applications. Tattooing is an art form that many practitioners and consumers aspire to. The procedure has gained new importance within the medical practice with greater application than just cosmetic tattooing. The reconstruction of a nipple areola, treatment for loss of pigment and filling in of 'hair' for alopecia areata have presented the physician with better options for those patients. The state laws vary as to who can perform these procedures and under what conditions, so be sure to check references or contact a professional organization, such as the Society of Permanent Cosmetics Professionals (www.spcp.org).

Microdermabrasion

Microdermabrasion, sometimes referred to as microabrasion, is one of the latest procedures for skin exfoliation. Like a miniature sand blaster, the moving handpiece impasses fine particles, known as corundum, against the face. (Corundum is an aluminum oxide mineral from which the gemstones ruby and sapphire and the abrasive material emery are made.) Corundum is an inert substance, lacking in any known active properties. Machine manufacturers make different models for use in the medical office and the salon.

The NCEA regulates microdermabrasion practice and licensing to include theoretical and practical applications as part of their core curriculum or as continuing education modules.

GENERAL CONSIDERATIONS

The NCEA recommends that aestheticians abide by federal, state and local regulations.

Presurgery Procedures

Aestheticians are the experts in cleansing and other techniques that create the best possible conditions for the skin. Every physician will have their own protocol for preparing patients for surgery, but the broad outline tends to be the same.

For facial cosmetic surgery, the regime commonly begins 3–6 weeks prior to surgery with a thorough, deep cleansing of the face and neck. If the treatment is performed far enough in advance of the surgery, exfoliation will be included as well. Lymphatic drainage has also been shown to have excellent outcomes when used preoperatively on a patient. These treatments may be performed manually or using a machine. Depending on the experience of the aesthetician, some physicians will allow treatment up until the day of surgery. Other types of treatments may be repeated at set intervals until about 2 days prior to surgery. The aesthetician will also advise patients about what skincare regime they should use during the weeks and days before surgery. The object is to keep the skin as healthy as possible.

The NCEA recognizes the following presurgery procedure treatments as appropriate for incorporation by the aesthetician:

1. skin treatments to hydrate and clear skin of blemishes – this may include microdermabrasion, chemical exfoliation treatments and more
2. manual or mechanical lymphatic drainage to improve circulation and lymphatic concerns
3. a product regimen that may include incorporation of retinoids, tretinoin and antipigmentation topicals
4. recommendation of antibruising herbal supplements or other homeopathic nutraceuticals.

Postsurgery Procedures

Postoperative skincare begins after receiving the green light from the surgeon. After surgery, the aesthetician may perform various procedures designed to hasten wound healing, such as hydration, and reduction of bruising and swelling via lymphatic drainage. When healing has progressed to the point where gentle manipulation can be performed, the aesthetician will give the patient new make-up and instruction on how to apply it and how to keep the skin clean and healthy. Here is where artistry becomes important. Cosmetic techniques the patient relied on before surgery may no longer be appropriate, either because a problem the patient had tried to cover up no longer exists or because the lines and contours of the face have changed. Naturally, patients who have just had cosmetic surgery have a strong interest in their new appearance and will turn to the aesthetician for advice about products and techniques that make the most of it. The aesthetician will, in essence, be responsible for putting the finishing touches to the whole experience.

For the reconstructive patient, the aesthetician's expertise will again serve to make the most of the medical procedure. Special care may be needed to promote healing and to minimize scarring, but the most important aspect of the work is often in the skilled use of make-up to camouflage scarring or discoloration. Since the deepest scars for the trauma patient or burn survivor may be the psychological ones that persist long after healing is complete, the aesthetician can play a very significant role in healing and even eliminating those psychological scars.

The NCEA recognizes the following postprocedure treatments as appropriate for incorporation in the work of the aesthetician:

1. skin treatments over intact skin, which could include microdermabrasion, chemical exfoliation treatments and more
2. manual or mechanical lymphatic drainage to improve circulation and lymphatic concerns
3. a product regimen that may include incorporation of retinoids, tretinoin, antipigmentation topicals, etc.
4. specific postprocedure products that may contain vitamins, essential oils, antioxidants, etc.
5. application of camouflage make-up to cover postoperative bruising and wounds.

Depending on the procedure performed the healing time will vary, and the basic prescribed regimen will also depend on the patient's skin type, postoperative complications (if any) and medications (i.e. postoperative antibiotics, herbals or nutritional supplements given by the physician or in some cases by wellness centers).

LEGAL AND LIABILITY ISSUES

Some recent unfavorable situations at medical and non-medical spas have caught the attention of state boards that regulate aesthetician licenses, as have some of the non-specialty physicians who start a business and begin performing laser light procedures, or what the dermatology community would call 'cutaneous medicine'. At the time of writing this chapter, it is still pretty much any physician's legal right to do just about anything – training or not! The American Medical Association has introduced more restrictive rulings on in-office dispensing and supervision requirements, including the physician's right to delegate procedures to staff members. All these developments have added to the burgeoning unrest of practicing physicians.

Ultimately, the first issue overlooked is simply this: is the facility actually a medical spa or is the word 'spa' being used to portray the sense of a non-clinical surrounding to the consumer? Two national organizations have issued position statements defining a medical spa and a day spa to help clarify the differences within this industry.

WHAT IS A MEDICAL SPA?

'A medical spa is a facility that during all hours of business operates under the on-site supervision of a licensed healthcare professional operating within their scope of practice, with a staff that operates within their scope of practice as defined by their individual licensing board, if licensure is required. The facility may offer traditional, complementary, and alternative health practices and treatments in a spa-like setting' (NCEA).

The proper licensing of your facility will ensure that those individuals working in the facility with you are working within their scope of practice. To refer back to the NCEA's definition, '... Practitioners working within a medical spa will be governed by their appropriate licensing board, if licensure is required.'

Proper licensing of the facility ensures that the licensed individual is working within a licensed facility, which then translates into liability insurance coverage. If a licensee – an aesthetician – is not working in a licensed facility (by the board issuing his/her license) then the possibility exists that should an 'incident' occur, the liability insurance policy will become null and void. Simply put, the licensee is in violation of a state licensing requirement that the licensee work in a licensed facility. The insurance company will deny the claim because the licensee was in violation of its license.

Perhaps more important than the industry definition of a spa is the connotation of 'medical' spa in the mind of the patient. The word 'medical' implies that there will be medical supervision or medical interaction of some kind. Also, there could be a belief that it is safer to have facials in this medical spa environment rather than a regular spa. Such a perception may or may not be true, depending on the amount of specific staff training that a licensee receives within the medical spa environment.

This would be a good time to mention that terms such as 'medical aesthetician' or 'clinical aesthetician' are meaningless and not recognized by state licensing boards anywhere in the USA as of this writing. NCEA's position is that:

'Estheticians should represent themselves according to their licensed title, as designated by their state licensing board or regulatory agency, and not promote themselves or allow any employer to market them otherwise.'

MEDICAL TREATMENTS VERSUS TRADITIONAL AESTHETIC SERVICES

What is the difference between a medical facial and a traditional facial? There is a vast difference of opinion on this subject, and it matters not only to the patient but also to the physician, in terms of liability. The laws on this matter vary considerably from state to state and are still in the process of being defined.

In over 28 states, the aesthetician license is not even valid or recognized in a medical setting. The important thing to remember is that an aesthetician's license to perform procedures varies according to whether the facility is licensed as a medical facility or spa/skincare (cosmetological) facility.

Insurance coverage for the aesthetician is often tied to the Cosmetology State Board that governs the aesthetician's license. Some state boards stipulate that the aesthetician must perform aesthetic skincare services in a licensed cosmetological facility. This statement precludes an aesthetician from practicing in a medical setting. In fact, in one case in which I became involved, the state board would not budge and insisted that the physician become a licensed master cosmetologist! Sometimes an ambiguous clause, stipulating that the aesthetician practice 'under the physician's supervision' is included, but this is subject to interpretation. What does supervision mean:

1. on the premises or in the building?
2. available by beeper/telephone?
3. physically in the room when the procedure is being performed?

NATIONAL CERTIFICATION STANDARDS FOR SKINCARE PROFESSIONALS

With so much ambiguity of terms, conflicting state regulations and the introduction of increasingly sophisticated technologies, the need for national standards becomes increasingly essential.

It is NCEA's goal to have all state regulatory boards recognize NCEA-certified professionals in their state. NCEA's certification goal is to raise the educational requirements of a skincare professional to a standardized 1200 hours across the country, in contrast to the current average state requirement of 600 hours, to include both theoretical and practical knowledge. The NCEA is also working toward international recognition of NCEA certification.

The NCEA Certification Program benefits the patients by:

1. providing patients with assurance that they are being treated by well-trained professionals with personal competence
2. identifying and controlling consumer (patient) risks
3. assuring the patient that the aesthetician is both maintaining and updating skills, by receiving training in new emerging technologies. (The NCEA Continuing Education Program has a requirement of 12 additional hours of credit every 3 years.)

THE ATTRIBUTES OF AN NCEA-CERTIFIED PROFESSIONAL

The attributes of an NCEA-certified professional include the following:

- serving the best interests of their clients at all times and providing the highest quality service possible
- maintaining client confidentiality, keeping treatment documentation records and providing clear, honest communication
- providing clients with clear and realistic goals and outcomes, and not making false claims regarding the potential benefits of the techniques rendered or products recommended
- adhering to the scope of practice of their profession and referring clients to the appropriate qualified health practitioner when indicated
- offering services only within the scope of their practice as defined by the state within which they operate, if required, and in adherence with appropriate federal laws and regulations.
- understanding of new techniques or procedures and obtaining adequate training before performing a treatment on the client
- representing their state licensure, education, training, qualifications and abilities honestly
- strictly adhering to all usage instructions and guidelines provided by product and equipment manufacturers, provided those guidelines and instructions are within their scope of practice as defined by the state, if required.

HOW TO FIND A QUALIFIED AESTHETICIAN

Look for professional attire. Aestheticians should 'walk the walk and talk the talk', i.e. have good skin, and be well groomed and well styled.

Get recommendations from people you respect, especially those who have obtained visibly good results. Make a surprise visit to the facility prior to making an appointment. Check to see their current license. Ask if they are NCEA certified (if so, they should have a valid certificate and certification card).

CONCLUSIONS

The career of the aesthetician is the fastest growing segment within the beauty industry. With the scientific advances in cosmeceutical ingredients and new device technologies, the state regulatory boards are scrambling to catch up. The aestheticians you trust to care for your patients' skin should have a 'never stop learning' attitude because the day they lose that desire to learn is the day they should stop being an aesthetician!

17 From the Inside Out: A Psychotherapist's Views on Aesthetic Enhancement

Michael Colberg

We have come to prefer a world where the distractable take Ritalin, the depressed take Prozac, and the unattractive get cosmetic surgery to a world ruled, arbitrarily, by those fortunate few who were born focused, happy, and beautiful. Cosmetic surgery is not "earned" beauty, but then natural beauty isn't earned, either. One of the principal contributions of the late twentieth century was the moral deregulation of social competition—the insistence that advantages derived from artificial and extraordinary intervention are no less legitimate than the advantages of nature.

Malcolm Gladwell[1]

INTRODUCTION

Technology has enabled people to seek facial rejuvenation and other cosmetic procedures. It has also helped to establish firmly the parameters of what it is they are seeking. It has created the illusion that they can become part of the 'focused, happy and beautiful' group that Gladwell writes of. Fortunately, or unfortunately, what they end up discovering, if they are conscious enough to notice, is that there is no group. There are other people whom the seeker perceives as being members of the group, but the quality of being safe and belonging is elusive. These qualities exist and develop only as people establish real relationships with themselves. We exist as individuals, and it is by developing what is special and unique within ourselves that we become whole and contributing members of society.

We happen to exist at a time when technology has both enabled us to alter our appearance and caused us to be connected in a much more immediate way than we have ever been connected before. Ironically, this has taken from us many of the tools we used to achieve intimacy. Television has replaced conversation. Email has replaced letter writing. Instant messages have replaced telephone conversations, and, in many instances, cell phone conversations have replaced time that was formerly used to gather our thoughts and to connect with ourselves. The internet has, arguably, removed the need to actually interact directly with other human beings. At the same time that we have gained the freedom to alter our appearance, to become 'who we want to be,' we have been isolated from having real contact with ourselves and with others. We are being inundated with images of those whose lives are lived in the glow of the public eye and those who will stop at nothing to get there. There are reality shows that document a reality that does not exist, there are talent shows featuring people without talent and there are makeover shows that highlight the degrees to which people will go to feel like they fit in without connecting to themselves. This has a numbing effect. The message is that, in order to be happy, we should abandon what causes us to be unique, thoughtful, creative and compassionate, and do what we can to conform to current trends. We are more in each other's faces but less in each other's hearts. Many of those who choose another path are banished to an invisible sideline.

Obviously, there are still many people for whom appearance is not particularly important. There is no body of information yet available that compares people who seek out cosmetic intervention with those who do not. In the end, it may be that the majority of people who seek cosmetic procedures simply place a higher emphasis on improving or maintaining their appearance than those who do not. It is possible that neither group represents the majority of pathology present in the population as a whole. We will need to wait for sound scientific data before we can move forward with that discussion.

The discussion in this chapter has several parts: a discussion of the psychological and emotional context in which the profession is operating, a look at cosmetic procedures from the physicians' perspective, a perspective on clients and some tools to help initiate some of the ideas presented. I want to begin by touching upon some of the major events that influenced how we have been thinking about and approaching the practice of cosmetic and minimally invasive plastic surgery.

A HISTORICAL PERSPECTIVE

Elizabeth Haiken did a particularly thorough job of discussing the history of the profession in her book *Venus Envy: A History of Cosmetic Surgery*.[2] There were attempts made to address disfigurement as early as the 16th century, but the first concentrated effort to address cosmetic reconstruction was made in response to wounds suffered on the battlefields of World War I. The medical community was both able and highly motivated to develop new ways to treat the disfiguring wounds suffered by soldiers during World War I. Although many of these wounds were not physically life threatening, they were psychologically life altering. By the beginning of the 20th century, the work of Freud, Hall, Jung and those who followed them began to explore what it means to have an internal life – a meaningful relationship with the self – and we entered the age of psychological awareness. Against this background, medicine's urge to 'make whole' seriously wounded World War I veterans takes on special meaning.

As society became aware of medicine's ability to alter appearance, other potential clients emerged. As author Christine Rose wrote, 'The greatest boon to modern cosmetic surgery was not the development of any particular technique or the creation of a miracle product. It was an import from psychology: the inferiority complex. Popularized by Viennese psychologist Alfred Adler in the early twentieth century, it reached an eager audience in the United States. The inferiority complex provided a crucial link: it joined individual mental health with physical appearance and thus "psychologized cosmetic surgery". People suffering from an inferiority complex because their breasts were small or their chins droopy were ill; they required medical intervention to alleviate their psychological suffering. As Haiken notes, by the 1920s and 1930s, Americans had made this link between physical appearance and mental health permanent; as a result "their demands for surgical attention became more insistent at the same time as the new language of psychology made these demands more persuasive". By 1940, *Good Housekeeping* magazine was asking, "why should anyone suffer under the handicap of a conspicuously ugly feature? Why not let modern science give him a normal face and an equal chance with other people?"'[3]

Cosmetic procedures came to occupy an established niche in the medical field, and people seeking cosmetic intervention became patients. This secured the fit between cosmetic procedures and the standard medical model. As the field of psychology has matured, each generation of studies has shown there to be less pathology among those seeking cosmetic intervention than the early studies suggested.

According to Sarwer et al., early reports of the psychological characteristics of rhinoplasty patients date back to the 1940s and 1950s. Many of these reports, as well as studies conducted into the 1960s, relied heavily on clinical interviews and observations of patients that suggested rhinoplasty patients were highly psychopathological. One group of investigators went so far as to state that *all* patients desiring rhinoplasty were mentally ill and described their sample of patients as suffering from a variety of psychiatric issues, ranging from feelings of inferiority to psychosis. In another study, 53% of patients received preoperative diagnoses of personality disorders.[4] More recent studies of patients who had rhytidectomies and blepharoplasties indicate that these patients are not as psychopathological as earlier studies suggested. In addition, results from body image studies indicate that patients seeking anti-aging procedures may place greater emphasis on their appearance and report less dissatisfaction with their overall body image than do patients who seek other procedures.[4]

Sarwer et al. concluded that, given the popularity of other minimally invasive facial procedures, there is a need for studies of the psychological characteristics of patients who seek these treatments.[4] I disagree. It is time for us to discard the pathology model, and for physicians who practice cosmetic and plastic surgery to understand the increasingly important role they have to play in helping their clients engage in self-care. This change in thinking can be seen elsewhere in the practice of western medicine. For example, the scientific community has begun to accept that meditation, acupuncture and other healing modalities contribute not just to healing but also to staying healthy. It is my belief that, in the coming years, our understanding of the connection between mind and body will change and play a different and increasingly important role in science and in the practice of medicine; the relationship between mind and body can be a source of health and well-being. People who feel good about themselves are often healthier than people who do not.

COSMETIC MEDICINE FROM THE PHYSICIAN'S PERSPECTIVE

Noting that the nature of medical education has not changed much in the last half century, Bloom writes, 'Until today ... this general form has persisted, producing an elite corps of highly trained specialists who are prepared to practice a science-based, technologically complex type of medicine'.[5] It would at first appear that this group of physicians is perfectly suited to enter a field where the use of technology is rapidly changing and expanding the very nature of cosmetic medicine. However, technological expertise is but one set of skills needed to practice minimally invasive cosmetic medicine.

According to the American Society of Plastic Surgeons (ASPS), over 13.5 million plastic surgical procedures were performed in 2004. Most of them were minimally invasive cosmetic procedures, many of which did not exist in 1992 when ASPS started tracking procedures.[6] As technology plays an increasingly important role in cosmetic practices, other professions have sought out and acquired the knowledge necessary to offer many of these procedures. The ASPS numbers are probably an underestimate because they do not account for the increasing number of non-plastic surgeon physicians, including cosmetic dermatologists, and trained aestheticians, who are also joining the pool of professionals offering minimally invasive cosmetic procedures. It would appear that the demand for these procedures is rapidly increasing, the kinds of procedures available are increasing and the number of practitioners is expanding.

Physicians practicing in the field of cosmetic surgery will be well served by acquiring interpersonal skills that are generally de-emphasized during their medical training. Sarwer et al. wrote, 'Plastic surgeons typically have not been provided with adequate training in how to better understand the emotional and interpersonal aspects of patient functioning'.[4] They go on to state, 'to obtain such training and integrate these skills into their everyday practice adds to the already demanding burdens that all surgeons experience. However, compared to their investments in developing their surgical skills, the amount of time and effort needed to develop a deeper understanding of the psychological functioning of their patients is relatively small'.[4]

I think that this last statement touches upon the very essence of what I hope to accomplish with this discussion. I believe that, as with those seeking to become surgeons, a certain amount of talent, and perhaps intuition, is needed to become an artful practitioner. Some people make gifted surgeons and others are gifted at helping people better understand themselves. Sometimes a person has both gifts and other times not. When surgeons find that they are not particularly skilled at client communication or assessment there is absolutely nothing wrong with reaching out and collaborating with someone who has been trained in those areas. It is important for surgeons to know and develop their strengths and to both acknowledge and respect their limitations.

Robert M. Goldwyn, writing in *Psychological Aspects of Plastic and Cosmetic Surgery: Clinical, Empirical and Ethical Perspectives*,[4] offers the following list of 'potentially problematic patients from a psychological perspective':

- the VIP patient
- the patient who appeals to the surgeon's ego
- the perfectionist patient
- the patient under psychiatric care
- the patient thought to be in need of psychiatric care
- the dishonest patient
- the disheveled patient
- the patient whose personality clashes with that of the surgeon.

I think the list suggests a problem associated with trying to standardize human behavior. Most of the judgments that need to be made when deciding whether or not a client is potentially problematic are subjective in nature. I personally feel that when a person is using a checklist to assess someone sitting across from them, they may be missing out on the best assessment tool they possess – themselves. The initial question for a surgeon to ask is: Am I comfortable moving forward with this person? If not, is there some conversation that can be had that would clarify whether client and surgeon could/should work together? Am I capable of having that conversation and, if not, can I collaborate with someone who is?

What are some of the things to look for and think about when trying to understand clients desiring cosmetic procedures? As Sarwer points out, 'These procedures are no longer reserved for the wealthy and elite; women and men across age, racial and socioeconomic groups seek cosmetic surgery to improve their appearance and ultimately their body image'.[7] In

2007, nearly 10 million minimally invasive procedures were performed in the USA, an increase of 81% from the number of procedures performed in 2000.[8] According to the American Academy of Cosmetic Surgery, between 1982 and 1992 the number of people surveyed who said that they approved of cosmetic surgery increased by 50% and the number who disapproved declined by 66%. With this decline in disapproval, consumer demand for surgery has skyrocketed.[3]

FROM THE PATIENT'S PERSPECTIVE

In a review of psychosocial outcomes for patients seeking cosmetic procedures, Honigman et al. found that, 'Most people seeking cosmetic surgery procedures appear psychologically healthy; however, some are not, and for these individuals, cosmetic procedures may have a negative outcome, creating problems for both patient and surgeon. The challenge that surgeons face is how to identify, before surgical intervention, those patients who may have a poor outcome in terms of psychological adjustment and psychosocial functioning despite a technically satisfactory result'.[9] Although pathology does exist within the plastic and cosmetic surgery seeking population, often in the form of body dysmorphic disorder, newer studies have shown that the majority of those undergoing procedures are not seriously impaired. This discussion will focus on that segment of the population.

My goal is to discuss cosmetic clients in a way that helps physicians better understand how to assess and guide clients, and to help them make intelligent decisions about whether the physician–client match is likely to be a good one. To do this, I am going to introduce an alternative to the traditionally used medical pathology model by borrowing from work originally written to help social workers move away from using this deficit-based lens. It introduces a 'strengths-based perspective' for use in client assessment and interaction. I find this approach to be useful for physicians seeking to improve their ability to assess and communicate more effectively with clients.

Dennis Saleebey describes the frame of the strengths-based perspective in three basic concepts:[10]

1. Given the difficulties they have, and the known resources available to them, people are often doing amazingly well, the best they can at the time.
2. People have survived to this point 'certainly not without pain and struggle' through employing their will, their vision, their skills and, as they have grappled with life, what they have learned about themselves and their world. We must understand these capacities and make alliance with this knowledge in order to help.
3. Change can only come when you collaborate with client's aspirations, perceptions and strengths, and when you firmly believe in them.

The strengths-based perspective embraces the world view of the client. It is truly starting where the client is, rather than starting where the theory is.

Viewed from a strengths-based perspective, we can say that the majority of clients seeking cosmetic consultations are functioning at a level that affords them the ability to make active choices about how they want to live. Stated simply, it is the physician's job to understand what their clients are hoping to accomplish, to decide whether they are comfortable helping their clients achieve that goal and, if the answer is 'yes', to help them refine their expectations so that they are aligned with all possible outcomes as they move forward together.

Although our ability to control extends only to making decisions about how to respond to what is actually happening, many people spend their time seeking to control as much of what is happening as possible. By definition, the thought of turning themselves over to a stranger who may alter their appearance puts patients out of control and may cause them to behave in ways that might appear pathological when, in fact, they are merely 'acting out' because they are feeling frightened. A question to ask is: Might the patient be experiencing vulnerability that has the appearance of instability? One way to check this out is to help the client try to access and express fearful feelings so that they can be addressed in a healthy way. Making use of a strengths-based model would help the client feel less out of control and powerless.

Dr Marian Cantisano-Zilkha wrote a manual entitled *Contemporary Guide to Aesthetic Enhancement*, which introduces and discusses minimally invasive modalities of facial periocular rejuvenation in a way that is intended to give a general education to doctors and the cosmetic industry.[11] Ultimately, it becomes a valuable tool for patients as they become as informed as possible and more able to take responsibility for, and to commit to, a course of action. This creates a sense of partnership, and working in this collaborative way helps clients take responsibility for the choices they make. The point I want to make is that having the guide available empowers the client and demystifies the procedures so that a more collaborative relationship can happen between the doctor and the client.

USING THE STRENGTHS-BASED MODEL

I think it is important to make it absolutely certain that patients are clear about the range of outcomes that are possible. This includes both how their appearance might and might not be changed by the procedure and what the downtime may be, and therefore be certain to be generous in your estimate of how long it might take for them to be ready to resume their lives. It is also important to explain the range of outcomes that are possible with each of the procedures under consideration and emphasize that results may differ among diverse individuals. If the client is following your lead and you are making an educated guess as to which path seems to be the best fit between their desire and what is possible, make sure that they know that this is an inexact science and that you cannot guarantee exactly how their body will respond. The goal is to form a collegial relationship. Remember, you are in charge of the procedure and they are in charge of the pre- and post-procedure care that may determine whether or not the procedure is a success. As the technology becomes more sophisticated, it is entirely possible that the strengths-based collaborative approach will help physicians to work with clients as their partners rather than experience them as the objects of their ministrations.

It is important to try to understand how each potential client looks at their aging process. It is entirely possible to grow in an age-appropriate way while seeking to avail oneself of the opportunities currently available to remain attractive and vital. As Sarwer pointed out, 'Using cosmetic surgery to bargain with the clock stirs deep emotions. Maturing faces (and our bodies) also confront us with our mortality, a reminder that no one lives forever. Our time is limited. At times, the emotional impact of these reminders is mistakenly experienced as a reaction to the skin and body changes themselves. Is the patient more upset about the wrinkles or the unalterable realities of aging?'[12] This is an important difference because even a successful surgical outcome will not address the fact that the client is aging. It is not possible to stay young. For those who are lucky enough to make it, being old is a natural part of being alive.

If a surgeon suspects that clients are struggling with the fact of aging, it may be useful to help them work through some of the normal emotional challenges that accompany aging. A surgeon might ask them if there is an age at which they imagine themselves putting a halt to cosmetic intervention. They may also ask them about how their family and friends negotiated, or are negotiating, the aging process. These inquiries may help give a physician a sense of whether the clients' expectations are realistic and, more importantly, whether these are the expectations with which the physician is comfortable. There is a difference between people seeking to look younger and people seeking to look good, refreshed and revitalized. As Jonathan Van Meter of *New York Magazine* observed, 'Even the most successful and beautiful result is entirely different from what a woman looked like when she was 30. Demi Moore, the gold standard of good plastic surgery, does not look at all like she did when she made *Ghost*. The *new new face* is a fantastic approximation! An uncanny resemblance! It is, at its best, a close copy of youthful beauty, not youthful beauty itself'.[13]

It can be difficult to distinguish between those who seek to remain vital looking and those for whom aging is so threatening as to pose the risk of serious destabilization. Although it is always possible that a previously invisible underlying instability may be triggered by a cosmetic procedure, the level of engagement needed to move through a procedure using a strengths-based collaborative gives both the client and the physician a greater opportunity to recognize and respond to any red flags before they become problems. This could spell the difference between a relationship ending in litigation or not.

When using a strengths-based perspective, clients must be approached as individuals. They should be respected as being the experts on who they are and how they want to live. On the other hand, the physician is the expert on how the body is responding to the aging process and how that process can be adjusted to suit the client's objectives. Special care must be taken when dealing with adolescents or young adults. There is now strong evidence that the brain does not cease to mature until the early 20s, particularly in the areas that govern impulsivity, judgment, planning for the future, foresight of consequences and other characteristics that make people morally responsible. In fact, the age of 21 or 22 years would be closer to the 'biological' age of maturity.[14] That being the case, extra thought should be given when considering working on an adolescent. Be thorough during the assessment process to make certain that it is the adolescent who wants the procedure and that the adolescent understands the nature of the procedure, the possible range of outcomes and the downtime involved. Obviously, agreeing to help a depressed teenager with severe acne scarring differs from enhancing the bust line of a depressed 14-year-old. It is important to make every effort to be alert to the whole person because the solution to their distress may not lie in changing their appearance, especially at that age.

People who want to look different may seek change for a variety of reasons. For example, a mysterious spy or crime figure seeks anonymity by changing his or her appearance, hoping to begin anew in a new locale. Can we wipe the slate clean by changing our wrapping or do we complicate matters when we do something to our outside without addressing the corresponding internal changes that need to be made? What about the person who goes through a life-altering tragedy? How important is it that they take time to reflect on the experience before turning to cosmetic surgery? The answers to these questions are complex and differ on a case-by-case basis. I imagine that, as a clinician, I would respond very differently to a client seeking to have breast reconstruction immediately following a mastectomy than I would to a person wanting complete facial rejuvenation a week after losing a child in a car accident.

Imagine persons who wish to have work done in order to resemble a celebrity in the hope that their lives may take on some of the 'sparkle' they attribute to that person. Would you, as a physician, be comfortable helping them to achieve their goal? Is their goal to look like that celebrity or to feel like they imagine that celebrity feels? Are you trained to be able to elicit that kind of information from a prospective client? Is one reason appropriate while the other is not? What about a second person who seeks the same goal for a completely different reason? They may regularly be mistaken for a particular celebrity and find that they can best support themselves and their families by building on this fluke of nature and want to further conform their features to and then find work impersonating the said celebrity. While the former person's motives may point toward the need for further evaluation, is that necessarily the case with the latter?

It is clear that looks do play an important role in the marketplace. There are apparently real economic harms and benefits tied to personal appearance. A 1993 study conducted by economists Daniel Hamermesh and Jeff Biddle, and published by the National Bureau of Economic Research, found that 'holding constant demographic and labor-market characteristics, plain people earn less than people of average looks, who earn less than the good-looking. The penalty for plainness is 5 to 10 percent, slightly larger than the premium for beauty. The effects are slightly larger for men than women; but unattractive women are less likely than others to participate in the labor force and are more likely to be married to men with unexpectedly low human capital'.[15]

A question to consider is whether we have arrived at a place where the presence of features such as gap teeth, an overly prominent nose, or elephant ears tends to identify someone as belonging to a lower socioeconomic class or undesirable ethnic group.

While some people seek to improve their body image by altering a feature they do not like, some may not really care that much about how they look but choose, or are pressured, to alter their appearance to make themselves more marketable. Others may find that something about their looks detracts from their ability to focus 100% on their job. Our environment also dictates what is appropriate for us. Traditionally, Europeans have been thought of as allowing themselves to age more naturally than those in the Americas.

CONCLUSION

What happens during an initial consultation is remarkably circumscribed. The patient is there to decide whether or not to receive care from the surgeon or to convince the surgeon to comply with his or her desire to have surgery. In turn, the surgeon is making a decision about whether or not to accept that person as a patient. This evaluative process puts the personality characteristics of both individuals on display.[4]

Goldwyn states, the surgeon is "making a decision about whether or not to accept that person as a patient."[4] The client is a patient from the moment the consultation begins. This may seem like a trivial point, but it undermines the creation of a collaborative stance by creating a power inequity. I believe that more is accomplished when the physician and the client work holistically. The entire person in their environment should be considered if necessary. The extent of this inquiry depends upon how comfortable the fit is between the client and the physician. If there is trust and understanding between them then the conversation can cover more ground with fewer words. If there is no innate connection, then it pays to take the time to cover all of the bases that need to be covered.

Recognizing that not all physicians have the talent to engage in these conversations and that some among those who do have the skills lack the time, I would like to make some suggestions. One possibility is for prospective clients to fill out questionnaires that are designed to get them to think about what they want to accomplish, why they are choosing to do it now, what their expectations of the physician and the procedure are, and whether there is any history that would contraindicate or complicate moving forward. Some sample questions are included at the end of this chapter. It might also be a good idea for physicians to form a relationship with a trained mental health professional who can offer input when needed.

Another idea borrowed from psychotherapy is the idea of a peer support and supervision group. It involves colleagues getting together to discuss what does and does not work as they try to develop their interpersonal skills further. A secondary benefit derived from forming a group of this type is that colleagues begin to get a sense of what types of clients are the best fit for them personally. This gives them an option to refer to a member of the group a client whose personality is not a good match for them.

We have arrived at an important moment in the practice of aesthetic enhancement and plastic surgery. In its infancy, cosmetic practice made the leap from addressing the needs of wounded veterans of World War I to those in the general population seeking to change their appearance. Now we have made a more subtle leap. We have entered an age when minimally invasive procedures have become available and highly sought after. In order to address the population of clients seeking treatment, physicians are best served by discarding the traditional pathology model and adopting a model more reflective of the times, one based on collaboration. Making use of a strengths-based model respects the fact that both physicians and clients have contributions to make to their interaction that can make their relationship more efficient and more satisfactory and, ultimately, optimizing the results.

We are moving into a time of uncertainty. We have many possibilities and few answers. I believe that we will have the best possible outcome if we learn to connect with each other and respect what each of us can and cannot bring to the table. I hope that those who read this chapter are better equipped and more motivated to connect, share and learn from both clients and colleagues.

SUGGESTED QUESTIONS FOR ASSESSING A PATIENT'S UNDERSTANDING AND READINESS FOR COSMETIC PROCEDURES

1. What is the goal?
2. Why now? What makes now feel like the right time for this procedure rather than a month or a year ago, or a month or a year in the future? (Do not stop with purely practical answers, like I have a vacation coming up or I just got a bonus check. Continue with 'Okay, but is there anything else?') (Sarwer/Grossbart)[12]
3. What are three wishes you have about the impact on your life from a successful outcome? Please answer on a pure fantasy level, do not be realistic. (Sarwer/Grossbart)
4. What are three realistic expectations you have for the impact a successful procedure will have on your life? Can you imagine any possible disadvantages to a successful outcome? (Sarwer/Grossbart)
5. How do you expect key people in your life will respond differently to you after the procedure? How about strangers? (Sarwer/Grossbart)
6. Does your target body part remind you of anyone you know, you have met, or any of your family members? Whose eyes or whose thighs do you have? (Sarwer/Grossbart)
7. Have you noticed that your readiness to have the procedure varies from day to day or from week to week? Is the desire greater with certain events, moods or the reactions of others? (Sarwer/Grossbart)
8. Have you noticed any unexpected emotional reactions to personnel, the doctor's office or talking about the procedure? (Sarwer/Grossbart)
9. Have you ever had any indications that others see you differently to how you see yourself? (Sarwer/Grossbart)
10. Do you ever have trouble following health or beauty guidelines that you agree with? (Sarwer/Grossbart)
11. What percentage of people's first impression of you do you believe your target body part accounts for? What percentage after they get to know you? (Sarwer/Grossbart)
12. Why are you choosing this procedure over another, more invasive surgical procedure?
13. Who are you telling about this procedure? Why and why not?

14. What about downtime?
15. How long do you expect this will it take to heal?
16. How long do you expect the desired effects of this procedure will last?

REFERENCES

1 Gladwell M. The sporting scene, "Drugstore athlete" *The New Yorker*. 2001;(10 September):52.

2 Haiken E. *Venus envy*. Baltimore: Johns Hopkins University Press; 1997.

3 Rose C. The Democratization of Beauty. *The New Atlantis*. 2004;(5):19–35.

4 Sarwer D, Pruzensky T, Cash T, et al., eds. *Psychological aspects of reconstructive and cosmetic plastic surgery: clinical, empirical, and ethical perspectives*. Philadelphia: Lippincott, Williams and Wilkins; 2006.

5 Bloom S. Structure and ideology in medical education: an analysis of resistance to change. *JHSB*. 1998;29(4):294–306.

6 Pruzensky T, Sarwer D, Cash T, et al. Multiple perspectives on the psychology of plastic surgery. In: Sarwer D, Pruzensky T, Cash T, et al., eds. *Psychological Aspects of Reconstructive and Cosmetic Plastic Surgery*. Philadelphia: Lippincott, Williams and Wilkins; 2006:13–22.

7 Sarwer D. Cosmetic surgery and changes in body image. In: Cash T, Pruzinsky T, eds. *Body image: a handbook of theory, research and clinical practice*. New York: Guilford Press; 2002:422–430.

8 American Society of Plastic Surgeons. *2008 Report of the 2007 National Clearinghouse of Plastic Surgery Statistics*. Arlington Heights, IL: American Society of Plastic Surgeons; 2008.

9 Honigman R, Phillips K, Castle DJ. A review of psychosocial outcomes for patients seeking cosmetic surgery. *Plast Reconstr Surg*. 2004;113(4):1229–1237.

10 Saleebey D. The strengths approach to practice. In: Saleebey D, ed. *The strengths perspective in social work practice*. Longman: White Plains; 1997:49–58.

11 Zilka M. *Contemporary Guide for Aesthetic Enhancement*. Newton, PA: Handbooks in Health Care Company; 2008.

12 Grossbart T, Sarwer D. Cosmetic surgery: surgical tools – psychosocial goals. *Semin Cutan Med Sur*. 1999;18(2):101–111.

13 Van Meter J. About face. *New York Magazine*. 2008;(August 11).

14 PBS Frontline. Inside the teen brain. Jay Geidd interview. Available at: www.pbs.org/wgbh/pages/frontline/shows/teenbrain.

15 Hamermesh DS, Biddle JE. Beauty and the labor market. *AER*. 1994;84(5):1174–1194.

18 The Future of Oculofacial Rejuvenation: A Perspective

Sterling Baker, Erin L Holloman

'Beauty is truth, truth beauty.'

Keats

This concept was studied by Keats while observing a painting on a Grecian urn. Keats further suggested that if we understand truth and beauty, we know all we need to know. As with many abstract concepts, we humans have a difficult time understanding this relationship. Truth is a concept that seems to defy definition. Yet, we seem to comprehend beauty on an intuitive basis, even though that intuition is greatly influenced by time and culture. To a major extent, we have historically and collectively equated beauty with youth. This youth portion of the equation frequently becomes the pursuit of vitality. With all of the hyperventilation we can muster, we enshrine vitality as a basic urge, if not a primal right, to live our allotted time as fully as possible. Then the beauty portion of the equation not so subtly suggests that the appearance of youth is as important – if not more so – than the possession of vitality. Keats and indeed many others remind us not to succumb to the myopic assertion that this generation and this time have somehow discovered a universal truth about beauty.

Even a cursory review of our history on the planet shows that we have long assumed appearance, which conceals chronologic progression, is a desirable goal, therefore are we now providing some new (and some not so new) methods that are mainly extensions of ancient practices? Perhaps lasers, which are arguably the newest set of our tools, are no more than sophisticated, high-tech ways to produce thermal damage to a graded depth in the relatively superficial dermis. Even if the aesthetic practitioners of ancient societies who used fire to singe the skin did not know the complexity of the target organ, they did know that they had to avoid full-thickness damage to prevent scarring. Some might contend that all modern practitioners should be so well informed.

Early efforts often were mechanical or thermal. These methods share a commonality with their modern equivalents. Energy is applied directly to the surface. Outer layers of the dermis are damaged. In a modern extension, these applications are altered to preserve the surface, usually by dynamic cooling delivered just prior to and immediately following the application of energy. Fractionated deliveries of energy leave areas of normal tissue between 'islands' of treated tissue to speed recovery. Rejuvenation is accomplished through regeneration of the damaged collagen in the papillary and upper reticular dermis. The efficacy of reepithelialization is a function in large part of the density of appendages in the treated area. In both of these applications, the skill of the practitioner is obvious to all. Knowledge of the territory and cultivation of a light touch can be summarized in the time-honored admonition to 'first do no (permanent) harm'.

Since early antiquity, rejuvenating lotions and potions have been concocted from all manner of secret ingredients. Early efforts involved cytotoxic and lytic agents that produced partial-thickness damage to the dermis. Understanding the target tissue, predicting the penetration depth and knowing the neutralization process were of critical importance if scarring was to be avoided. Surely, the exaggerated claims for the many proprietary agents and practices currently being promoted remind us of Bob Dylan's reference to his lost love in *Tangled Up in Blue*: 'The past is close behind.' If the past is indeed the recent prologue to our time, will the future be a refined version of the present? Or will it be unrecognizable?

So now we have arrived at the risky business of predicting. And, dear reader, you might be tempted to ask by what authority we represent our opinions as having value? Well, the authors of this book asked for our opinion and you acquired the book. In truth, our ability to see past our own noses is probably no better than yours. As you read this, do not take us (or yourself) too seriously! Enough already. What is out there?

Over the last two decades, we have learned that surgical wounds heal without scarring when cleft lips and palates are repaired intrauterine. The healing process occurs in an environment that lacks inflammatory cell proliferation. Histological analysis of these wounds shows increased deposition of hyaluronic acid. Perhaps, altering the wound environment with substances such as hyaluronics during surgery and postoperative recovery will decrease the presence of scarring.

Surely, somewhere in the future we will abandon the relatively gross insults to tissue that we now offer as therapeutic interventions. Patient complaints of prolonged side effects and lengthy recoveries do not now fit comfortably into our therapies and that is not likely to change in the future. Genomic studies may provide an early step in our understanding of how to arrest (or slow) the decline in peak performance as a result of the aging process by manipulating tissue to maintain maximum vitality. Understanding genetic coding could lead to ways to manipulate function at the cellular level. Or perhaps new cells will be developed from an as yet unknown source of stem cells. Given the ethical debate over embryonic stem cell use and the difficulty in obtaining those cells, an alternative source of resident cells with either inherent or inducible pluripotent potential may represent a more acceptable early effort. In fact, our initial efforts with fat autographs suggest that we may even now be at an early stage of grafting undifferentiated cells that will mature. At a more advanced cellular level, will specific specialized cells be reengineered by the insertion of new genetic information? For example, recombinant genetic technology has been utilized to 'teach' bacteria how to make human insulin. Early efforts to treat some forms of Leber's congenital amaurosis, an autosomal-recessive group of blinding retinal diseases, by inserting genetic material attached to an adenoviral vector into the eye have been encouraging.[1]

Our understanding of intercellular communication is limited. Pathways and transmitting agents are not clear. Some of the 'cross-talk' at the cellular level can produce effects that can be either beneficial or disastrous, depending on the tissue involved. Vascular endothelial growth factors (VEGF) have recently gained much interest, especially in the eye, because the neoangiogenesis they promote in hypoxic tissue can lead to new vessels that are not competent. In advanced cases of diabetes and macular degeneration, these new vessels tend to leak blood and serum that can obscure the visual axis, leading to irreversible damage of the retina. Anti-VEGF treatments are employed for targeted therapy in these diseases. However, VEGF has other modulating activities in vivo that can be useful in other locations. It affects a broad spectrum of neuronal and glial proliferation, cell migration, cell survival and proteolysis. Might it or other as yet unidentified modulating agents be useful in promoting rejuvenation locally at specified targets? Human growth hormone supplementation has been promoted rather vigorously as an antiaging agent. But many are concerned because of the possible proneoplastic potential of such activities. The goals of beauty and sustained youth seem direct enough, but what are the 'trade-offs'? Product liability is an issue that no one can ignore. Perhaps, viral stimulation will become a way to alter intracellular activity. Production of new collagen and elastin in the dermis is less important than the amount produced. Certainly, our early insights into modulators and receptor sites place us at the brink of an exciting and as yet poorly understood internal universe that seems to offer limitless possibilities. Will the beauty industry in its exponential and escalating growth modulate or be modulated by patient's needs and expectations in the search for the fountain of youth and vitality?

If the aging process is stopped or even reversed, what will the goal be? Who will decide what our allotted time is? Will we review the family album with succeeding generations who all are chronologically arrested at the same time in life? Who decides what are the optimal parameters for a prolonged existence? Will there be an ideal attainable by all of us? What sacrifice of individual phenotypic expression will we be willing to tolerate? A new organ (you specify which one) for someone who suffers with a failing one truly represents a medical miracle. New skin, forever youthful, may not be far behind. In his song *With Every Wish* Bruce Springsteen reminds us that we 'better think first, with every wish there comes a curse'. We cannot all live forever or even for a very long time – whatever that is.

REFERENCE

1 Bainbridge JW, Smith AJ, Barker SS, et al. Effect of gene therapy on visual function in Leber's congenital amaurosis. *N Engl J Med*. 2008;358(21):2231–2239.

Index

Note: Page numbers followed '*b*' indicate boxes; '*f*' indicate figures; '*t*' indicate tables

A

ablative lasers
- overview, 4
- thermal damage from, 43

accelerometer, 138–139
Accent XL®, 11, 70, 77
- *see also* radiofrequency volumetric heating technology

AcHyal, 99*t*
acne
- blue light treatment for, 60
- photodynamic treatment for, 63*t*
- scars *see* acne scars
- vitamin A for, 24

acneiform eruption after chemical peels, 36
acne scars
- carbon dioxide therapy for, 159–160, 167–168
- platelet-rich plasma for, 152, 152*f*, 153*f*

actinic keratoses
- alternatives to photodynamic treatment, 60
- photodynamic treatment for, 60–61, 61*f*, 62, 63*t*

adipose tissue, 143
adult mesenchymal stem cells (ADSCs), 125
aestheticians, 189–194
- attributes of an NCEA-certified professional, 194
- finding qualified, 194
- general considerations, 191–192
- legal and liability issues, 192–193
- medical spas, 193
- medical treatments *versus* traditional aesthetic services, 190
- national certification standards, 193–194
- patients and clients, 189–190
- physician benefits, 189
- skincare services beneficial in a cosmetic surgical setting, 190–191
  - chemical exfoliation, 190
  - comedone extraction, 191
  - cosmetic camouflage makeup, 191
  - dermal micropigmentation/permanent cosmetics, 191
  - lymphatic drainage, 191
  - microdermabrasion, 191
  - preoperative care, 190
  - tissue hydration, 190
- work in medical practice, 190

aging
- and dark circles, 127
- facial contour changes with *see* facial changes with age
- in the periorbital area, 29
- and platelet-rich plasma, 151–152, 151*f*
- process of, 97, 98*f*
- psychological effects of, 199

air, accidental injection of, 176, 176*f*
alexandrite lasers
- classification, 40*t*
- for dark circles, 130–131
- for hair removal, 44, 51
- indications, 43
- pigmentary changes, 48–49
- for tattoo removal, 49, 50*f*

Alloderm®, 99*t*, 101
allogenic collagen, 100–101
all-*trans* retinoic acid, 24
all-*trans*-retinol, 24
alopecia
- androgenic, 146
- frontal traction, 146
- mesotherapy for, 146–147, 147*f*
- treatment of, 147

alopecia areata, 147
alpha-hydroxy acids, 26
alpha-hydroxyl acid peels, 13
alpha-keto acids, 26
alpha receptors, 143, 144
alpha-tocopherol *see* vitamin E
altered passive eruption, 181–183
- complications and side effects, 185
- operative approach, 183–185, 184*f*, 185*f*
- optimizing outcomes, 185
- postoperative care, 185
- preoperative history and considerations, 183–185, 183*f*
- treatment
  - of type I A, 181–182, 182*t*
  - of type I B, 182, 182*t*
  - of type II A, 182*t*
  - of type II B, 182*t*
- type I, 181–182, 182*t*
- type II, 181, 182*t*

Aluma™, 77
amaurosis after fat transfer, 123
American Society of Aesthetic Plastic Surgery (ASAPS) procedures most frequently performed, 5, 5*t*
American Surgical Association classes for laser lipolysis, 134, 134*b*
aminoglycosides and botulinum toxin, 91
aminolevulinic acid methyl ester (Me-ALA), 58*f*, 57, 58, 59, 60–61
5-aminolevulinic acid (ALA), 58*f*, 57–59, 60–61
ammonium lactate in moisturizers, 22
analgesia
- in carbon dioxide therapy, 177
  - for acne/surgical scars, 168
  - for cellulite, 167*f*
  - for eye procedures, 171

analgesia *(Continued)*
for facial rejuvenation, 172
for localized fat, 165
for stretch marks, 169
in laser lipolysis, 135
androgenic alopecia, 146
androgens, 146
anesthesia
for chemical peels, 33
for injectable fillers/volumizers, 113
for laser lipolysis, 135, 137
sensation after carbon dioxide therapy, 175
animal collagen, 99–100
anterior uveitis after laser treatment, 47
anticoagulant drugs and platelet-rich plasma, 152–153
antihistamines in laser lipolysis, 135
antioxidants, 26
anxiolytics in laser lipolysis, 135
Aquamid®, 99*t*, 110
argon lasers
for aesthetic enhancement, 42, 42*f*, 43*f*
classification, 40*t*
pigmentary changes, 48–49
senile angiomas, 48
Artecoll®, 110
Artefill®, 99*t*, 110
arterial ulcers, carbon dioxide therapy for, 159, 177
artificial tears, after periorbital area chemical peels, 34
ascorbic acid *see* vitamin C
Asian eyelids, 18
Atelocollagen®, 100
Aurora™, 76–77
Autologen™, 99*t*, 101
autologous collagen, 101–102
autologous fat, 3, 97–98, 99*t*
see also fat transfer
autologous platelet-rich plasma rejuvenation, 149
combination treatments with, 154
contraindications, 152–153
controversies regarding, 150–151
for dark circles, 130
definition of, 149
growth factors in, 150*t*
indications, 151–152, 151*f*, 152*f*, 153*f*
physiological role of platelets in hemostasis, 149
post-treatment, 153–154
preparation and injection technique, 151
therapeutic effect of, 150

B

bag on a bag, 2
basal cell carcinomas (BCCs), photodynamic treatment for, 60–61, 61*f*, 62, 63*f*, 63*t*
beauty, 203
Belotero®, 99*t*, 105
beta-butanoic acid, 26
beta-hydroxy acids, 26
beta-lipohydroxyacid, 27
beta receptors, 143, 144
Bioalkamide®, 110
Bioinblue, 99*t*
Bioplastique®, 99*t*, 110
Biopolimero®, 111
biotin, 147
bipolar radiofrequency, 75, 75*f*, 76–77, 82
posttreatment care, 82
pretreatment care, 82
treatment parameters, 82*t*
treatment procedure, 82–83
bismuth subgalate after chemical peels, 33
bleeding after carbon dioxide therapy, 175
blepharochalasis, upper eyelid, 30, 30*f*, 32–33
blepharoplasty
combination of peeling with, 35
for dark circles, 132
number of procedures performed, 6*t*
blinking
after periorbital area chemical peels, 34
muscles for, 18
blistering after laser treatments, 47
blue light, 59, 60
Bohr effect, 156, 159
borage oil, 27
Botox®, 86, 87*t*
doses, 90
FDA approval, 86
in the glabella, 92
see also botulinum toxins
botulinum neurotoxin, 89–90, 89*f*
botulinum toxins, 1, 85–96
action, 6
after chemical peels, 36
areas generally targeted, 6
in combination therapy, 11–12
comparison of different, 87*t*
complications and side effects, 93–94
brow ptosis, 94
diplopia, 94
ecchymoses and bruising, 93
ectropion, 94
keratitis, 94
lip ptosis and oral incompetence, 94
ptosis of the upper eyelid, 93–94, 93*f*
that occur injecting the lower eyelid, 94
currently available, 86–89
dose of, 90, 92–93
economic impact of, 5, 6
FDA approval of, 11
history of the cosmetic use of, 85–86
indications, 85, 90–91
glabellar frown lines, 90, 90*f*, 91*f*
periorbicular area, 90–91, 91*f*
and injectable fillers, 12*t*
and intense pulsed light, 12*t*
mechanism of action, 89–90, 89*f*
for muscle relaxation and facial balance, 11
number of procedures performed, 6*t*
popularity, 5, 5*t*, 6
post-procedure care, 93
preoperative considerations, 91
as a pretreatment for other therapies, 12
rate of success, 6
summary, 85
techniques and doses, 92–93, 92*f*, 93*f*
type A, 3, 86
type B, 86
type C, 86
type D, 86

type E, 86
type F, 86
type G, 86
botulism, 85–86
bovine collagen, 99–100, 115*t*
Bowen's disease, 62, 63*t*
breast augmentation
with fat, 119
number of procedures performed, 6*t*
bruising
after botulinum toxin injection, 93
after carbon dioxide therapy, 175
burns after laser lipolysis, 138–139

C

cadaveric collagen, 100–101
calcium hydroxylapatite *see* synthetic calcium hydroxylapatite
camouflage, cosmetic, 129, 191
Cantisano-Zilkha, Dr. Marian, 198
Captique®, 102, 104, 109*t*
carbon dioxide insufflation *see* carbon dioxide therapy (CDT)
carbon dioxide lasers *see* CO_2 lasers
carbon dioxide tanks, 157
carbon dioxide therapy (CDT), 155–178, 155
complications and side effects, 175–177, 176*f*, 177*f*
contraindications, 158–161
general, 161
local, 161
temporary, 161
effects on the body, 156, 156*f*
equipment, 157–158, 157*f*, 158*f*
indications, 158–161
aesthetic, 159–161
dark circles, 131
vascular, 159
operative approach, 163
acne and surgical scars, 167–168
cellulite/orange peel skin, 166–167, 167*f*
crow's feet, 172, 172*f*
décolletage rejuvenation, 172–173, 173*f*
eye procedures, 169–171, 170*f*, 171*f*
hand rejuvenation, 172–173, 173*f*
localized fat, 164–166, 164*f*, 165*f*, 166*f*
nasogenian folds, 172, 172*f*
neck rejuvenation, 172–173, 173*f*
peri-oral wrinkles, 172, 172*f*
Raynaud's phenomenon, 163–164, 164*f*
stretch marks, 168–169, 168*f*, 169*f*
optimizing outcomes, 174–175, 174*f*
overview, 4
and platelet-rich plasma rejuvenation, 154
skin layers and CDT concerns, 161–163, 161*f*
intradermal injections, 163, 163*f*
subcutaneous injections, 162, 162*f*
cardiotoxicity, chemical peels, 36
Carruthers, Alistair, 86
Carruthers, Jean, 86
cellulite
carbon dioxide therapy for, 166–167, 167*f*, 177
description, 143
lipolysis for, 144
mesotherapy for, 143–144
pathophysiology of, 143
stages of, 143, 143*f*, 144*f*
treatment, 143–144
Cellu-M6®, 174
central fat pad, 19
chemical exfoliation, 190, 192
chemical peels, 1, 29–38
alpha-hydroxyl acid, 13
anaesthesia and patient monitoring, 33
as an alternative to photodynamic treatment, 60
categories/depth of, 32
choice of chemical agent, 32–33
combination therapy, 13, 35, 36*f*
complications, 35–36
for dark circles, 129, 129*f*
indications and contraindications, 29–30, 30*f*, 31*f*
long-term results, 36, 36*f*
and microdermabrasion, 12*t*
number of procedures performed, 6*t*
operative approach, 32
overview, 3–4
peeling technique, 33, 34*f*
postoperative care, 33–34
preoperative history and considerations, 31–32
pre-peel skin preparation, 32, 32*f*
repeated peelings, 35, 35*f*
special considerations for periorbital peelings, 34
trichloracetic acid, 13
cherry angiomas, 42
chromophores, 39, 130–131
lasers that use, 4
clients, 189–190
see also patient(s)
clonidine, 135
Clostridium botulinum, 11, 85
coenzyme Q-10, 146
coherent laser light, 39
Cohesive Polydensified Matrix®, 105
CO_2 lasers
for aesthetic enhancement, 42
classification, 40*t*
for dark circles, 130–131
development of, 16
for scar treatment, 52–53
for skin tightening, 10
thermal damage from, 44
collagen, 21
contraction *see* collagen contraction
definition of, 68
denaturing of the fibers, 71, 72*f*
for facial fillers (*see also specific types*)
complications, 115, 115*t*
evolution of, 98
FDA approved, 102*t*
types of, 98–102
stimulation of synthesis with carbon dioxide therapy, 156
type I, 68
type III, 68
collagen contraction, 71
cooling, 69–70
definition, 68–69
and neocollagenesis, 70
in radiofrequency, 77–78, 78*f*
sustained volumetric heating, 69, 69*f*

combining therapies, 9–20
benefits of specific therapies, 12*t*
deep level, 9–13
muscle relaxation and facial balance, 11–12
skin tightening, 10–11
surgical approach, 12–13
volume replacement, 10
platelet-rich plasma rejuvenation, 154
recommended techniques by facial area, 16*t*
superficial and medium levels, 13–16
chemical peels, 13
dermabrasion and dermaplaning, 13–15
fractioned laser devices, 16
Glogau photoaging classification, 13, 14*t*, 15*t*
intense pulsed light, 15
microdermabrasion, 13
non-ablative lasers, 16
photodynamic therapy, 15–16
comedone extraction, 191
computerized area, carbon dioxide therapy machines, 158, 158*f*
conjunctival wound during carbon dioxide therapy, 176
Conjunctyl®, 144, 145
continuous wave (CW) lasers
for aesthetic enhancement, 42, 42*f*
classification, 41*t*
energy, 41–42
for senile angiomas, 48
cooling collagen contraction, 69–70
copper, mesoglow/mesolift, 146
copper-selenium (CU-SE), mesoglow/mesolift, 146
copper vapor lasers
classification, 40*t*
senile angiomas, 48
corneal wound during carbon dioxide therapy, 176
corundum, 191
cosmetic camouflage, 129, 191
cosmetic dentistry, 179–188
altered passive eruption, 181–183
complications and side effects, 185
operative approach, 183–185, 184*f*, 185*f*
optimizing outcomes, 185
postoperative care, 185
preoperative history and considerations, 183–185, 183*f*
treatment of type I A, 181–182, 182*t*
treatment of type I B, 182, 182*t*
treatment of type II A, 182*t*
treatment of type II B, 182*t*
type I, 181
type II, 181
geometric parameters of harmony, 180–181, 180*f*
gingival contour, 179, 180*f*
indications and contraindications, 181–183
lips, 179, 180*f*
teeth, 180, 180*f*
vertical maxillary excess, 181–183, 185–188
complications and side effects, 188
operative approach, 186–187, 186*f*, 187*f*
optimizing outcomes, 187–188, 187*f*
postoperative care, 188, 188*f*
preoperative history and considerations, 185 188, 185*f*, 186*f*
treatment, 182–183, 182*t*
cosmetics, 23–24
classes of, 24
decorative, 24
definition of, 23–24
permanent, 191
regenerative-substitutive, 24
Cosmetics®, 87*t*
cosmoceuticals, 24–28
alpha-hydroxy acids, 26
beta-hydroxy acids, 26
beta-lipohydroxyacid, 27
dimethylaminoethanol, 26
essential fatty acids, 27
essential oils, 27
estrogens, 26
green tea, 27
hamamelis, 27
new developments, 27–28
new products, 27
soy, 26–27
spearmint, 27
vitamin A, 24
vitamin B_3, 25–26
vitamin C, 24
vitamin E, 25, 25*f*
vitamin K, 26
zinc, 26
CosmoDerm®, 99*t*, 100–101, 102*t*
Cosmoplast™, 99*t*, 100, 101, 102*t*
cranial nerves
III, 19
V, 19
VII, 18, 19, 138
croton oil, 32–33
see also phenol-croton oil-based solutions
crown-lengthening procedure, 183–184, 184*f*, 185–186, 187–188, 187*f*
crow's feet
causes of, 90–91
removal *see* crow's feet removal
crow's feet removal
botulinum toxin for, 29, 90–91, 92, 93*f*
carbon dioxide therapy for, 172, 172*f*
cryotherapy as an alternative to photodynamic treatment, 60
crystal lasers, 40*t*
cutaneous adnexa, 3*t*
cutaneous T cell lymphoma, 63*t*
cyclic AMP, 144, 156
Cymetra®, 99*t*, 100, 101

D

dark circles, 127–132
carbon dioxide therapy for, 131, 160, 170, 172*f*
causes of, 160
chemical peeling for, 129, 129*f*
contributing factors, 127, 128*f*
definition, 127
dietary supplement, 129
ethnic, 30
fillers for, 129–130, 130*f*
lasers for, 130–131
platelet-rich plasma rejuvenation for, 130, 152
research, 127
surgery (blepharoplasty) for, 132
topical therapy for, 127–129
dead hand after carbon dioxide therapy, 175

décolletage rejuvenation
carbon dioxide therapy for, 160, 172–173, 172*f*, 173*f*
mesoglow for, 146
platelet-rich plasma for, 151–152
decorative cosmetics, 24
deep intradermal injections, mesotherapy, 142
deep level combination therapies, 9–13
muscle relaxation and facial balance, 11–12
skin tightening, 10–11
surgical approach, 12–13
volume replacement, 10
Den-Hub, 142
deoxycholic acid, 144–145
dermabrasion
action of, 13–15
combination therapy, 13–15
overview, 13
DermaDeep®, 111, 112
Dermagen®, 111
dermal grafting, 99*t*
DermaLive®, 111–112, 111*f*, 112*f*
dermal micropigmentation, 191
Dermalogen™, 100, 101
dermaplaning
action of, 13–15
combination therapy, 13–15
Dermaplant, 99*t*
dermatitis papulosa nigra, 49
dermis, 21
composition of, 21
effects of aging on, 1–2, 3*t*
detergents, 23
dexpanthenol as a moisturiser, 22, 23*f*
DHN 1, 2, 3 and 4 devices, 142
diazepam, chemical peels sedation, 33
dietary supplements for dark circles, 129
dihydroxyacetone, 24
dihydroxyergotamine, 144
dimethylaminoethanol, 26
diode lasers
classification of, 40*t*
for hair removal, 44, 51–52
diplopia, following botulinum toxin injection, 94
disinfection protocol, 175
DMAE, 145, 146
DNA
mesoglow/mesolift, 145
repair mechanisms, 27–28
double chin, 145, 145*f*
D-pantethol, 147
Dutesteride, 147
dye lasers
for aesthetic enhancement, 42
classification, 40*t*
for senile angiomas, 48
Dysport®, 87*t*
doses, 90
in the glabella, 92

E

Eaton-Lambert syndrome, 91
ecchymoses
after botulinum toxin injection, 93
after fat transfer, 122, 124, 124*f*
economic impact of technologies, 4
minimally invasive procedures, 5
non-invasive procedures, 5–7
botulism toxin, 6
hyaluronic acid, 7
lasers, 6–7
microdermabrasion, 7
procedures most frequently performed, 5*t*
ectropion
contraindication for lower eyelid peeling, 30
following botulinum toxin injection, 94
edema
after fat transfer, 122, 124, 124*f*
after injectable filler, 115, 115*f*
elastic fibres, 21
electro-mechanical valve compartment, carbon dioxide therapy machines, 158
electro-optical synergy (ELOS), 82
electro-thermolysis, 10, 75
Elevess®, 99*t*, 102, 104, 109*t*
Ellman Dual RF Surgitron Unit device, 75, 76*f*, 79
compared with Thermage, 76*t*
Ellman RF cool gel, 79
Emla®, 168, 171, 172, 177
emollients, 22, 22*f*
emulsions, 23
Endermology®, 174
end filter, carbon dioxide therapy machines, 158, 159*f*
Endoplast 50, 99*t*
energy of lasers, 41, 41*t*
epidermal growth factor, 150, 150*t*
epidermal sliding in chemical peels, 33
epidermis, 21
composition of, 21
effects of aging on, 1–2, 3*t*
layers, 21
epilepsy triggering after carbon dioxide therapy, 175
Er-glass lasers, 40*t*
Er-YAG lasers, 42
classification, 40*t*
and platelet-rich plasma rejuvenation, 154
for scar treatment, 52–53
thermal damage from, 44
erythema
after infrared skin-tightening technique, 73
after injectable fillers, 114–115
after radiofrequency treatment, 81
erythema index (EI), dark circles, 127
essential fatty acids, 27
essential oils, 27
Esthelis®, 105
estrogens, 26
ethnic dark circles, 30
evening primrose oil, 27
Evolence®, 99*t*, 100, 102*t*
Evolution®, 99*t*, 112
exfoliation, 190, 192
external carotid artery, 19
eyebrows
anatomy, 17–18
clinical evaluation of, 2
ptosis, 94
recommended techniques for, 16*t*
eyelashes, 18

eyelids
  anatomy, 17
  anterior lamella, 18
  clinical evaluation of, 2
  evaluation of the, 17–18
  layers, 18
  lower *see* lower eyelids
  lymphatic drainage of the, 19
  nerves of the, 19
  persistent insufflation after carbon dioxide therapy, 176, 176*f*
  skin of the, 18
  structure of the, 18–19
  surgery *see* blepharoplasty
  upper *see* upper eyelids
  vessels of the, 19
eyes
  carbon dioxide therapy for, 169–171, 170*f*, 171*f*
  position of the, 18
  protection for infrared skin-tightening technique, 73

F

face
  balance, combining therapies for, 11–12
  changes with age *see* facial changes with age
  fat compartments, effect of aging on, 2
  segmentation, 73, 73*f*
facial changes with age
  contours, 1, 2, 2*f*
  by decades of life, 3*f*
  lower face, 2
  mid-face, 2
  skin, 1–2, 3*t*
  upper face, 2
facial fillers/volumizers *see* injectable fillers/volumizers
facial lipodissolve, 145, 145*f*
facial nerve, 18, 19
  marginal mandibular branch of the, 138
Fascian, 99*t*
fat
  localized *see* localized fat
  transfer *see* fat transfer
fat transfer, 119–126
  advantages of, 120*t*
  complications and side effects, 122–123
  for dark circles, 130
  donor sites, 122
  indications and contraindications, 119, 120*f*, 121*f*
  operative approach, 122, 122*f*, 123*f*
  optimizing results, 122, 124*t*
  postoperative care, 124
  preoperative history and considerations, 120–121
female eyelids, 17–18
festoons, 2
  botulinum toxin injection and, 94
  malar, 2
Fibrel®, 98
fibrin clot, 150
fibroblasts, 145, 150
fillers *see* injectable fillers/volumizers
filotov, 145
first filter, carbon dioxide therapy machines, 157–158, 158*f*
Fitzpatrick skin types, 15, 44–45
Fitzpatrick Wrinkle Classification System (FWCS), 79, 79*t*
flash-lamp pumped pulsed dye laser (PDL), 42–43
  for port-wine stains, 48
  for telangiectasias, 48
fluence of lasers, 39–41
5-fluorouracil as an alternative to photodynamic treatment, 60
folic acid in soy beans, 26–27
follicular melanosomes, 44
forehead, recommended techniques for, 16*t*
fosa caninae technique, 107, 108*f*
fractional photothermolysis, 52–53
fractioned lasers, 43–44
  combination therapy, 16
  development of, 16
  overview, 4, 16
  for scar treatment, 52–53
Fraxel™ laser, 16, 52–53
frenectomy, 186–187, 186*f*
frontal traction alopecia, 146
fruit acids, 26
future of oculofacial rejuvenation, 203–204

G

gas heater, carbon dioxide therapy machines, 158
gingival contour, 179, 180*f*
gingival line, 179, 180*f*
gingival zenith, 179, 180*f*
gingivectomy, 181–182, 182*t*
glabella
  injectable fillers, 114
  recommended techniques for, 16*t*
  use of botulinum toxin in, 90, 90*f*, 91*f*, 92
glabellar folds, 85
glabellar frown lines, botulinum toxin for, 90, 90*f*, 91*f*, 92
Glogau Wrinkle Scale, 13, 14*t*, 15*t*
glutathione, 145
glycerol as a moisturizer, 22
glycolic acid, 146
glycosaminoglycans, 21
Golgi apparatus pressure receptors, 156
Gore-Tex, 99*t*
granulomas
  after injectable fillers, 115
  after silicone injection, 108–110
  Artefill/Artecoll®-associated, 110, 110*f*
  DermaLive®-associated, 111–112, 111*f*, 112*f*
  poly-L-lactic acid injection and, 116–117
  polymethymethacrylate injection and, 116
green tea, 27
griseofulvin, 60*t*
ground substance, 21
growth factors, 149, 150, 150*t*
gummy smile *see* vertical maxillary excess

H

Haiken, Elizabeth, 196
hair, 21
hair removal lasers, 44, 51–52
hamamelis, 27
hand
  dead, after carbon dioxide therapy, 175
  rejuvenation *see* hand rejuvenation

hand rejuvenation, 172–173
  carbon dioxide therapy for, 160, 173*f*
  platelet-rich plasma for, 151–152, 152*f*
healing, 204
heart disease unmasking after carbon dioxide therapy, 175
heat
  Joule's law, 77
  in radiofrequency treatment, 77–78, 78*f*
heavy arm/limbs after carbon dioxide therapy, 175
hemangiomas, infantile, 48
heme biosynthesis, 57
He:Ne beam, 133
herpes simplex
  infection after chemical peels, 35
  reactivation after carbon dioxide therapy, 175
human growth hormone supplementation, 204
human placental collagen, 99*t*
human synthetic collagen, 100–101
Hyal system, 99*t*
hyaluronans, 102–106
  see also hyaluronic acid
hyaluronic acid, 99*t*, 102–106
  complications, 114–115
  for dark circles, 129–130, 130*f*
  in the dermis, 21
  economic impact of, 7
  general description of, 102
  gold standard, 97
  mesoglow/mesolift, 146
  non-animal-stabilized (NASHA), 129
  overview, 7
hyaluronic acid push, 130
hyaluronidase, 113–114, 114*t*
Hylaform®, 102, 104–105, 109*t*
Hylaform Plus®, 102, 104–105, 109*t*
hyperpigmentation after chemical peels, 35
hypodermal injection, mesotherapy, 142
hypopigmentation after chemical peels, 35

I

imiquimod, 60
impedance, 77
infantile hemangiomas, 48
infections
  after carbon dioxide therapy, 175
  after chemical peels, 35
  after injectable fillers, 116
  after laser lipolysis, 138–139
inferior oblique muscle, 19
informed consent
  for fat transfer, 121
  for laser lipolysis, 135
  for laser treatment, 45, 46*t*
infrared technologies, 4, 70–71, 67
  approaches to the treatment of skin laxity, 70–71
  basic concepts, 67–68
  definitions and terminology, 68–70, 68*f*, 68*t*
    collagen, 68
    collagen contraction, 68–69
    cooling, 69–70
    neocollagenesis, 70
    skin laxity, 68
    sustained volumetric heating, 69
  preparation and technique, 71–73
    optimizing outcomes, 71–72
    postoperative care, 73
    preoperative considerations, 71
    recommended technique, 73
    Titan™ treatment parameters, 72
  for skin tightening, 11
injectable fillers/volumizers, 1, 97–118
  allogenic, 10
  anesthesia, 113
  areas for, 98*f*
  autogenic, 10
  biodegradable, 10, 98–102, 99*t*
    allogenic collagen, 100–101
    animal collagen, 99–100
    autologous collagen, 101–102
    collagen products, 98–102, 102*t*
      complications, 115, 115*t*
    FDA approved, 109*t*
    non-FDA-approved xenogenic collagen, 100
    recombinant collagen, 102
  and botulinum toxin, 12*t*
  classification, 10, 98
  combination, 107–110
  combining therapies for, 10
  complications, 113–117
    collagen, 115, 115*t*
    hyaluronic acid, 114–115, 114*f*, 115*f*
    non-biodegradable fillers, 115–116, 116*f*
    poly-L-lactic acid, 116–117
    silicone, 117
  cross-hatching technique, 113, 114*f*
  for dark circles, 129–130, 130*f*
  economic impact of, 5
  evolution of, 97–98
  fanning technique, 113, 114*f*
  future of, 117
  general treatment techniques, 112–113, 113*f*, 114*f*
  hyaluronans, 102–106
  hyaluronic acid *see* hyaluronic acid
  ideal, 97
  inflammatory reaction to, 10
  and intense pulsed light, 12*t*
  keys to success/optimizing outcomes, 117
  linear threading technique, 113, 114*f*
  non-biodegradable, 10, 99*t*, 107–110
    complications, 115–116, 116*f*
    silicone, 108–110
      complications, 117
  non-FDA-approved permanent, 110–113, 110*f*, 111*f*, 112*f*
  overview, 3
  poly-L-lactic acid, 106–107
    complications, 107, 107*f*, 116–117
    contraindications, 107, 107*f*
    technique, 106–107
  selection of, 97
  serial puncture technique, 113, 113*f*, 114*f*
  synthetic, 10
  synthetic calcium hydroxylapatite, 107
  xenogeneic, 10
injection devices, mesotherapy, 141–142
insulin-like growth factor, 150, 150*t*
intense pulsed light (IPL), 1
  action, 15
  applications, 15

intense pulsed light (IPL) *(Continued)*
and botulinum toxin, 12*t*
botulinum toxin injections as a pre-treatment for, 12
classification, 40*t*
combination therapy, 15
comparison with laser treatment, 45*t*
dangers of, 45
indications, 47–53
acquired vascular lesions, 48, 48*f*, 49*f*
dark circles, 130–131
hair removal, 44, 51–52
photorejuvenation, 50–51
pigmentary disturbances, 48–49, 49*f*
port-wine stains, 48
scars, 52–53, 52*f*, 53*f*
tattoos, 49, 50*f*
and injectable fillers, 12*t*
and microdermabrasion, 12*t*
overview, 3, 15
sources, 44
test treatments, 45
intercellular communication, 204
internal carotid artery, 19
intradermal carbon dioxide therapy injections, 163, 163*f*
intradermal superficial injection, mesotherapy, 142
intraepidermal injection, mesotherapy, 142
isoflavones, 26–27
Isolaz, 154
Isologen®, 99*t*, 101–102
isovolemic degradation, 102–103

J

Joule's law, 77
Juvéderm 24 HV™, 109*t*
Juvéderm 30 HV™, 109*t*
Juvéderm™, 99*t*, 102, 104, 104*f*
Juvéderm 30™, 104, 109*t*
JuvédermUltra Plus™, 104
JuvédermUltra™, 104

K

Kaplan's interface, 141
keloids, carbon dioxide therapy for, 168
keratitis following botulinum toxin injection, 94
Kerner, Justinus, 86
kinetin, 27

L

lacrimal glands
function of, 19
inadvertent excision of, 19
lacrimal glands of Krause, 19
lacrimal glands of Wolfring, 19
lacrimal pump, 18
lactate dehydrogenase, 26
lactic acid, 26
L-ascorbic acid *see* vitamin C
laser-assisted liposuction, 53
laser lipolysis, 133–140
anesthesia, 135, 137
complications and side effects, 138–139
equipment and laser specifications, 133–134, 134*f*
general description, 133
indications and contraindications, 134–135
marking, 135, 136*f*
operative approach, 135–138, 136*f*, 137*f*
optimizing outcomes, 138
postoperative care, 139, 139*f*
preoperative history and considerations, 135, 136*f*
suctioning after, 138
lasers, 39–56
applications, 6–7
botulinum injections as a pre-treatment for, 12
classification of, 39–42
basic concepts, 39–42, 41*f*
by delivery type of energy, 41*t*
by emitted power, 40*t*
by emitted wavelength, 40*t*
energy, 41–42
fluence, 39
by optical medium, 40*t*
pulse width, 39
repetition rate, 41
spot size, 41
wavelength, 39
comparison with intense pulsed light, 45*t*
consent form for, 46*t*
dangers of, 45
economic impact of, 7
immediate post-treatment care, 47
indications, 47–53
acquired vascular lesions, 48, 48*f*, 49*f*
dark circles, 130–131
hair removal, 51–52
photorejuvenation, 50–51
pigmentary disturbances, 48–49, 49*f*
port-wine stains, 48
scars, 52–53, 52*f*, 53*f*
skin tightening, 70
tattoos, 49, 50*f*
number of procedures performed, 6*t*
optimizing outcomes, 47
overview, 4
preoperative history and considerations, 44–46
side effects, 47
test treatments, 45, 47
treatment, 47
types of, 42–44 (*see also specific types*)
use of, 44–47
see also specific laser types
lateral canthal tendon, 18
lavender oil, 27
legal issues, 192–193
leucocytes, 150
levator aponeurosis, 19
levator muscle, 19
liability issues, 192–193
lidocaine toxicity, 135
light-emitting diode devices, 1
lipase enzymes, 156
lip augmentation
Artefill/Artecoll®, 110
injectable fillers, 113, 113*f*
liplines, 179, 180*f*
lipodissolve, 144–145
facial, 145, 145*f*

lipolysis
for cellulite, 144
improvement, carbon dioxide therapy, 156
laser *see* laser lipolysis
liposuction, 133
number of procedures performed, 6*t*
popularity, 5, 5*t*
see also laser lipolysis; lipolysis
Lipotron®, 11, 75–76, 77*f*
see also radiofrequency volumetric heating technology
lip-repositioning, 184–185, 184*f*, 185*f*, 187*f*, 188
lips
augmentation *see* lip augmentation
in cosmetic dentistry, 179, 180*f*
ptosis following botulinum toxin injection, 94
recommended techniques for, 16*t*
repositioning *see* lip-repositioning
liver disease and laser lipolysis, 135
localized fat
carbon dioxide therapy for, 159, 164–166, 164*f*, 165*f*, 174, 177
mesotherapy for, 143, 144–145
loose skin, mesotherapy for, 145–146
lorazepam, chemical peels sedation, 33
lower eyelids
anatomy, 17
botulinum toxin injection in, 93, 94
chemical peels, 29, 35
clinical evaluation of, 2
dark circles *see* dark circles
fat deposits, 160, 170
marginal arterial arcade, 19
recommended techniques for, 16*t*
wound/tear due to moving during carbon dioxide therapy, 176
wrinkle removal, 29 (*see also specific procedure*)
lower facial contours, recommended techniques for, 16*t*
lower limb vascular diseases, carbon dioxide therapy for, 159
lymphatic drainage, 191, 192
of the eyelids, 19

M

malar eminences, recommended techniques for, 16*t*
malar festoons, 2
male eyelids, 17–18
male pattern baldness, 146
manual lymphatic drainage, 191, 192
marginal arterial arcade of the eyelids, 19
marionette lines, 2, 16*t*
matrix remodelling, 150
maxillary nerve, 19
mechanical syringe support, 141–142
medial canthal tendon, 18
medial canthi, 18
medial fat pad, 19
medical spas, 193
medications
interfering with botulinum toxin, 91
perioperative, in laser lipolysis, 135
meibomian glands, 18–19
melanin depositions
chemical peels for, 30
laser treatment for, 43
melanin index (MI), dark circles, 127
melanocyte pigment synthesis stimulation, carbon dioxide therapy, 156
melanocytes, 21
melanosomes, 48–49
melasma, 24
melomental folds, 2, 16*t*
mental health, 196
Mentha spicata, 27
Mesalyse I, 142
mesoglow, 145–146
mesolift, 145–146, 146*f*
Mesopen, 142
mesoperfusion, 142
mesotherapy, 141–154
aesthetic, 143–147
alopecia, 146–147, 147*f*
cellulite, 143–144, 143*f*, 144*f*
localized fat, 143, 144–145
loose skin, 145–146, 146*f*
complications, 148
contraindications, 147–148
deep intradermal injections, 142
hypodermal injection, 142
injection devices and mechanical syringe support, 141–142
intradermal superficial injection, 142
intraepidermal injection, 142
materials, 141–142
mechanism of action, 141
needles, 141
overview, 4
techniques and depths of injection, 142
Metacrill®, 99*t*, 112
microcirculation stimulation, 141
microdermabrasion, 191, 192
action of, 13
applications, 13
and chemical peels, 12*t*
combination therapy, 13
economic impact, 7
and intense pulsed light, 12*t*
overview, 7
microscopic epidermal necrotic debris (MEND), 44
microscopic treatment zones (MTZs), 43, 44
microstipling, 191
milia after chemical peels, 36
minimally invasive laser lipolysis *see* laser lipolysis
moisturizers, 22, 22*f*
after chemical peels, 34
monochromatic laser light, 39
monometilsianotriol salicylate *see* Conjunctyl®
Muller's muscle, 19
muscles
imbalance after fat transfer, 123
relaxation, combining therapies for, 11–12
Myobloc®, 86, 87*t*

N

nails, 21
nappage, 142, 143–144, 145, 146
nasal fat pad, 19
NASHA™ gels, 102–103
nasogenian folds, carbon dioxide therapy for, 161, 172, 172*f*

nasolabial folds
recommended techniques for, 16*t*
synthetic calcium hydroxylapatite, 107, 108*f*
national certification standards for skincare professionals, 193–194
National Coalition of Estheticians, Manufacturers/Distributors & Association (NCEA), 190
Certification Program, 194
postsurgery procedures, 192
presurgery procedures, 192
Natragel™, 113
Nd:YAG lasers *see* neodynium:yttrium-aluminium garnet (Nd:YAG) lasers
neck rejuvenation, 172–173
carbon dioxide therapy for, 160, 172*f*, 173*f*
laser lipolysis for, 134–135
needles
accidental fragmentation of in carbon dioxide therapy, 177
carbon dioxide therapy machines, 158, 159*f*
mesotherapy, 141
neo-angiogenesis effect of carbon dioxide therapy, 156
neocollagenesis, 70
neodynium:yttrium-aluminium garnet (Nd:YAG) lasers, 16
classification, 40*t*
combined with pulsed dye laser, 43
for dark circles, 130–131
for dermatitis papulosa nigra, 49
for hair removal, 44, 51
laser lipolysis, 133
for pigmentary changes, 48–49, 49*f*
for port-wine stains, 48
for scar treatment, 53, 53*f*
for skin tightening, 70
for tattoo removal, 49, 50*f*
for telangiectasias, 48
nerve damage
after fat transfer, 123
after laser lipolysis, 139
and platelet-rich plasma rejuvenation, 152–153
Neurobloc®, 87*t*
new developments, 27–28
NewFill® *see* poly-L-lactic acid (PLLA)
new products, 27
niacin *see* vitamin B_3
niacinamide, 25–26
nicotinamide, 25–26
nicotinamide adenine dinucleotide (NAD), 25–26
nicotinamide adenine dinucleotide phosphate (NADP), 25–26
nicotinic acid *see* vitamin B_3
non-ablative lasers
botulism injections as a pre-treatment for, 12
combination therapy, 16
overview, 4, 16
thermal damage from, 43–44
non-animal-stabilized hyaluronic acid (NASHA), 129
non-steroidal anti-inflammatory drugs (NSAIDs), 152–153

O

oculofacial aging concepts, 1
oculomotor nerve, 19
oral incompetence following botulinum toxin injection, 94
orange peel skin *see* cellulite
orbicularis oculi muscle, 18
orbital fat, 19
orthognathic surgery, 182, 182*t*, 183
Outline®, 112
owl monkeys, 105, 105*f*
oxygen, accidental injection of, 176, 176*f*
oxygenation index (OX), dark circles, 127
oxygen radical scavengers, 24

P

Pacinian corpuscles pressure receptors, 156
Paget's disease, photodynamic treatment for, 63*t*
pain relief/management *see* analgesia
palpebral conjunctiva, 19
palpebral fissure, 18
pantothenic acid in soy beans, 26–27
patient evaluation
chemical peels, 31–32
clinical evaluation of, 2
fat transfer, 120–121
first step in, 2
laser lipolysis, 134, 135
laser treatment, 44–45
patient monitoring, chemical peels, 33
patient(s)
definition of, 189–190
expectations, 189
perspective of cosmetic medicine, 198
relationship with, 189
time spent with, 189
understanding and readiness for cosmetic procedures, 201–202
PC/DC, 144–145
peer support groups, 201
Pellevè™, 75
energy levels, 78
technique, 79
pentoxyphylline, 144, 146
periocular vein, laser treatment for, 49*f*
peri-oral wrinkles, carbon dioxide therapy for, 161, 172
periorbicular area, botulinum toxin for, 90–91, 93
periorbital area
aging in the, 29
anatomy, 17
chemical peeling in the, 29, 34
see also chemical peels
pigmentation, chemical peels, 30, 30*f*
platelet-rich plasma rejuvenation, 152
see also eyelids
periorbital melanosis *see* dark circles
periorbital wrinkles *see* crow's feet
Perlane®, 99*t*, 102, 103–104, 105, 109*t*
Permacol®, 100
permanent cosmetics, 191
persistent eyelid insufflation after carbon dioxide therapy, 176, 176*f*
petroleum ointment after chemical peels, 33–34
phenol, 32–33
see also phenol-croton oil-based solutions
phenol-croton oil-based solutions, 32
phenothiazine, 60*t*
phentolamine, 144
phosphatidylcholine, 144–145
phosphodiesterase, 144
photoaging, 3, 23
Glogau Wrinkle Scale, 13, 14*t*, 15*t*
signs of, 13
therapy for, 13
photodynamic diagnosis (PDD), 60

photodynamic treatment (PDT), 1, 57–66
combination therapy, 15–16
contraindications and restrictions, 60, 60*t*
cure and improvement rates of various skin conditions with, 63*t*
definition of, 57–58, 58*f*
drugs used for, 58–59
5-aminolevulinic acid, 58–59
aminolevulinic acid methyl ester, 59
future of, 15–16
indications, 59*t*
lesion preparation and treatment, 60–62, 61*f*, 62*f*, 63*f*
light sources for, 59
overview, 15
patient selection, 60
for photorejuvenation, 62–65, 64*f*
requirements for effectiveness of, 58*t*
therapeutic alternatives, 60
photoepilation, 44
photography in laser lipolysis, 135
photomodulation therapy, botulinum injections as a pre-treatment for, 12
photorejuvenation
laser treatments for, 50–51
photodynamic treatment for, 62–65, 63*t*, 64*f*
photosensitizing drugs contraindicated in photodynamic treatment, 60*t*
phylloquinone, 26, 129
physician's perspective of cosmetic medicine, 197–198
phytonadione, topical, for dark circles, 129
piano massage, 174, 174*f*
pigmentary disturbances
dark circles, 127, 128*f*
laser treatments for, 48–49, 49*f*
pigmentation, 1
after chemical peels, 35
after laser treatment, 47
gender differentiation, 21
laser treatment for, 43
periorbital area, 30, 30*f*
see also hyperpigmentation; hypopigmentation
Piso 4 device, 142
Pistor, Dr Michael, 141
pixellated lasers *see* fractioned lasers
Pixel™ laser, 16
placental extract, mesoglow/mesolift, 145
platelet-derived growth factor (PDGF), 150*t*
platelet-rich plasma rejuvenation *see* autologous platelet-rich plasma rejuvenation
platelets, 130
activation of, 149
role in hemostasis, 149
see also autologous platelet-rich plasma rejuvenation
poikiloderma of Civatte, 23
point-by-point injection technique, 142
Polaris™, 76–77
pollinated laser light, 39
polyhydroxy acids, 26
poly-L-lactic acid (PLLA), 106–107, 99*t*, 109*t*
complications, 107, 107*f*, 116–117
contraindications, 107, 107*f*
technique, 106–107
polymethymethacrylate (PMMA), 110, 116
porcine collagen, 99–100
port-wine stains, 48
post-liposuction deformities, 119, 120*f*
postsurgery procedures, 192
potassium-titanyl-phosphate (KTP) laser, 160
preaponeurotic fat pad, 19
preoperative care, 190
pressure regulators, carbon dioxide therapy machines, 157, 157*f*
presurgery procedures, 192
procaine, 144, 147
professional error, 45
promyelocytic leukaemia, 24
Propionibacterium acnes, 60
Prosigne®, 87*t*
protoporphyrin IX (PpIX), 58*f*, 57, 58–59
psoriasis, carbon dioxide therapy for, 160
psychotherapist's views on aesthetic enhancement, 195–202
cosmetic medicine from the patient's perspective, 198
cosmetic medicine from the physician's perspective, 197–198
historical perspective, 196–197
strengths-based model, 199–200
ptosis
clinical evaluation of, 2
following botulinum toxin injection
brow, 94
lip, 94
upper eyelid, 93–94, 93*f*
pulsed dye laser (PDL), 42–43
combined with Nd-YAG laser, 43
port-wine stains, 48
stretch marks, 160
telangiectasias, 48
pulsed lasers, 42–43
classification, 41*t*
energy, 42
pulse width of lasers, 39
purified bovine collagen, 3
purpura after laser treatment, 42–43, 47
pyruvic acid, 26

Q

Q-switched lasers, 42–43
classification, 41*t*
for dark circles, 130–131
energy, 42
Nd:YAG, 43
ruby *see* Q-switched ruby lasers
tattoo removal, 49, 50*f*
Q-switched ruby lasers
classification, 40*t*
hair removal, 51
pigmentary changes, 48–49
tattoo removal, 49

R

Radiage® *see* Pellevè™
Radiance®, 107
Radiesse®, 99*t*, 107, 108*f*, 109*t*
radiofrequency technologies, 67, 74
approaches to the treatment of skin laxity, 70–71
basic concepts, 67–68
bipolar systems, 75, 75*f*, 76–77
complications and side effects, 81
definitions and terminology, 68–70, 68*f*, 68*t*

radiofrequency technologies *(Continued)*
collagen, 68
collagen contraction, 68–69
cooling, 69–70
neocollagenesis, 70
skin laxity, 68
sustained volumetric heating, 69
indications and contraindications, 78–79
mechanism of action, 77–78, 78*f*
monopolar systems, 75–76, 75*f*, 76*f*, 77*f*
optimizing outcomes, 81
postoperative care, 81
pre- and post-treatment, 80*f*, 81*f*
preparation and technique, 71–73, 79–81, 79*t*
optimizing outcomes, 71–72
postoperative care, 73
preoperative considerations, 71
recommended technique, 73
Titan™ treatment parameters, 72
skin-tightening technique, 79–81, 80*f*, 80*t*, 81*f*
unipolar systems, 75, 75*f*
see also radiofrequency volumetric heating technology
radiofrequency volumetric heating technology
applications, 10
FDA-approved devices, 10, 11
overview, 4
problems with, 10–11
skin tightening, 10–11
Raynaud's phenomenon
carbon dioxide therapy for, 159, 163–164, 164*f*
general description of, 159
reactive oxygen species (ROS), 57–58
receptor activation, carbon dioxide therapy, 156
recombinant collagen, 102
red light, 59
ReFirme™, 77, 82
treatment parameters, 82*t*
reflexive theory, 141
regenerative-substitutive cosmetics, 24
Regen PRP Kit®, 151
regional block for chemical peels, 33
Reloxin®, 87*t*
repetition rate of lasers, 41
resistance, 77
respiratory disease unmasking after carbon dioxide therapy, 175
Restylane®, 99*t*, 102, 103, 103*f*, 105, 109*t*
Restylane Lipp®, 103
Restylane push technique, 113, 114*f*
Restylane SubQ®, 103
Retin A™, 24
retinoic acid, 24, 146
retinol, 24, 129
Reviderm, 99*t*
rhytids *see* wrinkles
riboflavin, 26–27
Rioblush™, 154
Romberg's syndrome, fat transfer in, 119, 121*f*
rooster combs, 105
rosacea, increased with carbon dioxide therapy, 177
ruby lasers
classification, 40*t*
for dark circles, 130–131
indications, 43
Q-switched *see* Q-switched ruby lasers

S

scarring
acne *see* acne scars
after chemical peels, 36
lack of in intrauterine surgery, 204
surgical *see* surgical scars
traumatic scars, 160
treatment for *see* scar treatment/removal
scar treatment/removal
laser treatments for, 52–53, 52*f*, 53*f*
platelet-rich plasma for, 152, 152*f*, 153*f*
Scott, Alan, 86
Sculptra® *see* poly-L-lactic acid (PLLA)
sebaceous hyperplasias, photodynamic treatment for, 61–62, 62*f*
sedation for chemical peels, 33
selective photothermolysis, 39, 44
self-tanning agents, 24
senile angiomas, laser treatment for, 48
septum, 18–19
serum lipids after laser lipolysis, 139
silicone, 99*t*
complications, 117
evolution of, 98
as a facial filler, 108–110
silicone oil, 111
skin
care of *see* skincare
effects of aging on, 1–2, 3*t*
see also photoaging
eyelid, 18
function of, 21
irritability, 23
after laser treatment, 47
laxity *see* skin laxity
layers, 21 (*see also* dermis epidermis; subcutaneous fat)
and carbon dioxide therapy, 161, 161*f*
pigmentation *see* pigmentation
texture, 1
thickness, 21
tightening, 1, 10–11 (*see also specific treatments*)
types *see* skin type
washing and cleansing, 23
skincare, 21–28
basic, 22–23, 22*f*, 23*f*
cosmetic, 23–24
cosmoceuticals, 24–28
alpha-hydroxy acids, 26
beta-hydroxy acids, 26
beta-lipohydroxyacid, 27
dimethylaminoethanol, 26
essential fatty acids, 27
essential oils, 27
estrogens, 26
green tea, 27
hamamelis, 27
new developments, 27–28
new products, 27
soy, 26–27
spearmint, 27
vitamin A, 24
vitamin B_3, 25–26
vitamin C, 24
vitamin E, 25, 25*f*

vitamin K, 26
zinc, 26
products *see* skincare products; *specific products*
skincare products
moisturizers, 22, 22*f*, 23*f*
production of, 22–23
skin laxity
approaches to the treatment of, 70–71
definition of, 68, 68*f*
improvement following laser treatments, 67
radiofrequency technologies, 74–75, 78–79
skin tightening devices, 67–84
skin-tightening devices, 67–84
see also infrared technologies; radiofrequency technologies
skin type
in chemical peels assessment, 31
Fitzpatrick skin types, 15, 44–45
in laser treatment assessment, 45
in photorejuvenation assessment, 50–51
smile, 180–181, 180*f*
snap test, 94
SNARE proteins, 89–90
soaps, 23
sodium monomethyltrisilanol orthohydroxybenzoate, 144
soft fibroma, laser treatment for, 42, 42*f*
solar elastosis, 23
solid lipid nanoparticles, 22–23
Sommer, Herman, 86
soy, 26–27
spearmint, 27
spot size of lasers, 41
stem cells, 125, 204
ST Near Infrared handpiece, 11
stratum corneum, 21
dry, 22, 22*f*
storage of fat-soluble substances, 22
strengths-based model, 198, 199–200
Streptococcus equi, 104
stretch marks
carbon dioxide therapy for, 160, 168–169, 168*f*, 169*f*, 177
potassium-titanyl-phosphate (KTP) laser for, 160
pulsed dye laser (PDL) for, 160
striae albae, laser treatment for, 53
striae rubrae, laser treatment for, 53
subcutaneous carbon dioxide therapy injections, 162, 162*f*
subcutaneous fat, 21
function of, 21
thickness of, 21
subcutis *see* subcutaneous fat
subepidermal resurfacing *see* photorejuvenation
submental region laser lipolysis, 134–135, 138
submentonian fat tightening, 166, 166*f*
suborbital orbicularis oculi fat (SOOF), 18
sugar cane amino acids, 27
sulfonamides, contraindication in photodynamic treatment, 60*t*
sulfonylurea, contraindication in photodynamic treatment, 60*t*
sunscreens, 24
superficial and medium levels combination therapies, 13–16
chemical peels, 13
dermabrasion and dermaplaning, 13–15
fractioned laser devices, 16
Glogau photoaging classification, 13, 14*t*, 15*t*
intense pulsed light, 15
microdermabrasion, 13
non-ablative lasers, 16
photodynamic therapy, 15–16
superficial musculoaponeurotic system (SMAS)
effect of aging on, 2
insertion points, 78
supervision groups, 201
supraorbital nerve, 19
surgery
combination of peeling with, 35
combining therapies, 12–13
for dark circles, 132
surgical scars
carbon dioxide therapy for, 160, 167–168
platelet-rich plasma for, 152, 152*f*, 153*f*
Surgiderm®, 106
Surgilift, 99*t*
sustained volumetric heating, 69, 69*f*
see also infrared technologies; radiofrequency volumetric heating technology
syncope after carbon dioxide therapy, 175
synthetic calcium hydroxylapatite, 107, 109*t*
for dark circles, 130
synthetic collagen, 100–101
syringes, mesotherapy, 141–142
syringomas, laser treatment for, 42, 43*f*

T

tarsal plates, 18–19
tattooing, 191
tattoos, laser treatment for removal of, 43, 49, 50*f*
tear trough deformity, 127, 128*f*, 160
teeth, in cosmetic dentistry, 180, 180*f*
telangiectasias, 3
increased with carbon dioxide therapy, 177
laser treatment for, 48, 48*f*
Teosyal®, 99*t*, 106
testosterone, 146
tetracycline, contraindication in photodynamic treatment, 60*t*
Thermacool®, 70, 78
Thermage®, 10, 70, 76*t*
see also radiofrequency volumetric heating technology
thermal relaxation time (TRT), 39
thiamine, 26–27
thiazidics, contraindication in photodynamic treatment, 60*t*
thymidine dinucleotide, 27–28
thyroid, accidental puncture in carbon dioxide therapy, 177
tissue hydration, 190
Titan™, 70, 71, 71*f*
facial segmentation for, 73, 73*f*
pre- and post-treatment, 74*f*
treatment parameters, 72, 72*t*
topical therapy for dark circles, 127–129
tramadol, 33
transforming growth factor (TGF), 150, 150*t*
traumatic scars, carbon dioxide therapy for, 160
Trental®, 144
tretinoin, 24, 32
trichloracetic acid (TCA) peels, 13, 32, 33, 34, 129, 129*f*
trigeminal nerve, 19
tropic acid, 26
truth, 203
tubes, carbon dioxide therapy machines, 158

U

U225 device, 142
ulcers, carbon dioxide therapy for, 159, 177
ultraviolet (UV) rays
  and aging, 23, 97
  protection from, 22, 24
  UVA, 23
  UVB, 23
upper eyelids
  anatomy, 17
  blepharochalasis, 30, 30*f*, 32–33
  clinical evaluation of, 2
  marginal arterial arcade, 19
  ptosis, 93–94, 93*f*
  recommended techniques for, 16*t*
  skin crease, 18
urea as a moisturizer, 22

V

vagal reaction after carbon dioxide therapy, 175
van Emergen, Emile Pierre Marie, 86
vascular endothelial growth factor (VEGF), 125, 150, 150*t*, 204
vascular lesions, acquired, laser treatments for, 48, 48*f*, 49*f*
vasodilatation, effects of carbon dioxide therapy, 156
vaso-vagal syndrome after carbon dioxide therapy, 175
venous ulcers, carbon dioxide therapy for, 159, 177
vertical maxillary excess, 180–183, 185–188
  complications and side effects, 188
  operative approach, 186–187, 186*f*, 187*f*
  optimizing outcomes, 187–188, 187*f*
  postoperative care, 188, 188*f*
  preoperative history and considerations, 185–188, 185*f*, 186*f*
  treatment, 182–183, 182*t*
Visage®, 67, 70
Vistabel®, 87*t*, 92
vitamin A, 24, 26–27
vitamin A acid, 24
vitamin B_1, 26–27
vitamin B_2, 26–27
vitamin B_3, 26–27, 25–26
vitamin C, 24, 26
  after platelet-rich plasma rejuvenation, 153, 154
  alopecia, 147
  mesoglow/mesolift, 146
  topical, for dark circles, 129
vitamin E, 25, 25*f*
  in soy beans, 26–27
  topical, for dark circles, 129
vitamin K, 26, 129
volume replacement, 10
  see also injectable fillers/volumizers
volumizers *see* injectable fillers/volumizers

W

warm sensation with carbon dioxide therapy, 177
wavelength of lasers, 39, 40*t*
witch hazel, 27
Wood's light, 60
wrinkle removal, 1
  carbon dioxide therapy for, 160, 169, 172*f*, 177
  lower eyelids, 29
  radiofrequency resurfacing, 67
  see also specific procedure
wrinkles
  carbon dioxide therapy for, 161
  causes of, 85
  classification *see* Fitzpatrick Wrinkle Classification System (FWCS); Glogau Wrinkle Scale
  periorbital *see* crow's feet
  removal *see* wrinkle removal; *specific techniques*

X

xanthelasmata, laser treatment for, 42
xenogenic collagen, 99–100
xenon chloride excimer lasers, 40*t*
XEOMIN®, 87*t*

Z

zinc, 26
Zyderm®, 99–100, 99*t*, 102*t*
zygomatic arch, 94
zygomaticus major, 94
zygomaticus minor, 94
Zyplast®, 99–100, 99*t*, 102*t*